Laboratory techniques in biochemistry and molecular biology

4

LABORATORY TECHNIQUES IN BIOCHEMISTRY AND MOLECULAR BIOLOGY

Volume 4

Edited by

T. S. WORK – *N.I.M.R., Mill Hill, London*
E. WORK – *Imperial College, London*

NORTH-HOLLAND PUBLISHING COMPANY – AMSTERDAM · OXFORD
AMERICAN ELSEVIER PUBLISHING CO., INC. – NEW YORK

Part I A. N. Glazer, R. J. DeLange and D. S. Sigman

CHEMICAL MODIFICATION OF PROTEINS

Part II Hannah Gould and H. R. Matthews

SEPARATION METHODS FOR NUCLEIC ACIDS AND OLIGONUCLEOTIDES

1976

NORTH-HOLLAND PUBLISHING COMPANY – AMSTERDAM · OXFORD

AMERICAN ELSEVIER PUBLISHING CO., INC. – NEW YORK

ISBN North-Holland – series: 0 7204 4200 1
– volume 4: 0 7204 4215 X
ISBN American Elsevier: 0 444 10985 4
Library of Congress Catalog Card Number: 68-54514

Published by:
NORTH-HOLLAND PUBLISHING COMPANY – AMSTERDAM · OXFORD

Sole distributors for the U.S.A. and Canada:
AMERICAN ELSEVIER PUBLISHING COMPANY, INC.
52 VANDERBILT AVENUE, NEW YORK, N.Y. 10017

Printed in The Netherlands

Editors' preface

Progress in research depends upon development of technique. No matter how important the cerebral element may be in the planning of experiments, a tentative hypothesis cannot be converted into an accepted fact unless there is adequate consciousness of the scope and limitation of existing techniques; moreover, the results may be meaningless or even positively misleading if the technical 'know how' is inadequate.

During the past ten or fifteen years, biochemical methods have become specialized and sophisticated to such a degree that it is now difficult for the beginner, whether undergraduate, graduate or specialist in another field, to grasp all the minor but important details which divide the successful from the unsuccessful experiment. In order to cope with this problem, we have initiated a new series of Laboratory Manuals on technique. Each manual is written by an expert and is designed as a laboratory handbook to be used at the bench.

It is hoped that use of these manuals will substantially reduce or perhaps even remove that period of frustration which so often precedes the successful transplant of a specialized technique into a new environment. In furtherance of this aim, we have asked authors to place special emphasis on application rather than on theory; nevertheless, each manual carries sufficient history and theory to give perspective. The publication of *library volumes* followed by *pocket paperbacks* is an innovation in scientific publishing which should assist in bringing these manuals into the laboratory as well as into the library. In undertaking the editing of such a diverse series, we have become painfully conscious of our own ignorance but have been encouraged by our board of advisers to whom we owe many valuable suggestions and, of course, by our authors who have co-operated so willingly and have so patiently tolerated our editoral intervention.

T. S. & E. Work
Editors

Contents of part I and II

PART I

PART II

CHEMICAL MODIFICATION OF PROTEINS

Selected methods and analytical procedures

A. N. Glazer, R. J. DeLange and D. S. Sigman

Department of Biological Chemistry
U.C.L.A. School of Medicine, Los Angeles, California, U.S.A.

Contents

List of abbreviations

BNPS-skatole	2-(2-nitrophenylsulfenyl)-3-methyl-3-bromo-indolcninc
DFP	diisopropylfluorophosphate
DTNB	5,5′-dithiobis (2-nitrobenzoic acid)
DTT	dithiothreitol
EDTA	ethylenediaminetetraacetic acid
NEM	N-ethylmaleimide
NPS-	2-nitrophenylsulfenyl-
NPS-Cl	2-nitrophenylsulfenyl chloride
NTCB	2-nitro-5-thiocyanobenzoic acid
PMB	*p*-mercuribenzoic acid
SAEC	S-aminoethylcysteine
SCMC	S-carboxymethylcysteine
SMC	S-methylcysteine
THL	ε-N-trimethyl-L-δ-hydroxylysine
THLP	ε-N-trimethyl-L-δ-hydroxylysine phosphate
TNBS	2, 4, 6-trinitrobenzenesulfonic acid
TNM	tetranitromethane
TNP-	2, 4, 6-trinitrophenyl-
ε_M	molar extinction coefficient in litre mol^{-1} cm^{-1}
$\Delta\varepsilon_M$	change in molar extinction coefficient
φ	phenyl residue

Subject index p. 201

Introduction

Chemical modification of proteins is performed for a variety of reasons. In basic research, the two most widely used applications are in amino acid sequence analysis, and in the identification of residues at the catalytic and binding sites of proteins. There is a growing awareness of the fact that a large number of chemical modification reactions on proteins occur *in vivo*, and that such modifications have profound importance in affecting the biological functions of these macromolecules. Indeed, the naturally occurring amino acid derivatives in proteins offer valuable clues to the preparation of chemically related protein derivatives with potentially interesting biological activities.

The discussion of analytical procedures (ch. 2) includes methods for the quantitation of both chemically introduced and naturally occurring derivatives of amino acid residues. Since the amino- and carboxyl-terminal residues of proteins are frequent targets of chemical modification, methods for end-group analysis are presented. Methods for the analysis of amino sugars and carbohydrates are included in recognition of the rapidly growing interest in the modification of glycoproteins (e.g. pituitary glycoprotein hormones, constituents of cell membranes, etc.).

Procedures involving group-specific reagents, resulting in the modification of one type of amino acid side-chain (e.g. sulfhydryl), are discussed in ch. 3. Selection of methods for detailed presentation was based either on the high specificity of the modification, or on unique applicability to a general purpose, e.g. the preparation of biologically-active protein derivatives radio-labeled to a high specific activity. No complete coverage of all available methodology is intended, and many other experimental procedures may be found in the books and reviews referred to later in this chapter.

Group-specific reagents have been used often to achieve a site-specific modification of a native protein. Since the successful applications are largely the result of chance, experimental procedures are not given (but may be found in the review references listed below). Rather, attention is focussed on a consideration of the factors which lead to the frequently observed unexpected 'specificity' of such reagents.

A discussion of the various types of 'affinity' reagents for the binding and catalytic sites of proteins is presented in ch. 5 together with guidelines for the synthesis of typical compounds of each type. In affinity labeling, the information on the binding specificity of a protein for its normal ligand is exploited in the design of a substrate analogue bearing an active group.

There is an abundance of recent literature on the chemical modification of proteins. The laboratory-oriented treatment of the subject in Methods in Enzymology, vol. XI (Hirs 1967) and vol. XXVB (Hirs and Timasheff 1972) is particularly comprehensive and valuable. A monograph by Means and Feeney (1971) is also an excellent source of references and methods.

Affinity labeling has been reviewed in detail by Singer (1967), Baker (1967), and Shaw (1970a, b), and photoaffinity labeling by Knowles (1972).

Other recent reviews include those of Cohen (1968, 1970), Freedman (1971), Glazer (1970, 1975), Riordan and Sokolovsky (1971), Spande et al. (1970), Stark (1970), and Vallee and Riordan (1969).

The characterization of proteins and their derivatives is outside the scope of this monograph. It is necessary to emphasize, however, that modification of native proteins frequently gives rise to complex mixtures of products. The complexity of the situation is not immediately apparent solely from the stoichiometry of the modification reaction. The now classical case of the reaction of native bovine pancreatic ribonuclease A with iodoacetic acid at *p*H 5.5 may be cited in this context. One carboxymethyl group is introduced per molecule of ribonuclease, but this is the consequence of the formation of two products in unequal amounts, 1-carboxymethyl-his-12-ribonuclease and 3-carboxymethyl-his-119-ribonuclease (Crestfield et al. 1963).

There is a growing list of oligomeric enzymes which display the phenomenon of 'half-of-the-sites reactivity' (Levitzki et al. 1971), in which only half of the active sites react with chemically reactive substrate analogues. In such cases, it is necessary to discriminate between the case in which approximately half of the molecules fail to react because of prior denaturation, and cases in which *bona fide* 'half-of-the-sites reactivity' exists.

Finally, treatment with reagents such as tetranitromethane, may lead to products in which the expected tyrosine derivative is absent. The extent of formation of such derivatives is difficult to assess from amino acid analyses.

It is appropriate, therefore, to examine protein derivatives, following site-specific modification by electrophoretic and chromatographic methods. Acrylamide gel electrophoresis, both in the presence and absence of sodium dodecylsulfate (Gordon, this series, vol. 1), and isoelectric focusing on polyacrylamide gels offer convenient, rapid, and highly sensitive means of examining protein derivatives for homogeneity. Ion-exchange chromatography (Peterson, this series, vol. 2) and gel filtration (Fischer, this series, vol. 1) are powerful tools for the resolution of complex mixtures of derivatives. The following compendia summarize much of the relevant literature and references: polyacrylamide gel electrophoretic procedures (Maurer 1971); protein purification (Jakoby 1971); peptide fractionation (Hirs 1967).

Chemical characterization of proteins and their derivatives

2.1. *Amino acid analysis with special reference to problem amino acids and common derivatives*

In many studies of chemical modification of proteins (or peptides) it is essential to determine which amino acid residues have reacted with the reagent being investigated, and the extent of modification. It is not generally appreciated how difficult this can be, particularly for large proteins (or peptides) with multiple residues of the same type. Ideally, the amino acid sequence of the modified protein should be known, and peptides bearing the modified residues should be isolated and characterized. This is greatly facilitated if the modified residues have markers (radioactive, highly fluorescent, etc), which may be detected with high sensitivity. However, in many instances it is desirable as an initial or supplemental method to use amino acid analysis to monitor the results, and even in the ideal situation, peptides with modified groups must be analyzed.

Although the precision of analysis with our present technology is often 1 to 3%, the quantitative release of many amino acids and amino acid derivatives from proteins is often difficult and lowers the overall precision. For example, if constant-boiling HCl (about 5.7 N) is used to hydrolyze a protein *in vacuo* at 110°C for 24 hr (these conditions are those most commonly used), the amounts of aspartic acid, asparagine, serine, threonine, glutamic acid, glutamine, valine, isoleucine, methionine, tyrosine, tryptophan, cysteine and cystine present in the

Subject index p. 201

hydrolysate may be different from the amounts in the protein hydrolyzed. The differences are small for some of these amino acids (histidine and phenylalanine are sometimes also in this category), but large for others. Although some of these amino acids do not have side-chains that are usually modified in proteins, any amino acid can be the NH_2-terminal or COOH-terminal residue of a protein and have reactive α-amino or α-carboxyl groups; therefore, quantitative analysis of all amino acids is important. Fortunately, if control samples are hydrolyzed in the same manner as the experimental samples, many problems can be corrected. Some of the problems in preparing and analyzing protein hydrolysates will be discussed below.

2.1.1. Preparation of proteins for hydrolysis

It is essential that proteins, evaluated by amino acid analysis, are homogeneous as judged by several physical and chemical criteria (gel electrophoresis, column chromatography, end group analysis, etc.). The purified protein should be separated from substances of low molecular weight, such as inorganic salts, by dialysis against 0.1 M NaCl for at least 1 day (to displace other salts) and then against several changes of deionized water until chloride ions cannot be detected with $AgNO_3$ in the outer solution. Aliquots of the protein solution (or finely dispersed suspension) can then be lyophilized to dryness and used for the determination of ash content (combustion to constant weight in a platinum crucible over an open flame), water content (drying weighed, air-equilibrated samples to constant weight under vacuum at 105°C), nitrogen content (micro-Kjeldahl or Dumas procedures), phosphate determination, carbohydrate analysis (see §2.13), spectroscopy, metal analysis, amino acid analysis, etc. Alternatively, the entire protein preparation may be lyophilized to dryness, extracted with absolute ethanol and ether to remove any lipid material (Light and Smith, 1963), and weighed portions used for the determinations listed above. It is often desirable to separate prosthetic groups from the protein (if possible without modifying amino acid residues) prior to amino acid analysis. If an accurate extinction coefficient for the protein has been determined, it is often convenient to use it as a measure of protein content rather than the value determined by weighing.

After analysis of the protein, the dry weight (less ash) of the aliquot used for analysis should equal the combined weights of the amino acids recovered (calculated from the moles of amino acids found less 1 mole of water per mole of amino acid) plus any other known constituents (phosphate, carbohydrate, prosthetic groups, metal ions, etc.). If this is not the case (within experimental error), thorough examination of the protein for other unknown constituents should be made. Constituents of the protein may be expressed as moles per g (or 100 000 g) of protein, or if the molecular weight of the protein is known, as moles per mole of protein. In some cases moles per 100 moles of amino acids or molar ratios (based on one amino acid) are used.

2.1.2. Acid hydrolysis of peptides and proteins

Aliquots of the soluble or suspended protein, which has been suitably prepared for acid hydrolysis (§ 2.1.1), are lyophilized in appropriate glass containers that will withstand the hydrolysis conditions. For this purpose ordinary Pyrex or Kimax test tubes have been used, but many laboratories (including our own) prefer tear-drop glass bulbs with long stems that can be made easily in the laboratory or purchased commercially. The hydrolysis tubes should be cleaned with hot HNO_3 (concentrated HNO_3 diluted with an equal volume of water) or other appropriate glass cleaner, and then thoroughly rinsed with deionized water and dried before use. The amount of protein to be hydrolyzed will vary with the size, composition and availability of the protein. However, with most amino acid analyzers currently in use (e.g. the Beckman 120C), it is preferable to have at least 0.01 μmole (but less than 0.60 μmoles) of each amino acid for each column required for analysis, although amounts less than this can be determined less precisely. Therefore, for a protein with a molecular weight of 20 000 and having a single residue of histidine, a minimum of 0.4 to 0.5 mg of protein should be hydrolyzed for analysis with an analyzer which requires two columns for complete analysis.

The lyophilized protein is dissolved or suspended in 1 to 2 ml of 5.7 N HCl, which is usually prepared by glass distillation, repeated once or twice to form the constant boiling mixture. One drop of 5% (w/v) aqueous phenol is usually added for protective purposes. It is necessary to exclude oxygen from the tube during hydrolysis in order to recover maximum yields of the amino acids. Although this can be done by alternatively evacuating and flushing the tube with nitrogen, we have found that gradual evacuation of the tube with the aid of a high vacuum (mechanical) pump and then warming the tube for 30 sec in a 40°C bath with gentle agitation while it is still being evacuated, is an effective method of removing oxygen. Many protein samples will tend to froth under these conditions, and to prevent sample loss it may be necessary to freeze the samples in dry ice-acetone and gently thaw under vacuum, prior to warming. After this procedure the tubes are sealed under vacuum with an oxygen torch and placed in an oven at 110°C for the desired time. The sealing operation may be facilitated by having the hydrolysis tube connected through a short piece of rubber tubing to a stopcock which can be closed and removed from the vacuum system. The standard time of hydrolysis is 24 hr, but longer times may be necessary for quantitative estimation of some amino acids (see below).

After hydrolysis is complete the tubes are cooled, scored and opened, and the acid is removed, either by rotary evaporation or in a heated desiccator over NaOH at 40–50°C. In our laboratory it is standard procedure to examine 1/10 of each hydrolysate by high-voltage paper electrophoresis at *p*H 1.9 (see Appendix I) prior to analysis to ensure that appropriate amounts are analyzed. Some amino acid derivatives (oxidation products of methionine, methylated lysines, etc.) are also sometimes observed by this procedure. It is usually helpful to add an internal standard, either prior to hydrolysis to reveal hydrolytic losses or prior to analysis to reveal analytical losses. For this purpose we have used norleucine (0.03 μmoles). This amino acid elutes after leucine on the 60 cm column.

2.1.3. Analysis and calculations

The hydrolyzed samples, as prepared above, are dissolved in buffer and analyzed as recommended by the analyzer manufacturer. With a Beckman 120C analyzer we routinely dilute the samples to 1.0 ml with the recommended *p*H 2.2 buffer and 0.4 ml is used for each column. The amounts of each amino acid are determined by manual or automatic integration of the area under each amino acid peak. If automatic integration is used, the chart should be examined to be sure that the integration values correspond with the relative positions and peak heights obtained. The calculated amounts of the amino acids (usually in μmoles) can then be converted to moles of amino acid per mole of protein or per 100 000 g of protein by using the appropriate correction values for the amount of protein hydrolysate actually used for each column of the analyzer.

There has been a recent trend towards the use of high pressure systems and reagents other than ninhydrin to increase sensitivity and speed (e.g. see Moore 1972). Although not yet in general use, such systems hold considerable promise for the future. Expanded scales and one-column systems of analysis have also been used to boost sensitivity. However, in most of these more sensitive systems, the baseline is usually not as straight and free of drift as in the two-column systems, and there are often more problems encountered with interfering substances. At present we would recommend the use of the common commercial analyzers without special modifications (except for the possible inclusion of expanded scale modes) for the greatest accuracy in routine work. However, for situations where samples are obtained in limited amounts or where many samples need to be analyzed quickly, some of the newer systems may well be worthy of consideration. The application of fluorescamine to the quantitative fluorimetric determination of picomole quantities of amino acids, peptides and proteins is of particular interest in this context (Udenfriend et al. 1972).

It should be noted that for a protein having 20 residues of one amino acid (e.g. leucine), the precision of the results obtained by analysis of acid hydrolysates of this protein would usually indicate 20 ± 1 residues.

As mentioned in the introduction to ch. 2, if the procedures described in §2.1.2 and §2.1.3 are used with only one time of hydrolysis, quantitation of at least 13 of the 20 common amino acids may be in error. Special methods that may be utilized to obtain more accurate analyses of these 'problem amino acids' and their derivatives are given below.

Many of the details of analysis to be described in this article are based on procedures used in our own laboratory. An attempt will be made to give credit for other procedures. Beckman 120B and 120C analyzers have been used routinely in our own studies.

2.2. *Serine, threonine, tyrosine and derivatives*

2.2.1. *Analysis*

These 3 amino acids are often partially destroyed by acid hydrolysis with the amount of destruction dependent on the time of hydrolysis. With some proteins there is little or no loss of threonine or tyrosine, but serine destruction is rather constant in all proteins. It has been common practice to correct serine values by 10% for each 24 hr of acid hydrolysis, and sometimes threonine and tyrosine values are corrected by 5% as a first approximation of the extent of destruction.

The most accurate method of analysis for serine, threonine and tyrosine in proteins is to hydrolyze the proteins for several different times (e.g. 24, 48 and 72 hr) and extrapolate the values to '0' time. In general, the more times that are utilized, the more accurate will be the extrapolation. Extrapolation of the NH_3 content of these hydrolysates to 0 time will also give an estimate of the number of amides present in the protein, if care has been used to exclude NH_3 during purification of the protein. The inclusion of phenol in the hydrolysates has generally decreased the rates of destruction, particularly for tyrosine. If serine phosphate (§ 2.12.4) or similar derivatives are present, the extrapolated curve will be more complex due to different rates of destruction.

Since most derivatives of serine and threonine are not stable to acid hydrolysis, they will not be discussed here. However, those occurring naturally in proteins are described in § 2.12.4. It should be noted that 0-maleylated derivatives and similar derivatives of serine and threonine have been found as side-products of reactions used to modify other residues in proteins (e.g. ch. 3).

2.2.2. *Halogenated and nitrated derivatives of tyrosine*

A common finding, if proteins are hydrolyzed with undistilled HCl or in the absence of phenol, is the conversion of some tyrosine to halogenated derivatives or 'tyrosine-X', which is usually the 3-chloro-derivative (see Sanger and Thompson 1963). Exposure of certain peptides or peptide hydrolysates to polluted air ('smog') has also caused some of the tyrosine to be converted to a substance which elutes in the nitrotyrosine position on the analyzer. It is conceivable that this substance is indeed nitrotyrosine, produced from nitrogen oxides or other pollutants in the air. Halogenated and nitrated derivatives of tyrosine may also be prepared by specific chemical modification reactions (§ 3.7).

The halogenated and nitrated derivatives of tyrosine may be analyzed by continuing elution of the 60 cm column past the elution of phenylalanine. Elution volumes, determined for one run with a Beckman 120C analyzer, were 204 ml for phenylalanine, 223 ml for nitrotyrosine and 264 ml for tyrosine-X. The various halogenated derivatives of tyrosine would undoubtedly elute from this column at different positions as was found for elution from a 15 cm column operated according to Spackman et al. (1958): tyrosine 17.5 ml; 3-chlorotyrosine, 26.0 ml; 3.5-dichlorotyrosine, 33.3 ml; 3-bromo-tyrosine, 31.5 ml; 3,5-dibromotyrosine, 47.5 ml; 3-iodotyrosine, 42.7 ml; 3,5-diiodotyrosine, 87.5 ml; 3-chloro- 5-bromotyrosine, 39.5 ml; lysine, 52 ml; NH_3, 77.5 ml (see Sanger and Thompson 1963). In a regular 2-column analysis of a peptide or protein, the presence of peaks on the short column between the positions of phenylalanine and tryptophan is often indicative of halogenated or nitrated derivatives of tyrosine, but further confirmation in other systems should be obtained. We have found that a 60 cm column, eluted with the usual short column (basic) buffer gives excellent separations of many of these derivatives.

Sanger and Thompson (1963) also reported the high voltage electrophoretic migrations of the halogenated derivatives at *p*H 1.85 (2% formic acid, 8% acetic acid, 1 hr at 4000 volts; this system should be comparable to the *p*H 1.9 electrophoresis described in the Appendix). All migrate slower than tyrosine in this system: tyrosine, 22.5 cm; 3-chlorotyrosine, 19.3 cm; 3,5-dichlorotyrosine, 16.5 cm; 3-bromo-tyrosine, 18.0 cm; 3,5-dibromotyrosine, 14.8 cm; 3-iodotyrosine,

17.0 cm; 3,5-diiodotyrosine, 13.0 cm; and 3-chloro-5-bromotyrosine, 15.7 cm. The migrations in *p*H 8.9 electrophoresis are also reported. Nitrotyrosine has a migration of 0.87 compared to 1.00 for tyrosine in *p*H 1.9 electrophoresis. It should be noted that these derivatives have lower color values than tyrosine and that quantitation is generally not good after acid hydrolysis.

2.3. *Valine and isoleucine*

During acid hydrolysis of proteins, valine and isoleucine are often released more slowly than other amino acids due to steric hindrance of hydrolysis by the β-branched sidechains. The Ile–Ile bond is particularly resistant to hydrolysis and is cleaved to the extent of about 50% in 24 hr at 110°C. This could mislead an investigator into the belief that one residue of isoleucine was present in a given peptide rather than two. The Val–Val, Val–Ile and Ile–Val bonds are also slowly hydrolyzed, being 60–75% cleaved in 24 hr at 110°C. Therefore, if the amounts of valine and isoleucine appear to reach a plateau after 72 hr of hydrolysis, these values may be used; otherwise, hydrolysis for 120 hr may be required to obtain quantitative values. Small amounts of *allo*isoleucine, which elutes from most analyzer columns just before isoleucine, should be included in the isoleucine determination.

2.4. *Aspartic acid, glutamic acid, asparagine and glutamine*

The amounts of aspartic acid, asparagine, glutamic acid and glutamine in a protein cannot be determined by analysis of acid hydrolysates alone. In order to obtain these values it is necessary to determine the complete sequence or to analyze enzymic hydrolysates which have been prepared by successfully hydrolyzing quantitatively all peptide bonds in the protein (see § 2.11). Since this is often impractical or difficult to do, it has been customary to report the combined values of aspartic acid and asparagine as Asx (or aspartic acid) and glutamic acid and glutamine as Glx (or glutamic acid). These values can be obtained after acid hydrolysis by the usual procedures outlined above, since the amides are quantitatively converted to the acids under these conditions. If the amide content has been estimated by extrapolation of the NH_3 content of the hydrolysates to 0 time (see § 2.2.2), the combined content of the aspartic acid plus glutamic acid can be estimated, but the amount of either individual component cannot be determined. The combined content of glutamine and asparagine can also be estimated after treatment of the protein with concentrated HCl in a closed container for 10 days at 37°C (Rees 1946) or with 2 N HCl for a few hours at 100°C (Leach and Parkhill 1955). In this latter procedure, it is necessary to do timed hydrolyses with extrapolation to 0 time for accurate results. In these and other procedures which depend on the production of NH_3, controls should be run to determine the amount of free NH_3 before hydrolysis.

A complex procedure for determining the content of asparagine and glutamine separately in proteins has been described (see Chibnall et al. 1958). This procedure makes use of esterification of the protein, reduction of the resulting esters of aspartic acid and glutamic acid with lithium borohydride and hydrolysis of asparagine and glutamine to the acids in which form they are analyzed. Despite the side reactions for which corrections must be made, this method, in conjunction with total enzymic hydrolysis, may be useful to those who must quantitatively estimate these 4 amino acids.

It should be noted that if asparagine and glutamine are released from a protein (e.g. by enzymic hydrolysis § 2.11.4), methods are available for analyzing them separately (see Benson et al. 1967; Tower 1967).

2.5. *Cysteine, cystine, methionine and derivatives*

These 3 sulfur-containing amino acids and their derivatives are susceptible to oxidation and other destructive reactions. Even when great care has been taken to remove all oxygen from hydrolysis tubes, considerable losses of cysteine and cystine are found after acid hydrolysis, and this usually prevents direct quantitation of these amino acids in proteins. However, total cysteine plus half-cystine content may be determined as cysteic acid after performic acid oxidation (§ 2.5.1) or as S-sulfocysteine. Estimation of cysteine or half-cystine individually may be made by making other derivatives (§ 3.8), some of which may be analyzed spectrophotometrically and others by amino acid analysis (see below). Since cysteine elutes in the same position as proline, it may be necessary to convert any free cysteine to cystine by air oxidation or to S-sulfocysteine (see below) after acid hydrolysis in order to obtain good results for proline.

It should be noted that total cysteine plus half-cystine can also be determined as S-sulfocysteine after acid hydrolysis in the absence of oxygen (Inglis and Liu 1970). This is apparently possible because derivatives of cystine and cysteine that form during acid hydrolysis can be reduced with dithiothreitol to cysteine which is then converted to the S-sulfo derivative by tetrathionate (§ 3.8.8). For proteins which contain tryptophan, tetrathionate ($Na_2S_4O_6$) should also be included in the 6 N HCl prior to hydrolysis. S-sulfocysteine elutes from a 60 cm column of a Beckman 120C analyzer in the same position as cysteic acid (unretarded position) and other substances like O-phosphoserine, and therefore it is necessary to run control samples to detect interfering substances. S-sulfocysteine has a lower 570 nm/440 nm ratio than cysteic acid and has a color value of 74% that of aspartic acid under the described conditions of formation. The most widely used procedure for the determination of the half-cystine and cysteine content of proteins is carboxymethylation or carboxyethylation.

If appropriate precautions have been taken in the preparation of a protein, and if oxygen is completely removed before hydrolysis, methionine will usually be recovered from acid hydrolysates in yields greater than 95%. However, in some proteins (particularly those that are chemically modified) and in many peptides the methionine may be at least partially oxidized to the sulfoxide or sulfone forms, and even though these may be analyzed with amino acid analyzers (see below), the total yield of methionine (and oxidized products) is usually somewhat low. A good check on total methionine content in a peptide or protein is obtained by analyzing for methionine sulfone after performic acid oxidation, since methionine and its sulfoxides are quantitatively converted to the sulfone by this procedure.

2.5.1. *Performic acid oxidation (for analytical work)*

After oxidation of unmodified proteins with performic acid (§ 3.8.1) the methionine will all be present as methionine sulfone, and the cysteine and cystine will be present as cysteic acid. The method for oxidizing proteins with performic acid on a preparative scale (§ 3.8.1) has been modified for analytical studies (Moore 1963), to allow rapid destruction of excess performic acid. However, tryptophan is still destroyed by the performic acid in this modified procedure, and quantitation of tyrosine may be complicated by the formation of halogenated derivatives (§ 2.2.3).

The performic acid is prepared in the usual manner by allowing a mixture of 1.0 ml of 30% (w/v) H_2O_2 and 9.0 ml of 88% (w/v) formic acid to stand at room temperature for 1 hr, after which it is cooled to 0°C. A known amount of protein, usually the amount used for routine hydrolysates, is dissolved in 1 to 2 ml of the reagent in a cooled hydrolysis tube. If the protein does not dissolve readily in the cold reagent, it can usually be dissolved first in 0.1 ml of 100% formic acid at room temperature. The mixture is kept at 0°C for 4 hr after which performic acid is destroyed by the addition of 0.15 ml of cold 48% (w/v) HBr per ml of performic acid reagent used. The bromine which forms, as well as the formic acid solution, can best be removed from the hydrolysis tube by rotary evaporation under high vacuum (mechanical pump) at 40°C with NaOH pellets in the condenser trap; the condenser should be cooled with dry ice in ethanol. Acid hydrolysis of the oxidized sample and analysis of the resulting hydrolysates are performed in the usual manner (§2.1.2).

2.5.2. *Cysteic acid*

Cysteic acid is the major product of performic acid oxidation of cysteine and cystine in proteins, and is usually produced in yields of more than 90%. Cysteic acid is not retarded by the resins generally used in amino acid analyzers and therefore elutes at the breakthrough volume (about 42% of the elution volume of aspartic acid). However, since other substances such as O-phosphoserine can also elute in this position, it is essential to analyze hydrolysates made both before and after performic acid oxidation of the protein to determine if interfering substances are present. Cysteic acid has a color value of 101% that of aspartic acid (Spackman et al. 1958), and in electrophoresis at *p*H 1.9 it has a mobility of 0.47 towards the anode compared to 1.00 towards the cathode for aspartic acid.

2.5.3. *S-Carboxymethylcysteine (SCMC) and S-carboxyethylcysteine*

S-Carboxymethylcysteine is prepared by alkylation of cysteine with iodoacetic acid (§3.8.2). Iodoacetamide gives the amide derivative, which is converted to SCMC by acid hydrolysis. Since SCMC (and other derivatives of cysteine) is especially susceptible to oxidative and other destructive reactions, it may be helpful in some instances, to include one drop of 5% mercaptoacetic acid (or some other reducing agent) in addition to the phenol in the 6 N HCl prior to hydrolysis. However, blanks should be run (no protein) to correct for any interfering ninhydrin-positive substances derived from the reducing agent. SCMC elutes from the 60 cm column of a Beckman 120C analyzer at a volume of 46 ml compared to 52 ml for aspartic acid. The color value for SCMC is 92% that of aspartic acid (Spackman et al. 1958).

It has recently been observed that SCMC can cyclize, particularly at acid *p*H (optimally at *p*H 3) to give a thiazine derivative which is ninhydrin-negative (Bradbury and Smyth 1973) (§ 3.8.3). For this reason it may often be preferable to make the S-carboxyethylcysteine derivative in proteins (§ 3.8.3) as it does not readily undergo this type of reaction (Bradbury and Smyth 1973). S-carboxyethylcysteine elutes from a 60 cm column of a Beckman 120C analyzer between serine and glutamic acid; its color value should be similar to that of SCMC.

2.5.4. *S-Aminoethylcysteine (SAEC)*

This positively-charged derivative is prepared from cysteine and ethylenimine (§ 3.8.4) and is often used to introduce additional sites of tryptic hydrolysis into proteins. SAEC has a mobility of 2.07 compared to 1.00 for aspartic in *p*H 1.9 electrophoresis, and elutes from a 20 cm (basic) column of a Beckman analyzer at 82 ml compared to 74 ml for lysine and 96 ml for histidine (Schroeder et al. 1967). SAEC has a color value of 92% that of lysine and 88% that of leucine, if losses due to acid hydrolysis are included (Hofmann 1964).

2.5.5. *S-Methylcysteine (SMC)*

S-Methylcysteine, which is a neutral derivative produced by alkylating cysteine with methyl-p-nitrobenzenesulfonate (§ 3.8.6) has a mobility of 1.04 compared to 1.00 for aspartic acid in *p*H 1.9 electrophoresis and elutes from the 60 cm column at the trailing edge of the proline peak (Heinrikson 1971). This often prevents accurate estimation of proline, but if the proline content is low, there is little problem in quantitating the SMC derivative. If better separations are desired, the investigator suggests the use of a 150 cm column, but it also seems likely that changes in ionic strength or *p*H of the buffer or changes in the temperature of the column would also allow better separations with the 60 cm column. The color values for SMC are 98% (unhydrolyzed) or 89% (including correction values for losses during acid hydrolysis) that of alanine. A decomposition product (possibly the sulfone) is formed during the first 22 hours of acid hydrolysis, but not thereafter, and elutes at the position of the leading edge of aspartic acid. Perhaps the amount of this decomposition product could be reduced if phenol or a reducing agent is included during hydrolysis (§ 2.1.2).

2.5.6. *Thialaminine*

Thialaminine, or the basic ethyltrimethylammonium derivative of cysteine, is prepared from cysteine and (2-bromoethyl)trimethylammonium bromide (§ 3.8.5). Thialaminine is stable to acid hydrolysis for periods of at least 72 hr at 106°C, elutes from a 10 cm column of PA-35 resin on the Beckman analyzer between lysine and histidine and has a color value 86% that of lysine (Itano and Robinson 1972).

Another basic derivative of cysteine, S-(4-pyridylethyl)-L-cysteine has also been characterized. It elutes from the short column of the analyzer just before arginine and has a color value of 102% that of leucine (Friedman et al. 1970).

2.5.7. *S-Succinylcysteine (S-1,2-dicarboxyethyl-L-cysteine)*

S-Succinylcysteine is the product formed from the reaction of cysteinyl

Methionine sulfoxide may be released essentially quantitatively by hydrolysis with 15% (~4.4 M) NaOH (see Neumann et al. 1962). The procedure described by these investigators calls for hydrolysis of 5 mg of protein in special vapor-tight, screw-cap Telfon vials, but it is possible to hydrolyze 1 mg or less if the hydrolysis is carried out in hydrolysis tubes with small volumes and containing a polypropylene liner to hold the sample in a manner similar to that described by Hugli and Moore (1972). Convenient liners for these small amounts of protein and NaOH are small conical plastic tubes (such as the micro sample tube, Dynalab Corp., Rochester, N.Y.). The dried sample is dissolved in 0.2 ml of 15% NaOH (freshly made from 50% NaOH each time) for each mg of protein, and after evacuating the tube cautiously to remove bubbles without loss of sample, the tube is sealed and placed in an oven at 110°C for 16 hr. Alternatively, the tube may be successively evacuated and flushed with nitrogen several times before sealing. After hydrolysis the tube is cooled before opening, and the solution is acidified with 0.19 ml of 6 N HCl and 0.1 ml of 1.1 M citric acid (containing 0.05 ml of thiodiglycol per ml) per 0.2 ml of 15% NaOH used, to give a final *p*H lower than 2.2. The solution is diluted to 1.0 ml for each mg of protein hydrolyzed, and aliquots of 0.5 to 1.0 ml are analyzed (e.g. on the 60 cm column of a Beckman 120C analyzer). The 150 cm column system described by Moore et al. (1958) may also be used.

The method described above gives direct analysis of methionine sulfoxide content in proteins. Another method makes use of carboxymethylation of methionine at acid *p*H to give the carboxymethylsulfonium derivative (§ 3.5). Methionine sulfoxide, which is not affected by the carboxymethylation reaction, is then oxidized to the sulfone which is stable to acid hydrolysis and can easily be quantitated. This is possible because methionine carboxymethyl-sulfonium salts are not affected by performic acid oxidation, although they are degraded by acid hydrolysis. Therefore, the methionine sulfone content is equal to the methionine sulfoxide content plus any sulfone that may have been initially present (shown by analysis before oxidation).

2.5.10. Methionine carboxymethylsulfonium salts

These derivatives of methionine (isomers) are prepared by treating proteins with iodoacetic acid; the reaction is most specific for methionine at acid *p*H (§ 3.5). These derivatives are not affected by performic acid oxidation (see under methionine sulfoxide), but are degraded by acid hydrolysis to give methionine, carboxymethylhomocysteine, homoserine and homoserine lactone (Gundlach et al. 1959).

Carboxymethylhomocysteine elutes from most analyzer columns just after proline, and the other two derivatives are discussed below. It should be possible to quantitate the carboxymethylsulfonium derivative after complete enzymic hydrolysis (see § 2.11), since it has been shown that they elute as two peaks just prior to aspartic acid (Gundlach et al. 1959). The amount of carboxymethylsulfonium derivative present can best be quantitated by oxidizing the non-carboxymethylated methionine to methionine sulfone (§ 2.5.9) and subtracting the amount of methionine sulfone from the total methionine content of the protein to obtain the amount of methionine carboxymethylsulfonium salts.

2.5.11. Homoserine and homoserine lactone

Treatment of proteins with cyanogen bromide results in cleavage of the peptide chain COOH-terminal to methionyl residues with concomitant conversion of the methionine to homoserine lactone which is in equilibrium with homoserine. In certain instances (e.g. -Met-Ser- or -Met-Thr-) some of the methionine is converted to homoserine without peptide bond cleavage (see Schroeder et al. 1969). Homoserine and its lactone are also products of the breakdown of the carboxymethylsulfonium salts of methionine (§ 2.5.10).

Homoserine elutes from the 60 cm column of a Beckman 120C analyzer just prior to glutamic acid and has a color value 95% that of leucine (Hofmann 1964). Better separation of homoserine and glutamic acid can be achieved by lowering the *p*H of the eluting buffer to 3.20 (Ambler 1965) or to 2.80 (Schroeder et al. 1967). Homoserine has a mobility of 1.37 compared to 1.00 for aspartic acid in *p*H 1.9 electrophoresis.

Homoserine lactone elutes from the short column (basic) immediately after NH_3 and has a color value of 57% that of lysine (Hofmann 1964). The mobility of the lactone in electrophoresis at *p*H 1.9 is 2.45 compared to 1.00 for aspartic acid. The lactone gives a yellow-brown color with ninhydrin (homoserine gives a blue color).

Solutions of homoserine and its lactone slowly reach equilibrium under most conditions at room temperature. As a result, samples of these derivatives prepared for analysis often gradually change in concentration even during the chromatographic steps, and color values usually reflect such losses. Acidic conditions favor lactone formation, and trifluoroacetic acid at 20°C for 1 hr can be used to convert essentially all of the homoserine (free or in peptides) to the lactone form (Ambler 1965). Alkaline conditions favor homoserine formation, but may often be too harsh for many peptide procedures (see Ambler 1965).

2.6. *Tryptophan and derivatives*

Little or no tryptophan will usually be found in protein hydrolysates prepared with acid in the usual manner. Mercaptans added to the 6 N HCl usually increase the yields of tryptophan (Matsubara and Sasaki 1969), and substitution of p-toluenesulfonic acid (with added 3-(2-aminoethyl) indole) in place of the HCl has been used to good advantage (Liu and Chang 1971).

At the present time the hydrolytic methods of choice for tryptophan analyses appear to be with methanesulfonic acid in the presence of added 3-(2-aminoethyl) indole (see Moore 1972) or with NaOH in the presence of starch (Hugli and Moore 1972). Both methods will be described below, but it should be noted here that hydrolysis with NaOH has the advantage that carbohydrate in the protein sample does not affect the yields of tryptophan as it does in the acid hydrolysates. Other methods of tryptophan analysis involving spectrophotometry (Goodwin and Morton 1946; Edelhock 1967), titration with N-bromosuccinimide (Spande and Witkop 1967), or the formation of colored derivatives (Spies and Chambers 1948; Barman and Koshland 1967;

Spies 1967; Scoffone et al. 1968) may be used to give initial estimates or verification of tryptophan content. It should also be possible to obtain good tryptophan analyses after complete enzymic hydrolysis (§ 2.11).

Hydrolysis of proteins with methanesulfonic acid is carried out in the usual type of hydrolysis tube with 4 N methanesulfonic acid, containing 0.2% 3-(2-aminoethyl) indole, at 115°C for 24 hr (Liu; see Moore 1972). The acid mixture is available in sealed vials from Pierce Chemical Corp. The usual precautions to remove oxygen should be followed. Since the acid is not volatile, it is necessary partially to neutralize the cooled hydrolysate with an equal volume of 3.5 N NaOH and dilute with water to a volume 5 times the volume of acid used for hydrolysis. The procedure recommends the use of 1 ml of the methanesulfonic acid mixture (for about 2–5 mg of protein), which would result in 5 ml of diluted hydrolysate. Since 1-ml aliquots are analyzed (see below), only 20% of the protein hydrolyzed is utilized for each analysis. However, where the amount of protein available for hydrolysis is limited, it should be possible to scale down the amounts of materials used to levels such as 0.2 ml of the acid mixture for 0.5 mg of protein if appropriately smaller hydrolysis tubes are used.

Aliquots of 1 ml of the hydrolysate are used for analysis with the short (basic) column of a Beckman analyzer; elutions from a 10 cm column of PA-35 resin being: tryptophan, 30 ml; lysine, 37 ml; histidine, 45 ml; and arginine, 82 ml. However, mannosamine and galactosamine coelute with tryptophan in this system and if they are present (determined by extending a 60 cm column run for 60 ml past phenylalanine; see also § 2.13.1), a 20 cm column of the same resin at 55°C, eluted at 50 ml per hr with 33 ml of 0.2 N sodium citrate buffer at *p*H 4.25 and then with 230 ml of 0.35 N buffer at *p*H 5.28, should be used (Liu and Chang 1971). The elution volumes in this system are: tyrosine, 42 ml; phenylalanine, 46 ml; glucosamine, 82 ml; mannosamine and galactosamine, 90 ml; tryptophan, 98 ml; lysine, 125 ml; histidine, 136 ml; arginine, 250 ml. The color value obtained for tryptophan in this system is 78% that of lysine. With proteins hydrolyzed with HCl (or in the presence of some HCl), an acid decomposition product may be observed at 94 ml in this system.

Hydrolysis of proteins (1 to 5 mg) with 4.2 N NaOH (0.6 ml) in the presence of partially hydrolyzed starch (25 mg) has been reported by Hugli and Moore (1972) to give yields of tryptophan greater than 97% for several proteins. These investigators used the bottom portions of polypropylene centrifuge tubes as liners in regular glass hydrolysis tubes to avoid silicate formation. It is also possible to hydrolyze smaller amounts of protein in smaller volumes if small conical plastic tubes (such as the micro sample tube, Dynalab Corp., N.Y.) are used in smaller hydrolysis tubes. Care should be taken not to melt the plastic liners when sealing the tubes. In practice, the protein (in 0.1 ml of 0.005 N HCl or NaOH is added to a 10.9 × 50 mm liner inside a 16 × 150 mm thin-walled Pyrex test tube, and 0.5 ml of 5 N NaOH (freshly prepared from 50% NaOH) is added after adding 25 mg of partially hydrolyzed starch. The addition of 1-octanol (5 μl of a 1% solution in toluene) aids in preventing frothing during evacuation. A constriction (to about 2 mm) is made in the glass tube near the middle, and the lower portion is cooled in a dry ice acetone bath for 1.5 min (do not freeze). The tube is evacuated with a high vacuum pump by repeatedly opening and closing a stopcock while tapping the tube to dislodge air bubbles. When the pressure has stabilized between 25 and 50 microns of mercury, the tubes are sealed and placed in an oven for hydrolysis at 110°C for 16 hr. If Val–Trp or Ile–Trp bonds are present, (or if it is not known if they are present) it is necessary to hydrolyze one sample for at least 98 hr at 110°C or 48 hr at 135°C, since these bonds are only slowly hydrolyzed. After carefully cooling the hydrolysates (to prevent loss of sample), the tubes are opened and 0.5 ml of 0.2 M citrate buffer at *p*H 4.25 (without Brij 35) is added and mixed. The solution is then transferred with several rinses of buffer to a chilled (dry ice) 2.5 ml (or 5 ml) volumetric flask, containing 0.42 ml of 6 N HCl, and diluted to volume with the *p*H 4.25 buffer. The precautions of using *p*H 4.25 buffer and the chilled HCl are for the purpose of avoiding losses of tryptophan, known to occur in most acidic solutions.

Aliquots of 1.0 ml of the diluted hydrolysates are analyzed on the short column (Beckman analyzer), eluted at 50 ml per hour with a buffer prepared by diluting the usual *p*H 5.3 buffer to give a final Na^+

concentration of 0.21 M (the final *p*H is 5.4) (Hugli and Moore 1972). This buffer separates tryptophan from lysinoalanine, which is a product formed from lysine and dehydroalanine during alkaline hydrolysis of many proteins (Bohak 1964); tryptophan, 37 ml; lysinoalanine, 55 ml; lysine, 68 ml; and histidine, 79 ml. These results are for a 0.9×8 cm column of Beckman PA-35 resin, but better results are often obtained on a 12 cm column, which allows more time for the baseline to be established after the neutral and acidic amino acids are eluted. Any ornithine formed from arginine during alkaline hydrolysis will elute just prior to lysine. Hexosamines (see § 2.13) are destroyed by alkaline hydrolysis, and neither they nor hydroxylysine (see § 2.12.1.3) interfere with the tryptophan analysis. The color value for tryptophan in this particular system was determined to be 79% that of lysine (Hugli and Moore 1972).

1-Formyltryptophan. This derivative of tryptophan, which is formed in proteins by formylation in anhydrous formic acid saturated with gaseous HCl (§ 3.6.1), is not stable to acid or alkaline hydrolysis, but could be obtained after complete enzymic hydrolysis of derivatized proteins (§ 2.11). With a 0.9×7 cm short (basic) column on a Beckman 120B Analyzer, 1-formyltryptophan elutes in 53 ml compared to 37 ml for tryptophan (Previero et al. 1967a). In paper chromatography with 1-butanol : acetic acid : water (4 : 1 : 5, v/v) tryptophan has an R_f of 0.50 and 1-formyltryptophan has an R_f of 0.58. The amount of derivative formed in proteins may be determined by lyophilization of the solution after the formylation reaction has ceased (usually by 40 min as measured by change in absorbance at 298 nm) and measuring the absorbance at 298 nm of an aliquot of the protein dissolved in 8 M urea at *p*H 4. The molar extinction coefficient of 1-formyltryptophan has been calculated as 4880 at 298 nm, and the change in absorbance at 298 nm can be used as a measure of tryptophan content in proteins where this is not known (Previero et al. 1967b).

Other derivatives of tryptophan which may also be obtained after enzymic hydrolysis of derivatized proteins are those obtained by reaction with sulfenyl halides (Scoffone et al. 1968) and 2-hydroxynitrobenzyl bromide (Barman and Koshland 1967) (§ 3.6.2).

2.7. *Lysine derivatives*

Analyses for lysine after acid hydrolysis of proteins are usually quantitative and reliable, unless the lysines have been exposed to certain types of reagents (e.g. cyanate, nitrous acid). In a few proteins some lysines are ε-N-methylated (see § 2.12.1.2); the methyllysines are stable to acid hydrolysis and emerge from many analyzer columns as a shoulder on the trailing edge of lysine, thus making lysine quantitation less precise (see § 2.12.1). Methyllysine may also be formed in proteins by chemical modification (§ 3.1.1.3). Many derivatives of lysine are not stable to acid hydrolysis (e.g. ε-N-acetyllysine) and will not be discussed here, but those which occur naturally in proteins are discussed in § 2.12.1.

2.7.1. ε-N-Carboxymethyllysines

Both the ε-N-monocarboxymethyl and the ε-N-dicarboxymethyl derivatives of lysine are formed by reaction of proteins with iodoacetate at alkaline *p*H values at which lysyl residues are at least partially unprotonated (§ 3.8.2). Both derivatives are stable to acid hydrolysis under the usual conditions.

Both the mono- and di-derivatives are analyzed with the longer column used for analysis of the acidic and neutral amino acids. In the original studies of Gundlach et al. (1959), the 150 cm column was used: ε-N-dicarboxymethyllysine, 90 ml; aspartic acid, 122 ml; ε-N-monocarboxymethyllysine, 335 ml; and methionine, 341 ml. The dicarboxymethyl derivative elutes after cysteic acid but before methionine sulfoxides. To our knowledge other analytical systems have not been used, but the 60 cm column may not give adequate separations, especially for the mono-derivative, since it elutes prior to methionine which is already close to the buffer change peak. It seems likely that by appropriate manipulation of times of buffer change, the *p*H or ionic strength of the buffer, or the temperature of the column, good separations could be obtained with the 60 cm column.

2.7.2. Homoarginine

Homoarginine is the product of guanidination of lysyl residues with either 0-methylisourea or reagents such as 1-guanyl-3,5-dimethylpyrazole nitrate (see §3.1.1.2). Like arginine, homoarginine is stable to acid hydrolysis, but not to alkaline hydrolysis.

Homoarginine elutes from the short (basic) column of the analyzer after arginine; e.g. with one system homoarginine has an elution volume 1.33 times that of arginine (Habeeb 1960). The color constant should be similar to that of arginine. The migration of homoarginine in a number of chromatographic systems has been described (Bell 1962). Homoarginine has a mobility of 2.20 compared to 1.00 for aspartic acid in *p*H 1.9 electrophoresis.

2.7.3. Deamination products of lysine

Treatment of proteins with nitrous acid can lead to deamination of the lysyl residues as well as of the NH_2-terminal residues. Kurosky and Hoffmann (1972) have identified three products of lysine deamination which elute from the 60 cm column of a Beckman 120C Analyzer at (1) the position of glutamic acid, (2) 7 min before glycine and (3) 10 min before tyrosine. Products (2) and (3), which are the major products formed, are believed to be ε-hydroxynorleucine and its lactone respectively. The most accurate method for analyzing for lysine deamination is to measure the loss of lysine rather than to measure the three derivatives.

2.7.4. Homocitrulline

The ε-amino groups of lysyl residues in proteins may be carbamylated by cyanate to give homocitrulline residues (§ 3.1.2.1). It should be noted that some carbamylation of proteins can occur in urea solutions that have not been deionized to remove cyanate. The extent of modification is often difficult to assess, however, since acid hydrolysis of fully carbamylated proteins under the usual conditions gives homocitrulline plus 17–33% free lysine (Stark and Smyth 1963). Although the lysine recovery (in %) is variable, depending on the protein studied, for a given protein the lysine recovery is apparently constant.

If accurate quantitation of homocitrulline content of a protein is necessary, complete enzymic hydrolysis (§ 2.11) might be tried.

Homocitrulline elutes from most analyzer columns just prior to valine. Alternatively, the unreacted lysines can be converted under denaturing conditions to other acid-stable derivatives (homoarginine, methyllysines, carboxymethyllysines) which can be quantitated after acid hydrolysis (above and § 2.12). The homocitrulline content can then be assumed to be the difference between the total lysine content and the content of the acid-stable derivative. Alkaline hydrolysis of carbamylated proteins gives quantitative conversion of homocitrulline to lysine (Stark and Smyth 1963), and this can be used to check the homocitrulline content of the protein in which the other lysines have been converted to another derivative that does not give lysine by alkaline hydrolysis (see also § 3.1.2.1.).

2.8. *Histidine and derivatives*

Although analyses for histidine after acid hydrolysis are usually satisfactory, the values found may be slightly low, particularly after chemical modification of other residues. This has often led to estimates of the number of residues in a protein that are too high, when histidine has been used to calculate a one-residue value.

Naturally-occurring derivatives of histidine (methylhistidines and phosphohistidines) are described in § 2.12.2. The carboxymethylhistidines are the best characterized derivatives of histidine formed in proteins *in vitro*.

2.8.1. *Carboxymethylhistidines*

Nitrogens 1 and 3 in the imidazole ring of histidyl residues in proteins may be alkylated with iodoacetic acid (generally in a much slower reaction than alkylation of cysteinyl residues) to give three carboxymethyl derivatives: 1-carboxymethylhistidine, 3-carboxymethylhistidine and 1,3-dicarboxymethylhistidine (§ 3.4). In general, the 3-carboxymethyl derivative is formed most rapidly. These derivatives are stable to acid hydrolysis under the usual conditions (but excess reagent must be removed) and may be analyzed on the long column of most analyzers as described below.

Using the 150 cm column of Spackman et al. (1958), Crestfield et al. (1963) showed that 1,3-dicarboxymethylhistidine elutes about 55 ml before aspartic acid (124 ml), 1-carboxymethylhistidine elutes about 9 ml after glutamic acid (177 ml) and 6 ml before proline (193 ml), and 3-carboxymethylhistidine elutes about 16 ml after alanine (264 ml). The color values of the dicarboxymethyl- and monocarboxymethyl-derivatives were determined as 96% and 99% that of serine respectively, and 97% and 100% that of glycine respectively.

The dicarboxymethyl derivative has been characterized in electrophoretic and chromatographic systems, and all three derivatives were separated by ion exchange chromatography in pyridine-formic acid buffer at *p*H 3.25 (Banaszak and Gurd 1964).

2.8.2. Other derivatives of histidine

Many derivatives of histidine are not stable to acid hydrolysis and are not discussed here (however, see § 2.12.2 for those that occur naturally in proteins). Brief mention should be made of the iodination of histidyl residues by HOI (§ 3.7.2). The mono- and diiodohistidines can be identified and distinguished from the iodinated tyrosines by high voltage paper electrophoresis in 1 M formic acid (Roholt and Pressman 1972) after complete enzymic hydrolysis of the protein or peptide (§ 2.11; Roholt and Pressman 1972). Quantitation and identification are facilitated by the use of radiolabeled reagent.

2.9. Arginine and derivatives

There is usually little difficulty in obtaining satisfactory analyses for the arginine content of proteins hydrolyzed with acid under the usual conditions. There are few derivatives of arginine that are included in the scope of this treatise. Derivatives of arginine obtained by treating proteins with diketones appear to be the best described to date (see § 3.2), but acid hydrolysis destroys these derivatives with 12% regeneration of arginine noted in at least one instance (Yankeelov 1970).

2.10. *Other amino acids*

As stated previously, any amino acid may be the NH_2-terminal or COOH-terminal residue of a protein and be subject to destructive reactions during chemical modification studies. In general in addition to some of the amino acids described above, analyses for glycine, alanine and leucine are usually very satisfactory. Values for phenylalanine are sometimes slightly low, and due to its lower color value, proline gives less precise results than other amino acids, particularly for proteins with low proline contents.

2.11. *Complete enzymic hydrolysis of proteins and peptides*

Because of the lability of several amino acids and many of their derivatives under conditions generally required for quantitative hydrolysis of peptide bonds, a number of attempts have been made to use enzymes under mild conditions to hydrolyze proteins and peptides completely. In theory this seems possible, but in practice it has been difficult to achieve.

In retrospect some of the major difficulties encountered in attempts to hydrolyze proteins completely with enzymes are: (1) inability to maintain proteins (or regions of proteins) in a completely denatured state under the mild conditions employed for enzymic hydrolysis (it has been demonstrated that many native proteins are highly resistant to proteolysis); (2) the formation of peptide aggregates which are resistant to proteolysis; (3) the presence of certain bonds (e.g. those involving proline) or sequences (e.g. several acidic residues in a cluster) which are poorly hydrolyzed by most enzymes; (4) the presence of blocking groups (e.g. α-N-acetyl) and large prosthetic groups (e.g. covalently bound heme in cytochrome *c*) which restrict proteolysis in certain regions; (5) the formation of α, β- or β-peptide bonds from aspartyl residues (these are not hydrolyzed by most proteases); and (6) the cyclization of glutamine which often causes low yields of glutamine in hydrolysates; if glutamine occurs as the NH_2-terminal residue of peptides, it is difficult to hydrolyze these peptides completely. In addition, it should be noted that proteins containing disulfide bonds are often not hydrolyzed completely by enzymes unless the disulfide bonds are reduced (and preferably alkylated, § 3.8.2). In general each protein must be examined as an individual case, since a procedure successful for one protein may not work well for another. Peptides are generally hydrolyzed more successfully by enzymes than are proteins.

Some recommended procedures that may be tried are described below. Regardless of the method used, the important criterion for success is the quantitative recovery of those amino acids or derivatives in which one is interested. For example, if one has made a radiolabeled derivative of cysteine in a protein, all of the radioactivity must be demonstrated to elute in the position of this derivative after complete enzymic hydrolysis; if it does not, it is not certain whether the enzymic hydrolysis was incomplete or if other residues have also been modified.

Although any of several combinations of proteases can be used, ideally, one or more non-specific endopeptidases should be used first to convert the protein into many small peptides. These small peptides can then be degraded to amino acids by aminopeptidases and prolidase (hydrolyzes X-Pro bonds). Sometimes, carboxypeptidases are also used. Although leucine aminopeptidase has been used as the aminopeptidase (see Hill and Schmidt 1962), it may be preferable to use aminopeptidase M (Rohm and Haas, supplied by Henley and Co. of N.Y.), since this enzyme removes most residues at acceptable rates. Leucine aminopeptidase removes hydrophobic residues most rapidly, whereas some other residues are removed very slowly. Most procedures should probably include the use of prolidase (Miles) since many aminopeptidases do not cleave X-Pro bonds at appreciable rates. If it is found that proline is not released quantitatively by these procedures, the use of citrus leaf carboxypeptidase C (Rohm and Haas) can be tried after the initial endopeptidase hydrolysis and before the addition of aminopeptidase M and prolidase. Carboxypeptidase C (also yeast carboxypeptidase Y – see Hayashi et al. 1973) hydrolyzes proline bonds (as well as all others), but if proline is at or adjacent to the NH_2 terminus of a peptide, it would probably not be released. In all procedures a control consisting of the enzymes only should be run in parallel with the hydrolyzed sample, and corrections should be made for any amino acids found by analysis of the control. *Subject index p. 201*

2.11.1. Procedure 1: pepsin, subtilisin, aminopeptidase M, prolidase

This method may often be useful with proteins that can be maintained in a largely denatured state at acid *p*H. The protein (usually about 10 mg per ml) may be denatured in solvents like 6 M guanidinium chloride or 8 M freshly deionised urea and dialyzed exhaustively against 5% formic acid at room temperature at about *p*H 2. If cysteine or cystine residues are present, these should be reduced and alkylated (§ 3.8.2) prior to enzymic hydrolysis.

Pepsin* (1% by weight) is added to the protein in 5% formic acid at *p*H 2 and hydrolysis is allowed to proceed at 40°C for at least 6 hr (overnight is often preferable). The peptide mixture is lyophilized and redissolved or suspended in 0.2 M NH_4HCO_3 to give a final *p*H between 7.5 and 8.0 (adjust with NH_3 if necessary). The pepsin is denatured by the high *p*H.

Subtilisin* (1% by weight) is added, and hydrolysis is allowed to proceed at 40°C for at least 6–8 hr (or overnight). The subtilisin is subsequently inhibited by incubation with 0.1% (v/v) diisopropylfluorophosphate (DFP) for 1 hr at 40°C. In some instances it may be possible to omit the use of subtilisin after pepsin, or pronase or papain may be found to give better results.

$MnCl_2$ (0.025 M) is added to the peptide mixture obtained by the above procedure (at *p*H 7.5 to 8.0) to a final concentration of 0.005 M and aminopeptidase M (2000 mU per ml of peptide mixture) and prolidase (imidodipeptidase; 100–200 units per ml of reaction mixture) are added; hydrolysis is allowed to proceed for at least 16–24 hr. The enzymic hydrolysate is lyophilized to dryness over P_2O_5, redissolved in 5% acetic acid and lyophilized again. This procedure is usually sufficient to remove most of the NH_3, so that analysis for the basic amino acids can be made. Repeated additions of water (or 5% acetic acid) and lyophilization can be used to reduce the NH_3 content further, if desired.

The times of hydrolysis and the amounts of enzymes added (2 or more additions of pepsin or subtilisin may sometimes prove beneficial)

* See Appendix II.

may be increased to give better hydrolysis if evidence is obtained for incomplete hydrolysis. Preliminary evidence for incomplete hydrolysis may be obtained by a peptide map of the hydrolysate (use at least 0.05 μmoles of the protein) using electrophoresis at *p*H 1.9 in the first direction (see Appendix) and chromatography in 1-butanol-acetic acid-water (200:30:75, v/v) as the second direction. Comparison of this map with a map of a standard mixture of amino acids (plus any derivatives that may be present) may demonstrate additional ninhydrin-positive spots that may correspond to unhydrolyzed peptides. Unhydrolyzed peptides are sometimes also detected as additional peaks eluting from the columns of amino acid analyzers. Peptides frequently have poor color values and are not detected as easily as the amino acids.

2.11.2. Procedure 2: use of insoluble enzymes

A newly described procedure for complete enzymic hydrolysis of proteins and peptides (Brown and Wold 1973) makes use of several proteases which are covalently attached to insoluble supports (Cuatrecasas et al. 1968). The advantages of using these enzymes in the insoluble form are that the enzymes may be easily removed from the products, and there is little or no hydrolysis of the enzymes themselves which reduces the corrections for controls. One disadvantage of the insoluble proteases may be that the size of the insoluble particles introduces steric factors hindering the hydrolysis of large peptides or proteins.

Although the details of the hydrolysis procedure are yet to be published in detail (see Brown and Wold 1973), the first hydrolysis is with agarose-bound aspergillopeptidase A* at *p*H 1.5–2.0 for 18 hr. The resulting peptide mixture is then hydrolyzed simultaneously with agarose-bound pronase* and aminopeptidase M* for 16 hr in borate buffer at *p*H 7.6, and finally with agarose-bound prolidase* for 2 hr in the same buffer. It may prove helpful (not indicated in the procedure) to add the prolidase at the same time as the aminopeptidase M, since it

* See Appendix II.

has been demonstrated that X-Pro dipeptides are often found in aminopeptidase M hydrolysates as diketopiperazines which are resistant to the action of prolidase (e.g. see Waley et al. 1970). The proteases are presumably removed by filtration or centrifugation (with washing).

2.11.3. Procedure 3: papain, leucine aminopeptidase, prolidase

This early procedure for enzymic hydrolysis of proteins was reported by Hill and Schmidt (1962) to be successful for hydrolysis of several proteins. Papain was found to be superior to subtilisin or a combination of trypsin and chymotrypsin for the initial hydrolysis. The method might be improved if aminopeptidase M (discovered after the method was developed) is used in place of the leucine aminopeptidase, but to our knowledge this has not been tested. The problem with diketopiperazine formation from X-Pro dipeptides in aminopeptidase M hydrolysates of peptides (see above) may make this substitution less desirable than it would seem at first.

In this procedure, 1–2 μmoles of protein (0.1–0.5% in water) at *p*H 7.0 is heated at 95°C for 3 min to denature the protein. After cooling, buffer (0.2 M sodium acetate at *p*H 5.2) is added to a final concentration of 0.03 to 0.05 M, and the mixture is incubated at 40°C for 10 min. Sodium cyanide (0.1 M, neutralized to *p*H 7.0) is added as activator to a final concentration of 0.01 M, and papain (C_1 of 1.2 to 1.5)* in a 0.5 to 1.0% solution is added to give a final weight equal to 1 to 5% that of the protein. After hydrolysis for 18–24 hr at 40°C in a closed container, the *p*H is adjusted to 2 to denature the papain, and a measured aliquot is lyophilized to dryness.

The dried peptide mixture is redissolved in 1–2 ml H_2O and adjusted to *p*H 8.4–8.6 with dilute NaOH. Tris buffer (other buffers can be substituted to prevent interference with any subsequent analyses) (0.5 M at *p*H 8.5) and $MnCl_2$ (0.025 M) are added to give final con-

* The specific activity (C_1) is expressed as K_1 (first-order rate constant calculated in decimal logarithms) per ml of protein N per ml of reaction mixture and is determined at a substrate concentration of 0.05 M α-N-benzoyl-L-argininamide at *p*H 5.5 and 39°C in the presence of 0.005 M cysteine and 0.001 M EDTA.

centrations of 0.005 M. Leucine aminopeptidase (4 to 6 mg, $C_1=88$) and prolidase (0.5 to 1.0 mg, $C_1=20$) are added, and hydrolysis is allowed to proceed for 15 to 24 hr at 40°C. The enzymes are inactivated by adjusting the *p*H to 2 with 1 N HCl, and prior to analysis the amino acids are removed from the proteins by dialysis, gel filtration or other methods.

2.11.4. Analysis of enzymic hydrolysates

Tryptophan, asparagine, glutamine and any other acid-labile derivatives will be the major components which are present in enzymic hydrolysates but not in acid hydrolysates. If cysteine and cystine are converted to S-carboxymethyl cysteine (§ 3.8.2), this will be present in both the acid and enzymic hydrolysates. Tryptophan may be analyzed as indicated in §2.6. Asparagine and glutamine can be quantitated together as a single peak in many common analyzer systems employing a temperature change which separates the amides from the serine position where they elute in most routine systems. The color values for asparagine and glutamine are 93% and 87%, respectively, that of aspartic acid (Spackman et al. 1958). By the use of a lithium buffer system, asparagine and glutamine can be separated from each other and from other amino acids, thus allowing them to be quantitated individually (Benson et al. 1967).

Acid-labile derivatives may elute from analyzer columns in the positions of other amino acids, and therefore, may be missed and interfere with accurate quantitation of the other amino acids. Modification of column temperature, buffer *p*H, buffer ionic strength, etc. may often be necessary to give good resolution of some of these derivatives.

2.12. Naturally-occurring amino acid derivatives in proteins

An ever-increasing number of amino acid derivatives is found to occur naturally in proteins. These include ε-N-methyllysines, ε-N-acetyllysine, α-N-acetyl derivatives of various residues, N-methylhistidines, N-phosphohistidines, N-methylarginines, phosphoserine, phosphothreonine, hydroxyproline, hydroxylysine, trimethylhydroxylysine, tyrosine sulfate, iodotyrosines, carbohydrate moieties and coenzymes covalently bound to various residues, lysine condensation products in proteins like elastin, adenyl groups covalently bound to tyrosine residues, covalently bound ADP-ribose moieties, etc. Many of these derivatives are acid-labile and would not be detected after acid hydrolysis of the proteins.

To the investigator studying chemical modification of proteins, derivatives like those listed above are of interest for two primary reasons: (1) some derivatives are sites of modification and (2) complete modification of a particular class of amino acid functional groups with a reagent may not be possible because of the presence of these derivatives. For any protein being investigated by chemical modification and containing these types of derivatives, any results and conclusions must account for the effects of these derivatives.

2.12.1. Lysine derivatives

2.12.1.1. ε-N-Acetyllysine

This derivative of lysine has thus far been identified only in histones (see DeLange and Smith, 1971, 1974), but may also be produced in other proteins by chemical acetylation, e.g. with acetylimidazole, or acetic anhydride. Since the ε-amide bond is acid-labile, this derivative may be present in other proteins, which have not been hydrolyzed and analyzed by enzymic methods (see § 2.11).

ε-N-Acetyllysine may be identified (see DeLange et al. 1969a) by paper electrophoresis at *p*H 1.9 (migration of 0.7 compared to 1.0 for alanine), paper chromatography in 1-butanol : glacial acetic acid : H_2O (200 : 30 : 75 v/v) (migration is 0.85 that of tyrosine) or 1-butanol : pyridine : glacial acetic acid : H_2O (90 : 60 : 18 : 72 v/v) (migration is 0.89 that of valine). With the 60 cm column of a Beckman 120B analyzer, ε-N-acetyllysine elutes at 77 min compared to 86 min for glycine and 92.5 min for alanine. We have used the average color value, calculated as indicated by the analyzer manufacturer, as the color value for estimating the amount of this derivative. (The average color value is obtained by averaging the color values for the amino acids resolved on the long column of the analyser with the exception of proline and cystine).

2.12.1.2. ε-N-Methyllysines

The ε-N-methyllysines have been found in histones (see DeLange and Smith, 1971, 1974), cytochromes *c* (see DeLange et al. 1970), flagellin (see Glazer et al. 1969), ribosomal proteins (Comb et al. 1966) and muscle proteins (see Paik and Kim, 1971 for a review). In some proteins (e.g. calf thymus histone III) ε-N-monomethyllysine, ε-N-dimethyllysine and ε-N-trimethyllysine are all three present, whereas in other proteins only one derivative (e.g. cytochromes *c*) or two of the derivatives (e.g. calf thymus histone IV) are present. Methylated lysines can also be formed in proteins by chemical modification *in vitro* (§ 3.1.1.3).

The ε-N-methyllysines are stable to acid hydrolysis and may be identified with the aid of an amino acid analyzer. With many routine analyzer systems ε-N-monomethyl- and ε-N-dimethyllysine elute as a shoulder or a partially resolved peak on the trailing edge of the lysine peak. If a 60 cm column is eluted with the buffer usually used for the 15 cm column these two methylated lysines are well resolved from lysine but not from each other. ε-N-trimethyllysine usually elutes with lysine or slightly ahead of it in these systems (15 cm or 60 cm column eluted with *p*H 5.28 buffer).

Paik and Kim (1967) developed a method utilizing the 60 cm column, eluted at 30°C with a citrate buffer (0.2 M) at *p*H 5.84, which resolved all three methyllysine derivatives from each other and from other basic amino acids. It has been found that the separations are sensitive to slight changes in *p*H, column temperature, ionic strength and the type of resin used. In our own laboratory we have used a 48 cm column of Durrum DC-2 resin (Appendix II) (DeLange et al. 1970) which gives excellent resolution, but requires at least 7 hr (18 hr if arginine analyses are required). Seely et al. (1969) have used a column (0.9 × 15 cm) of Aminex A-5 resin (Appendix II), eluted at 25°C with buffer at *p*H 6.48 (prepared by adding NaOH to the usual *p*H 5.28 buffer) to give resolutions in 2 hr (or even less) that should be adequate for many purposes. In this system at a flow rate of 34 ml per hr. the elution volumes and color constants (in parentheses) were: lysine, 47.5 ml (43.5); ε-N-monomethyllysine, 55 ml (39.7); ε-N-dimethyllysine, 59.5 ml (39.2); and ε-N-trimethyllysine, 63 ml (35.5). Histidine elutes just before lysine and NH_3 elutes just after ε-N-trimethyllysine. All of the acidic and neutral amino acids elute before 28 ml.

Benoiton et al. (1971) have found that lysine and ε-N-monomethyllysine have similar 570/440 nm ratios after reaction with ninhydrin as measured with the analyzer, and that ε-N-dimethyllysine and ε-N-trimethyllysine also have similar 570/440 nm ratios, but the 570/440 nm ratios of the two pairs are different. This provided a method for estimating from the 570/440 nm ratio the content of ε-N-monomethyllysine and ε-N-dimethyllysine in hydrolysates that are analyzed in systems in which these two derivatives are not separated. For other analyzer systems that have been used to study methylated lysines, see the references cited above and also Deibler and Martenson (1973).

The methylated lysines can also be separated and identified by paper chromatographic systems. However, in electrophoresis at *p*H 1.9 all three derivatives migrate similarly to arginine. They also migrate with lysine during chromatography in 1-butanol:glacial acetic acid:water (200;30:75 v/v), but are partially resolved in 1-butanol:pyridine:glacial acetic acid:water (90:60:18:72 v/v) for 40 hr: lysine and ε-N-trimethyllysine, 1.00; ε-N-monomethyllysine and ε-N-dimethyllysine, 1.18; and arginine, 1.38 (see DeLange et al. 1969b).

The best paper resolutions of the methyllysines are obtained by descending chromatography for 16–18 hr at room temperature (21°C), using *m*-cresol: 88% phenol:borate buffer (190:165:45 v/v) with papers dipped (and then dried) in 0.1 M EDTA (adjusted to *p*H 7.0 with NaOH) essentially as described by Stewart (1963) except that Whatman No. 3 paper (57 cm in length) can be used in place of No. 52 paper, and the papers do not need to be dipped in acetone. The borate buffer is prepared by dissolving 3.944 g of boric acid in water, adjusting the *p*H to 9.3 with NaOH and diluting to 1 liter. Because of the *p*H 9.3 buffer used, better colors are obtained with a ninhydrin reagent buffered at a lower *p*H (e.g. 0.1% ninhydrin in 95% ethanol: glacial acetic acid: collidine (50:15:2)). The R_f values are lysine, 0.18; arginine, 0.30; histidine, 0.43; ε-N-monomethyllysine, 0.44; ε-N-dimethyllysine, 0.76; ε-N-trimethyllysine, 0.88 (DeLange et al. 1969b).

Histidine and ε-N-monomethyllysine can be distinguished by their different colors with ninhydrin (supplemented by the use of Pauly reagent) or by using two-dimensional separations (e.g. *p*H 1.9 electrophoresis, followed by the cresol–phenol system). ε-N-Monomethyllysine has a color with the ninhydrin reagent similar to that of lysine (blue-grey) whereas the other two derivatives give colors similar to arginine (blue-violet), and histidine gives a yellow-brown color.

2.12.1.3. Hydroxylysine

Hydroxylysine is found in collagen and gelatin and possibly some other other proteins (see Vickery 1972). It is formed *in vivo* by oxidation of lysyl residues in these proteins at the δ-carbon. Hydroxylysine is stable to acid hydrolysis, but undergoes racemization under the usual conditions of hydrolysis to give a mixture of the natural hydroxylysine and *allo*-hydroxylysine.

Several analytical systems appear to be satisfactory for the resolution and quantitation of hydroxylysine. If a protein is suspected of having hydroxylysine, perhaps several systems should be used. Spackman et al. (1958) resolved the hydroxylysines from a number of other components on a 50 cm column of Amberlite IR-120, eluted at 30°C with 0.38 N sodium citrate buffer at *p*H 4.26; hydroxylysine, 131 ml; *allo*-hydroxylysine, 137 ml; and lysine 218 ml. The hydroxylysines elute after the amino sugars in this system. Knox et al. (1970) showed that hydroxylysine is eluted just before lysine from a 0.9 × 7 cm column of PA-35 resin, eluted with 0.255 M sodium citrate buffer at *p*H 5.0 (see also Hugli and Moore 1972). An early system developed by Piez and Morris (1960) was later modified (Miller and Piez 1966) to give an accelerated method for analyzing for all of the constituents of collagen. The resins (PA 28 at 55°C or AA-15 at 60°C) were eluted in a column (0.9 × 51 cm) at 80 ml/hr with a gradient established with a Varigrad containing various amounts of *p*H 2.91 citrate buffer and 0.4 M sodium citrate in the chambers. Hydroxylysine elutes at about 213 ml, between phenylalanine (197 ml) and ammonia (246 ml). The color value for hydroxylysine is about the same as that of lysine (Spackman et al.

1958). Hydroxylysine has a mobility of 2.26 compared to aspartic acid in *p*H 1.9 electrophoresis.

2.12.1.4. Trimethylhydroxylysine (THL) and its phosphate (THLP)
These two derivatives have been identified in proteinacious material from cell walls of diatoms (Nakajima and Volcani 1970). In *p*H 1.9 electrophoresis they migrate 2.4 cm (THLP) and 6.1 cm (THL) towards the negative electrode, respectively, at 33.3 volts/cm for 20 min. In the analyzer system of Dus et al. (1966), THLP elutes in about the same position as threonine, and THL elutes between NH_3 and arginine (a buffer peak also elutes in this region). In the complex analyzer system of Hamilton (1963), THLP elutes at a volume about 2.4 times that of cysteic acid and 0.58 that of aspartic acid.

2.12.1.5. Desmosine, isodesmosine and related derivatives
Lysine (and hydroxylysine) residues in collagen and elastin are

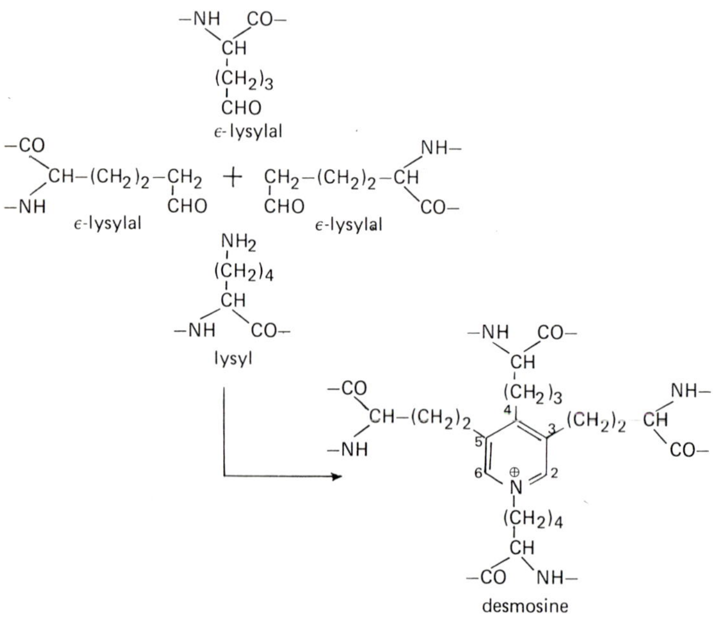

converted to a variety of aldehyde and aldol products which can condense to form desmosine (derived from four lysines) or other types of cross-links (see Traub and Piez 1971; Piez 1968). Desmosine and isodesmosine are the best characterized of these derivatives, and they may be analyzed after acid hydrolysis. In the analyzer system of Piez and Morris (1960), which was later modified by Miller and Piez (1966), these two derivatives elute in the order isodesmosine-desmosine between phenylalanine and hydroxylysine and have color values 3.6 times that of leucine (see also Miller et al. 1965).

2.12.1.6. Other lysine derivatives

The ε-amino groups of lysyl residues serve as attachment sites of a number of coenzymes in proteins (e.g. biotin in pyruvate carboxylase, pyridoxal phosphate in phosphorylase, lipoic acid in lipoate acetyl-transferase) and form covalent intermediates in several enzymic reactions (e.g. transaldolase, aldolase, etc.). Discussion of all of these naturally-occuring derivatives of lysine will not be attempted in this treatise, but the investigator using chemical modification of proteins should be aware of their possible presence and effect on the results of his experiments. It should be noted that ε-N-phospholysine has been reported in nucleoside diphosphate kinase (Wålinder 1968).

2.12.2. Histidine derivatives

3-*Methylhistidine.* This derivative, but not the 1-methyl or 1,3-dimethyl derivatives, has been reported in myosin and actin (Asatoor and Armstrong 1967; Johnson et al. 1967; Elzinga 1971; Huszar and Elzinga 1971) and histones (Gershey et al. 1969).

The 3-methylhistidine is easily distinguished from the 1-methyl derivative (formed by alkylation, § 3.4) by electrophoresis at *p*H 6.5 (Johnson et al. 1967) as well as with automatic analyzers (Spackman et al. 1958; Johnson et al. 1967; Elzinga 1970). In general a longer short column (0.9 × 15 cm or 0.9 × 20 cm) is required for good separations of 3-methylhistidine from histidine (the 3-methyl derivative elutes between histidine and NH_3 in these systems). The color value of 3-methylhistidine is 85% that of histidine (Spackman et al. 1958).

N-Phosphohistidine. Histidyl residues, phosphorylated at either nitrogens 1 or 3 in the ring, have been reported in enzymes like succinate thiokinase (Kreil and Boyer 1964; Hultquist et al. 1966) and nucleoside diphosphate kinase (Norman et al. 1965; Wålinder 1968, 1969) and in histone (Smith et al. 1973). These derivatives are unstable to acidic conditions, but stable under alkaline conditions. Therefore, analyzer systems have not been employed, but chromatography on columns (1.2 × 44 cm) of Dowex 1-X8 with $KHCO_3$ (gradient of 250 ml of 0.2 M $KHCO_3$ to 250 ml of 0.8 M $KHCO_3$) has been used (see Wålinder 1968).

2.12.3. Methylarginines

Arginyl residues in which the nitrogens of the guanidine group are methylated have been reported in nuclear acidic protein (Friedman et al. 1969), histone (Paik and Kim 1970), myosin (Reporter and Corbin 1971) and in the basic protein of myelin (Carnegie 1971; Baldwin and Carnegie 1971; Brostoff and Eylar 1971). Three derivatives, N^G-monomethylarginine, N^G,N^G-dimethylarginine (unsymmetrical) and N^G,N'^G-dimethylarginine (symmetrical) have been identified (not all in each protein) in the different proteins.

The analyzer system described by Deibler and Martenson (1973) is probably the most effective method for separating the methylarginines from each other and from other methylated amino acids. However, ε-N-trimethyllysine was not studied in this system which utilizes Durrum DC-2A resin in a column (0.9 × 30 cm) eluted at 45 ml/hr with sodium citrate buffer (0.35 M in sodium ion) at *p*H 5.80 or 5.835. The initial elution is at 28°C, but at 200 min the temperature is changed to 55.5°C and the buffer to *p*H 4.70 (0.35 M in Na^+). Under these conditions the following elution times (in min) are obtained with the *p*H 5.835 buffer: lysine, 142; ε-N-monomethyllysine, 161; ε-N-dimethyllysine, 171; histidine, 187; 3-methylhistidine, 203; 1-methylhistidine, 220; ammonia, 222; N^G, N^G-dimethylarginine, 345; N^G,N'^G-dimethylarginine, 365; N^G-monomethylarginine, 416; arginine, 434. Similar results are obtained with the *p*H 5.80 buffer.

Several electrophoretic and chromatographic systems have also been used to separate and identify the methylarginines (see Reporter and Corbin 1971 and Nakajima et al. 1971).

2.12.4. O-Phosphoserine and O-phosphothreonine

O-Phosphoserine has been reported in a number of proteins in which it appears to function as an intermediate in enzymic reactions (e.g. phosphoglucomutase), as a regulator of enzymic activity (e.g. phosphorylase) or protein function (e.g. histones), and as a nutritive component (e.g. casein). O-Phosphothreonine has been reported in some of these proteins, but generally to a much more limited extent and only in those which also contain O-phosphoserine.

These derivatives are not stable to complete acid hydrolysis of proteins, but may be recovered in limited amounts after partial acid hydrolysis. For example, after 90 min of hydrolysis at 100°C in 5.7 N HCl about 30% of the covalently-bound phosphate in phosphoglucomutase was recovered as O-phosphoserine (Milstein 1964), but after 20 hr of hydrolysis at 105°C in 5.7 N HCl, no O-phosphoserine was found (Murray and Milstein 1967). The amount liberated at a certain time will depend on the nature of the residues around the phosphoserine residues in each protein. Hydrolysis of peptides containing O-phosphoserine may often give low yields of serine (e.g. see Nolan et al. 1964). Complete enzymic hydrolysis of proteins or peptides containing O-phosphoserine is the only presently available method for quantitative recovery of this derivative.

In most analyzer systems O-phosphoserine and O-phosphothreonine elute at the same volume as cysteic acid (the unretarded position) and can, therefore, interfere with analyses for cysteic acid (and *vice versa*). The color value for O-phosphoserine is 1.04 times the average value calculated for the amino acids (except proline and cystine) eluted from a 60 cm column in a two-column system (Beckman manuals). It should be noted that O-serine sulfate and O-threonine sulfate, which can be formed during preparation of hydrolysates in the presence of sulfate (Moore 1963; Murray and Milstein 1967), also elute in this position. Electrophoresis at *p*H 3.5 is an effective means of separating O-phosphoserine from other amino acids, since it migrates further than aspartic acid towards the positive electrode (see Murray and Milstein 1967). O-Phosphothreonine has a migration slightly less than O-phosphoserine in this system. O-Phosphoserine has a mobility of 0.21 towards the anode as compared to a mobility of 1.00 for aspartic acid towards the cathode on *p*H 1.9 electrophoresis.

2.12.5. Derivatives of tyrosine

Tyrosine O-sulfate is present in fibrinogen of certain species (Jevons 1963) and in gastrin (Gregory et al. 1964). It is not stable to acid hydrolysis (62% is converted to tyrosine in 0.5 N HCl at 100°C), but is stable to alkaline hydrolysis (e.g. 0.2 M $Ba(OH)_2$ at 125°C for 24 hr). Although it has apparently not been determined with analyzers, tyrosine-O-sulfate may be identified by column chromatography on Dowex 2 (Hill and Schmidt 1962) and by several electrophoretic and chromatographic systems (Jevons 1963; Doolittle 1965). At *p*H 3.9 tyrosine O-sulfate migrates slightly faster than aspartic acid toward the positive electrode.

The thyroid protein, thyroglobulin, contains 3-monoiodotyrosine, 3,5-diiodotyrosine and several iodinated thyronine derivatives (Salvatore and Edelhoch 1973). Iodohistidines may also be present in this protein. 3-Bromotyrosine has been reported in serum proteins (Firnau and Fritze 1972). Methods for separating and analyzing these and other halogenated tyrosines are presented in § 2.2.3.

2.12.6. Hydroxyprolines

Hydroxyproline has long been known to be a constituent of collagen and gelatin (see Harrington and von Hippel 1961) and thought to be a constituent of elastin (see Piez 1968). Only recently has it been verified that peptides obtained from elastin do contain hydroxyproline (Foster et al. 1973). Until 1962 only the 4-hydroxy derivative had been identified in collagen, but in that year the 3-hydroxy derivative was also reported to be present in small amounts (Ogle et al. 1962; Irreverre et al. 1962a). More recently, 3,4-dihydroxyproline has been found in diatom cell walls (Nakajima and Volcani 1969).

Hydroxyprolines usually elute before aspartic acid in most analyzer systems (e.g. see Spackman et al. 1958; Miller and Piez 1966; Hamilton 1963). The *cis* or *allo* isomers, which are rarely found in proteins, elute later near the position of threonine; in some systems 3-hydroxyproline (*trans*) elutes just prior to methionine sulfoxides, and 4-hydroxyproline (*trans*) elutes between methionine sulfoxides and aspartic acid (Hamilton 1963; Irreverre et al. 1962b; Glimcher et al. 1964). With a 150 cm column system, 3,4-dihydroxyproline elutes in a position similar to the *trans*-3-hydroxyproline (Nakajima and Volcani 1969).

2.12.7. *Other derivatives of amino acids*

In addition to those derivatives given above it should be mentioned that many other derivatives have been reported in proteins. A partial listing of these is given here to make the investigator aware of the types of derivatives that may play some role in chemical modification experiments. Some of these derivatives are dehydroalanine (e.g. Girot et al. 1969), covalently-bound pyruvate (e.g. Wickner et al. 1970), covalently-bound lipid (Braun and Bosch 1972), ε-(γ-glutamyl)lysine (Pisano et al. 1969; Harding and Rogers 1971), γ-carboxyglutamic acid (Stenflo et al. 1974; Magnusson et al. 1974), citrulline (Steinert et al. 1969), pyrrolidone carboxylic acid (Doolittle and Armentrout 1968), flavin covalently bound to histidine (Walker and Singer 1970), pantotheine covalently bound to histidine (Vanaman et al. 1968). Carbohydrate can be covalently attached to asparagine (Hunt and Dayhoff 1970), serine and threonine (Traub and Piez 1971), lysine (Braun and Bosch 1972), hydroxylysine (Traub and Piez 1971) and α-amino groups (Bookchin and Gallop 1968).

2.13. *Analysis of carbohydrates in glycoproteins*

Many proteins of various types have been shown to be glycoproteins, which are defined as those proteins containing covalently-bound carbohydrate. Various neutral carbohydrates (glucose, mannose, galactose, fucose), N-acetylated hexosamines (N-acetylglucosamine, N-acetylgalactosamine) and sialic acids (N-acetylneuraminic acid, N-glycolylneuraminic acid) have been identified in the carbohydrate moieties of glycoproteins, and the attachment sites have been shown to be through the side chains of asparaginyl, seryl, threonyl, hydroxylysyl, hydroxyprolyl and lysyl residues (Spiro 1970; §2.12). Since carbohydrates in glycoproteins represent highly specific, natural chemical modifications, and since the carbohydrates may be modified by certain chemical modifications in the laboratory, it is of value to the investigator to be able to analyze for the carbohydrates in glycoproteins.

2.13.1. Identification of a protein as a glycoprotein

Many glycoproteins (but not all) contain N-acetylhexosamines which may be converted in about 50% yield to the hexosamines by acid hydrolysis in 6 N HCl for 24 hr at 110°C (§ 2.1). The hexosamines may be identified with the analyzer, using either the 15 cm column (elution between phenylalanine and lysine, Spackman et al. 1958) or the 60 cm column (elution after phenylalanine, Beckman Technical Bulletin A-TB-008, 1964). The use of the 60 cm column generally seems preferable, since tryptophan, halogenated tyrosines, etc. are more likely to interfere with analyses on the short column. Depending on the resin being used, glucosamine may coelute with phenylalanine on the 60 cm column unless the buffer change is made at an earlier time than usual. In one analysis the buffer change was made at 78 min, just before glycine (elution time, 84 min), and phenylalanine eluted at 164 min, glucosamine at 174 min and galactosamine at 184 min (DeLange 1970). Quantitative analysis of hexosamines should be made after cleavage as described in § 2.13.2.

If a protein does not contain hexosamines, one other test for the presence of neutral sugars should be made. This can be done by paper chromatography (Carsten and Pierce 1963; Spiro 1965) or gas chromatography (§ 2.13.3) after appropriate hydrolysis (§ 2.13.2), or a simple colorimetric reaction, such as the orcinol method (below), may be used.

Proteins to be analyzed for hexoses by the orcinol method (Winzler 1955) should be free of extraneous carbohydrate. The protein (2–10 mg) is dissolved in 0.1 N NaOH (1.0 ml), and a blank of 0.1 N NaOH (1.0 ml) and a standard of galactose and mannose (0.1 mg of each in

1.0 ml of 0.1 N NaOH) are also prepared. To all 3 tubes orcinol-H_2SO_4 reagent (8.5 ml) is added, and the contents of the tubes are mixed. The orcinol-H_2SO_4 reagent is freshly prepared from 7.5 volumes of Reagent A (60 ml of concentrated H_2SO_4, 40 ml of H_2O) and 1 volume of Reagent B (1.6 g of orcinol, recrystallized from benzene, in 100 ml of H_2O). The tubes are capped with glass marbles to minimize evaporation and placed in a water bath at 80°C for exactly 15 min. The tubes are cooled in tap water, and the absorbances at 540 nm are determined. For qualitative testing, greater sensitivity may be obtained at 420 nm, but more substances interfere at this wavelength, and quantitation is less precise because the color values for the various hexoses differ much more at the lower wavelength. Sialic acids do not react with orcinol and hexosamines do not interfere at 540 nm. The optical density is linear to a total amount of 0.5 mg of hexose. If the protein is colored, another blank should be run with protein but no orcinol present.

An alternate colorimetric method for hexoses is the anthrone procedure (Spiro 1965).

2.13.2. Release of carbohydrates from glycoproteins

In order for quantitative analyses to be made of the carbohydrates present in glycoproteins, it is necessary to cleave the carbohydrate under conditions where destruction is minimized. Fucose and the sialic acids are particularly susceptible to destructive reactions, and this may often necessitate cleavage of the carbohydrate under more than one condition to obtain quantitative results for all constituents present. Most methods of cleavage (other than total enzymic hydrolysis, which is usually very difficult to achieve) (see Spiro 1972) lead to partial or total loss of the N-acetyl groups. In general higher yields are obtained if reagents are of high purity (e.g. redistilled HCl, if used), oxygen is excluded, etc. The procedures to be described below may need to be modified to suit the particular protein being studied. It is usually recommended that preliminary experiments utilizing varying times, temperatures, etc., be conducted to determine optimum conditions of release.

Sialic acids can usually be liberated from glycoproteins with 0.1 N

H_2SO_4 at 80°C for 1 hr (Spiro 1965). This is probably because of the terminal positions of these substances in the carbohydrate moieties of glycoproteins, and the lability of the particular glycosidic bond. Complex polysaccharides containing sialic acids, may require more stringent conditions of hydrolysis such as 2 N methanesulfonic acid in anhydrous methanol (Liu 1972). However, more stringent hydrolysis in aqueous media usually leads to greater destruction of sialic acids. Neuraminidases may also be used to release sialic acids (see Liu 1972).

The neutral sugars can usually be released from glycoproteins with 1 N HCl (or H_2SO_4) at 100°C for 4–6 hr, although in some instances 2 N HCl or longer times may be required (see Spiro 1972). Since fucose is in terminal positions in the carbohydrate chains of glycoproteins, and since it is more susceptible to destruction, 0.5 N HCl or shorter times of hydrolysis will usually improve the yield of this sugar. Fucose may be determined by a specific colorimetric test (Spiro 1965).

The N-acetylhexosamines can usually be quantitatively released (as the hexosamines) from glycoproteins with 4 N HCl at 100°C for 6 hr (Spiro 1972). However, under these conditions the other carbohydrate components will undergo varying amounts of destruction.

From the comments above it is obvious that no single condition of cleavage is generally satisfactory for the quantitative release and recovery of all carbohydrates in glycoproteins. Two procedures are described below which may be satisfactory for many purposes. In the first, sialic acids are lost, but the procedure lends itself to the later formation of the alditol acetates of the neutral sugars and their analysis by gas chromatography (§ 2.13.3). This is an excellent method of analysis, since only one product for each sugar is obtained. After this procedure the hexosamines may also be determined with the analyzer. In the second procedure sialic acids are also obtained, but the methyl derivatives formed are best analyzed after further derivatization which results in more than one peak for many of the carbohydrate derivatives during gas chromatography (§ 2.13.3).

Method 1 (Kim et al. 1967). The glycoprotein (usually 1–2 mg) is hydrolyzed for 24 hr with 1.5 ml of 0.25 N H_2SO_4 and 200 mg of

Dowex 50-X12 (200–400 mesh, H^+ form) with continuous rotation in an oven at 100°C. Inositol (50 μg; replaces glucose in original method) and norleucine (25 μg) are added in 0.2 ml H_2O as internal standards (50 μg of galactosamine may also be used if none is present in the protein). After cooling, the mixture is placed on a small column (e.g. disposable pipette, 0.6 × 10 cm with a glass wool plug) and washed with glass-distilled water. The filtrate is adjusted to *p*H 5.0–5.5 with saturated $Ba(OH)_2$, and the precipitate is collected by centrifugation and washed with hot H_2O twice. The combined washes and supernatant fraction are passed through another column of Dowex 50, H^+ (100 mg), then a column of Dowex 2-X8 (200–400 mesh, formate form), and finally lyophilized to dryness. This fraction (neutral sugars) may be converted to alditol acetates and analyzed by gas chromatography (§ 2.13.3). The combined resins from all 3 columns are eluted in a small column with 10 ml of 6 N HCl. Aliquots (e.g. 5 ml) are taken to dryness and analyzed for hexosamines by the procedure described in § 2.13.1. The yield of hexosamine was generally 85–89% as judged from recovery of internal standard (galactosamine).

Method 2 (Clamp et al. 1967). The glycoprotein (0.1–0.5 mg), together with an internal standard (0.05–0.1 mg of D-mannitol), is refluxed in a 10 ml pear-shaped flask with 1 N HCl (from dry gas) in anhydrous methanol (2–5 ml) at 80°C (oil bath) for 24 hr. After cooling, the solution is neutralized with silver carbonate and 0.05–0.1 ml of acetic anhydride is added to the mixture which is left at room temperature for 6 hr. This step is to reform the N-acetyl derivatives which are partially deacetylated during methanolysis. The mixture is filtered; the filtrate is evaporated under reduced pressure at 40°C and finally dried in a vacuum desiccator over P_2O_5 for 12 hr. This carbohydrate material is suitable for forming the trimethylsilyl derivatives which may be analyzed by gas chromatography (§ 2.13.3.2) (Clamp et al. 1967). However, more than one peak for most carbohydrates is obtained. The recovery of sialic acids is a definite advantage of this procedure.

2.13.3. *Analysis of carbohydrates in glycoproteins*

Although several systems have been developed for analysis of carbohydrates in proteins, only 2 will be given here to illustrate 2 approaches which are rather different despite their common use of gas chromatography. Other methods, particularly anion exchange chromatography of the borate-complexes of the neutral sugars, may be of special interest (see Spiro 1972). The two methods that follow are those used to analyze the carbohydrates obtained by cleavage as described in § 2.13.2 (Methods 1 and 2).

Method 1 (Kim et al. 1967). The dried filtrate obtained after hydrolysis and passage through 3 small columns (Method 1 § 2.13.2) is redissolved in 0.5 ml of H_2O and treated with $NaBH_4$ (5 mg/mg of monosaccharide) at 4°C overnight. Glacial acetic acid is added to acidify (to *p*H 4.5) and destroy excess reagent. The reduced mixture is passed through a column of Dowex 50 (50 mg, H^+ form) and rotary evaporated to dryness. Absolute methanol (3 ml) is added, and the mixture is heated to 50°C for 30 sec and evaporated to dryness at room temperature. The treatment with methanol is repeated twice more to remove borate as methyl borate.

The sugar alcohols from above are acetylated by refluxing at 100°C for 20 min in 0.3 ml pyridine and 0.2 ml glacial acetic acid. After drying over NaOH pellets and concentrated H_2SO_4, the alditol acetates are dissolved in pyridine (1 μl/10–20 μg of carbohydrate) and 0.3 to 0.5 μl is injected for each gas chromatographic run. The instrument used was a Model 1609 (F+M Scientific Corp., Avondale, Penn.) equipped with a hydrogen flame detector and a column (0.125 inches by 10 feet) of Gas Chrom Q (60–80 mesh), precoated with 3% ENCSS-M (Applied Science Laboratories, State College, Penn.). It was operated at 175°C with a port temperature of 300°C, a detection temperature of 215°C and at 45–50 ml/min. Fucose is detected at about 6 min, mannose at 20 min, galactose at 23 min, and glucose at 26 min. For further details of this system see Laine et al. (1972). The overall recovery of the neutral sugars was in excess of 85%. The hexosamines are analyzed as described in § 2.13.2 (Method 1) and § 2.13.1; glucosamine has a color value 1.02, and galactosamine 0.89 of the average color value for the long column which is calculated as described in § 2.12.1.1. Sialic acids, if present, should be analyzed as described below or after milder cleavage conditions as described in § 2.13.2. It should be noted that after methanolysis with 2 N methanesulfonic acid as catalyst and subsequent saponification, the methoxyneuraminate product can be analyzed with an analyzer (Liu 1972). Methoxyneuraminate elutes from the 60 cm column at a volume of about 0.61 that of aspartic acid and has a color value 58% that of aspartic acid.

Method 2 (Clamp et al. 1967; Laine et al. 1972). The dried mixture of carbohydrates (2–2000 μg of sugar) obtained by methanolysis (Method 2, § 2.13.2) is triturated with pyridine (redistilled): hexamethyldisilazane: trimethylchlorosilane (5:2:1) at room temperature for 30 min. The NH_4Cl that forms is settled out, and 1 μl of the supernatant is injected for gas chromatography. Alternatively, the supernatant may be dried in a stream of nitrogen and redissolved in CS_2 for injection. The instrument used was a F&M Hewlett-Packard 402 gas chromatograph with flame ionization detectors. It was operated at a nitrogen gas flow of 35 ml/min with a detector temperature of 280°C. The column (3 mm × 2 m) contained 3% SE-30 on 100/120 Supelcoport (Supelco, Inc.), and was operated with a temperature gradient of 150°C to 250°C with a change of 3°C per min. L-Fucose elutes as 3 peaks at about 4–6 min, D-mannose as 2 or 3 peaks at about 9–11 min, D-galactose as 3 peaks at about 9–11 min, D-glucose as 2 peaks at about 12–13 min, 2-acetamido-2-deoxy-D-galactose as 3 peaks at about 15–17 min, 2-acetamido-2-deoxy-D-glucose as 3 peaks at about 15–18 min and N-acetylneuraminic acid as 3 peaks at about 25–27 min. In all cases one or two of the peaks represent the bulk of the material and all peaks can be assigned with the exception of overlap between some of the peaks of D-mannose and D-galactose.

2.14. *End-group methods*

Procedures for the determination of NH_2-terminal and COOH-terminal residues in proteins and peptides can be utilized to assess the presence and extent of modification of α-amino and α-carboxyl groups in addition to side-chain modifications. These procedures are especially useful in pinpointing the exact residues in the sequence which have

Subject index p. 201

been modified. In many instances this will require cleavage of the protein to smaller fragments which may then be isolated and examined by these methods. However, in some instances (see example in § 2.15) the modified residues are sufficiently close to the ends of the polypeptide chain to be determined without cleavage of the protein.

2.15. Sequential degradation and determination of amino-terminal residues (Edman degradation)

With the development of automated instruments (sequenators) for the sequential degradation of proteins and polypeptides from the amino terminus (Edman and Begg 1967) the problem of identifying modified residues in proteins has been greatly simplified. However, if the modified residues are not sufficiently near the amino terminus (usually within 30 residues), the protein must be cleaved to obtain peptides containing the modified residues near enough to the NH_2-terminal ends that their identities and positions can be determined. Although considerable progress has been made in the technology of sequencing smaller peptides with sequenators, this is not always practical or possible. The major problem has been the extraction of smaller peptides into the solvents used to extract excess reagents or the derivatives of the NH_2-terminal residues. For this reason and also because many investigators do not have access to a sequenator, a method for degrading peptides manually will be given below. This method works best for peptides which dissolve in the reagents indicated. For proteins or even very large peptides, a method such as that described by Schroeder (1972a) will usually give better results, especially if more than one degradative step is necessary. Where the quantitation of only the NH_2-terminal residue is desired, the cyanate method (Stark 1967a, 1972a) can be used in addition to the manual or automated release of the NH_2-terminal residue by the Edman procedure and its quantitative estimation by gas–liquid chromatography (see below).

Although it is not within the scope of this treatise to describe the methodology used with sequenators, an example of their usefulness in studying chemical modification will be described. Histones are modified *in vivo* by acetylation (also methylation and phosphorylation, see DeLange and Smith 1971, 1974). In some histones the α-amino groups are acetylated (in addition to lysine residues) and this precludes direct examination of the internal sites of acetylation by the Edman procedure. However, histones IIb2 and III have free α-amino groups and this enabled Candido and Dixon (1972) to examine these histones (from trout testis) which had been acetylated intracellularly with ^{14}C-labeled acetate. Each residue that was released by the Edman procedure (using a sequenator) was examined for radioactive material and it was found that lysyl Residues 14 and 23 (major sites) and 9 and 18 (minor sites) were partially acetylated in histone III and lysyl Residues 5, 10, 13 and 18 were partially acetylated in histone IIb2. This type of approach should be applicable to many other studies of chemical modification.

Manual Edman degradation. Although there are many variations in procedure that can be used to achieve satisfactory Edman degradations of proteins and peptides, all of them make use of the same basic

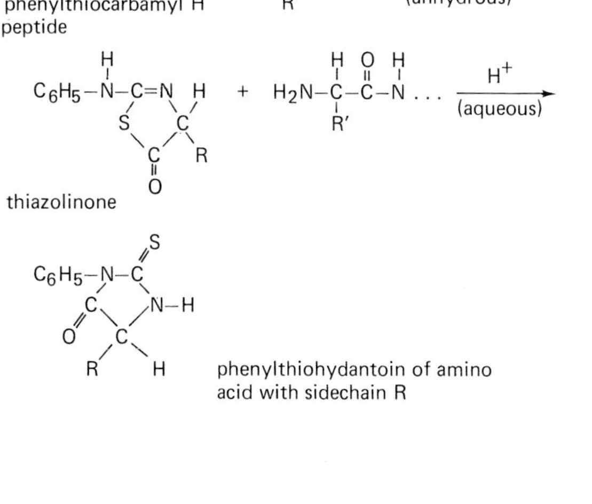

reactions. In order to repeat this procedure over many steps, it is important that all reagents and solvents be highly purified (e.g. sequenator-grade chemicals, Beckman or Pierce Chemical) and that oxygen or other oxidants be excluded to allow high yields at each step. One such procedure that has been used in our own laboratory is described below. It is essentially as described by Peterson et al. (1972). All reagents are sequenator grade.

The peptide (usually 50–250 nmoles) is dissolved in 100 μl of coupling buffer (0.4 M dimethylallylamine in 1-propanol:H_2O, 3:2 (v/v) adjusted to *p*H 9.5 with trifluoroacetic acid) in a 3 ml conical glass stoppered centrifuge tube. After replacing the air with nitrogen by briefly evacuating the tube in a desiccator under vacuum and re-pressurizing with nitrogen, phenylisothiocyanate (5 μl) is added under a stream of nitrogen and the tube is stoppered as the nitrogen stream is withdrawn. The tube is mixed and placed in a 50°C heating block for 20 min, after which the contents are dried at 40°C with a stream of nitrogen (in a fume hood) until the liquid is gone and then in a desiccator under high vacuum (mechanical pump) for 15 min over $CaCl_2$. After repressurizing with nitrogen, the dry, derivatized peptide is extracted under nitrogen with 100 μl and then 50 μl of benzene. The last traces of benzene are removed with a stream of nitrogen and finally in a desiccator under high vacuum for 15 min. After repressurizing with nitrogen, the derivatized peptide is ready for cleavage as described below.

To the derivatized peptide is added 100 μl of trifluoroacetic acid under nitrogen, and the tube is stoppered and placed in a heating block at 50°C for 7 min. The trifluoroacetic acid is evaporated with a stream of nitrogen at 25–40°C in such a way that a thin film is formed for several cm up the sides of the tube, and finally in a desiccator under high vacuum. The dried peptide film is then extracted 3 times with ether (50–200 μl each depending on the solubility of the peptide). The ether must be free of peroxides (absence of yellow color 5–10 min after mixing equal volumes of ether and 4% (w/v) aqueous KI). Storage of ether over $FeSO_4$ crystals and under nitrogen is usually effective in preventing peroxide formation. The last traces of ether are removed from the peptide with a stream of nitrogen, and the peptide can be stored at this stage until the next degradative cycle is started. If it is necessary to hydrolyze a sample of peptide for analysis, this is done by removing an aliquot of the peptide after dissolving it in the coupling buffer.

The combined ether extract (which may be washed with 0.01 N HCl to remove peptide material) is evaporated to dryness with a stream of nitrogen and 50 μl of 1 N HCl is added. After mixing, the thiazolinone derivative of the NH_2-terminal residue is converted to the phenylthiohydantoin by incubation at 80°C (temperature block) for 10 min. If Asx or Glx residues are expected, 80°C for 3 min may give better results and for threonine, proline and serine, 50°C for 10 min may be better (Li and Yanofsky 1972). After cooling, the phenylthiohydantoin is extracted into ethyl acetate (100–200 μl for each of 3 extractions), which is then evaporated with a stream of nitrogen. The phenylthiohydantoins of arginine, histidine and cysteic acid will usually remain in the aqueous phase and may be recovered by lyophilization and dissolving the residue in methanol.

The phenylthiohydantoins may be identified directly by thin layer chromatography or gas-liquid chromatography (see below). Alternatively, they can be hydrolyzed at 140°C in 5.7 N glass-distilled HCl *in vacuo* (see § 2.1.2 for other details) in the presence of phenol (1 drop of 5% phenol in water) to regenerate the amino acid, which can be identified with an analyzer or by *p*H 1.9 electrophoresis. The regeneration is not quantitative, and several amino acids, particularly serine and threonine, are usually destroyed completely.

Thin layer chromatography of phenylthiohydantoins can be carried out on Eastman K301R plates with fluorescent indicator (Jeppsson and Sjöquist 1967) or on sheets of Eastman 6060 silica gel (Peterson et al. 1972).* In either case 2 solvents are used routinely for development, and if positive identification of the phenylthiohydantoin has not been made with these systems, other solvents are used (Jeppsson and Sjöquist 1967). With smaller peptides the use of either Solvent V (heptane : propionic acid : ethylene chloride, 58 : 17 : 25 v/v) or Solvent IV (heptane : *n*-butanol : 75% formic acid, 50 : 30 : 9 v/v) may be adequate

* A useful thin layer chromatography system has been described by Inagami and Murakami (1972).

for identification. In other instances it is necessary to develop with Solvent V first (requires about 1 hr) and, after drying, with Solvent IV (requires about 2 hr) to give better separations. The sheets are equilibrated for 30 min in a tank lined with Whatman 3MM paper, which is saturated with solvent, prior to ascending chromatography in the same tank. After drying at 100°C for 15 min the phenylthiohydantoins of tryptophan, tyrosine, asparagine and histidine are slightly yellow and those of glycine, threonine and serine are slightly pink. These colors are often helpful in making identifications.

For gas-liquid chromatography of phenylthiohydantoins of amino acids we routinely use a Beckman GC-65 instrument as recommended by the manufacturer, but many other instruments can also be used. The nature of the packing material in the columns is of critical importance, and usually more than one type is required for positive identifications (see Pisano 1972). Silylation of some of the phenylthiohydantoins is important in order to obtain a good response and to allow identification by shifting the elution position (analyses for the phenylthiohydantoins of aspartic acid, glutamic acid, lysine, serine, threonine, S-carboxymethylcysteine and cysteic acid are all improved after silylation). Although several solvents can be used, we routinely dissolve the phenylthiohydantoin in ethyl acetate (usually 20 μl) and inject 1 μl aliquots. If silylation is necessary, this is usually carried out directly on the column by injecting 1 μl of the sample which has been 'sandwiched' between two 1 μl aliquots of silylating reagent in a Hamilton syringe. Any sample remaining is usually hydrolyzed with HCl (see above) to regenerate the amino acid which is identified by electrophoresis at *p*H 1.9 or with an analyzer for confirmation. The phenylthiohydantoin of arginine is usually identified (from the aqueous phase) by the Sakaguchi reaction after electrophoresis at *p*H 1.9 (with a standard). For other details of gas-liquid chromatography of phenylthiohydantoins see Pisano and Bronzert (1969) and Pisano (1972).

2.16. Determination of COOH-terminal sequences

Although the COOH-terminal residues of proteins and peptides may be determined after hydrazinolysis (see Fraenkel-Conrat and Tsung 1967; Schroeder 1972a), and it is possible to degrade sequentially many proteins and peptides from their COOH termini (see Stark 1972b), most COOH-terminal sequence information is derived from hydrolysis of proteins and peptides with carboxypeptidases. Until recently, carboxypeptidases A and B were those usually utilized for this purpose, but recently carboxypeptidase C (citrus leaf, Rohm and Haas) and carboxypeptidase Y (yeast, see Hayashi et al. 1973) have been used, since either of these enzymes shows limited variation in the rates of hydrolysis of various peptide bonds and even hydrolyzes those bonds involving proline at appreciable rates. This is to be compared with carboxypeptidase B which hydrolyzes only bonds involving COOH-terminal lysine and arginine, and carboxypeptidase A which hydrolyzes bonds involving COOH-terminal hydrophobic residues much faster than bonds with other COOH-terminal residues. Neither carboxypeptidase A nor B usually hydrolyzes bonds involving proline in the penultimate position at appreciable rates. However, the greater specificity of carboxypeptidases A and B can be used to great advantage with certain peptides or proteins, and because of this and their commercial availability (and cheaper price), it is anticipated that carboxypeptidases A and B will continue to be used at least initially until it can be demonstrated whether satisfactory results can be obtained with the more recently introduced enzymes.

Proteins or large polypeptides can be conveniently hydrolyzed with carboxypeptidases inside dialysis tubing. The released amino acids are easily collected by removing the dialysate (or aliquots) at prescribed times. To illustrate how this can be done, the following example is given.

The protein (0.55 μmoles, 22 mg) is dialyzed against 0.1 M NH_4HCO_3 at *p*H 8.0 to give a final solution that is 4.0 mg/ml. Carboxypeptidase B (0.22 mg, treated with diisopropylfluorophosphate (DFP), see below) is added and after gentle mixing, 1.0 ml is dialyzed against 20 ml of 0.1 M NH_4HCO_3 (*p*H 8.0) for 30 min at 40°C with stirring of the dialysate. The remainder of the mixture is incubated at 40°C during this time, and at the end of the 30 min, carboxypeptidase A (0.18 mg, treated with DFP, see below) is added. Four aliquots of 1.0 ml each are dialyzed separately against 20 ml of 0.1 M NH_4HCO_3 (*p*H 8.0) at 40°C with stirring for an additional 15 min (sample 1), 1 hr (sample 2), 4–6 hr (sample 3) and overnight (sample 4). At the designated times the dialysates are frozen and lyophilized until most of the fluffy salt has disappeared. Each sample is then redissolved in 5% acetic acid (10 ml) and lyophilized to dryness over P_2O_5. This procedure usually reduces the NH_3 content of the dialysates to acceptable levels for amino acid analysis of the basic residues, but the last step (5% acetic acid) can be repeated several times if NH_3 levels are found to be too high. Prior to analysis of the dialysates, it is often advisable to dissolve each sample in 0.25 ml of H_2O and examine 25 μl by electrophoresis at *p*H 1.9 to be sure that hydrolysis proceeded satisfactorily. Since 0.1 μmole of protein was used for each sample, this is the maximum amount that can be found upon amino acid analysis of the total sample for 1 residue of amino acid released. Smaller amounts of material can be utilized, but if the volume of protein solution is not reduced appropriately (which makes the dialysis procedure more cumbersome), the rate of hydrolysis will be slower (this can be advantageous for some proteins). The purpose of adding the carboxypeptidase B initially was to determine whether any basic residues released were at the COOH terminus. With many proteins, carboxypeptidase A alone or carboxypeptidase A with carboxypeptidase B added later may be better. The dialysis tubing should be thoroughly washed (boiling in water for 5 min is often used) before use and should be handled only with gloves to prevent contamination with amino acids from sweat, etc. The conditions of hydrolysis (temperature, time, concentration of enzyme, etc.) may be varied to suit the protein being hydrolyzed. Some proteins may not be hydrolyzed unless they are denatured, and denaturation may cause them to be insoluble. However, dissolving the protein in 8 M urea or 100% formic acid and dialyzing against several changes of the NH_4HCO_3 buffer will usually allow satisfactory results to be obtained. It is very important that carboxypeptidase preparations are free of endopeptidase activity, since this can lead to erroneous results. Trypsin and chymotrypsin are the most common endopeptidases found in preparations of carboxypeptidases A and B, and they can both be inhibited by DFP. Carboxypeptidase B is usually stored as a frozen solution, but carboxypeptidase A is stored at 4°C as a suspension in water. It is necessary to wash the carboxypeptidase A by pelleting the protein by centrifugation and resuspending to volume with cold H_2O. This procedure should be repeated once or twice if the preparation has been stored for more than a few days. Aliquots of the washed suspension of carboxypeptidase A (e.g. 10 μl containing 200 μg of enzyme) are treated with 0.1 N NaOH (3–5 μl), and as soon as the protein has dissolved, it is immediately diluted with 0.1 M NH_4HCO_3 (e.g. 0.4 ml at *p*H 8.0). To inhibit any trypsin and chymotrypsin present, DFP (20 μl of a 1–2% solution in anhydrous isopropyl alcohol) is added, and the reaction mixture is incubated at 40°C for 1 hr. Carboxypeptidase B is treated in a similar manner, except that it is not necessary to dissolve it with NaOH. These solutions of carboxypeptidase may be used in place of some of the buffer in the hydrolysis mixtures to prevent further dilution.

For hydrolysis of smaller peptides it is necessary to carry out the reaction in tubes (e.g. 3 ml conical glass tubes). As an example, a decapeptide (0.15 μmole) was dissolved in 0.25 ml of 0.1 M NH_4HCO_3 (*p*H 8.0) containing 50 μg of carboxypeptidase B, treated with DFP (see above). After 15 min an aliquot of 20 μl was removed and added to 1 drop of 50% acetic acid, and 0.1 ml of 0.1 M NH_4HCO_3 buffer containing 50 μg of carboxypeptidase A (treated with DFP as described above) was added to the reaction mixture. Aliquots of 0.1 ml were removed at 10 min, 1 hr and 5 hr and added to 2 drops of glacial acetic acid to stop the reaction. The samples were dried over P_2O_5 and 1/10 of each was examined by electrophoresis at *p*H 1.9. The remainder of each sample was analyzed on both columns of the analyzer.

Hydrolysis with carboxypeptidase C or carboxypeptidase Y can be performed in a similar manner to that described above except that a buffer at *p*H 5.3–5.5 should be used (0.1 M pyridine adjusted to *p*H with glacial acetic acid has been used). We have generally used 300 units of carboxypeptidase C per 0.1 ml of reaction mixture containing up to 0.1 μmole of peptide.

Modification of protein side-chains: group-specific reagents

The protein derivatives described in this chapter are in the main used in amino acid sequence analysis, or for the purpose of determining the content of a given residue in a protein. For such purposes, quantitative modification of the residue in question is mandatory. Consequently, some of the methods described below specify the inclusion of high concentrations of denaturing agents in the reaction mixtures. This is not always essential. For certain functional groups, e.g. amino groups, complete modification is frequently attained with the native protein.

Group-specific reagents have been used extensively for site-specific modification of native proteins. For such a purpose, the modification is performed on the native protein (or in a solvent which does not *irreversibly* alter the conformation of the protein). The concentrations of the modifying reagents are generally considerably lower than those used for the total modification of a given side-chain, and the conditions of reaction, e.g. *p*H, temperature, organic solvent concentration, are suitably chosen, bearing in mind the stability characteristics of the protein under study. Ch. 4 is devoted to the consideration of the factors governing site-specific modification with group-specific reagents.

Because of the individual nature of the problems encountered, we have made no attempt to present detailed methodological information on site-specific modification. This is available in abundance in the books and reviews cited in ch. 1.

3.1. Modifications of amino groups

3.1.1. Modifications of amino groups leading to retention of positive charge

3.1.1.1. Amidination

$$R{-}NH_2 + C_2H_5O{-}\overset{\overset{\displaystyle NH{\cdot}HCl}{\|}}{C}{-}R' \longrightarrow R{\cdot}NH{-}\overset{\overset{\displaystyle NH{\cdot}HCl}{\|}}{C}{-}R' + C_2H_5OH$$

The selective conversion of the amino groups of proteins to the amidine derivative proceeds smoothly at mildly alkaline *p*H. The modification leads to little alteration in the charge, solubility, and physical properties of proteins (Ludwig and Hunter 1967; Hunter and Ludwig 1972). The ease of preparation of imidoesters with a variety of R′ groups has been of particular advantage in the design of cross-linking reagents for the study of the subunit structure of oligomeric proteins (e.g. Davies and Stark 1970), or ribosomes (Bickle et al. 1972). The reagents utilized for such purpose have included diimidoesters of the general formula

$$CH_3O{-}\overset{\overset{\displaystyle NH{\cdot}HCl}{\|}}{C} - R - \overset{\overset{\displaystyle NH{\cdot}HCl}{\|}}{C}{-}OCH_3 \quad \text{where} \quad R = (CH_2)_n, \quad \text{where} \quad n = 1{-}8$$

Certain of these reagents are available commercially; all may be synthesized by the method of McElvain and Schroeder (1949). The synthesis of an interesting imidoester derivative, methyl-4-mercapto-butyrimidate has been described by Traut et al. (1973) (see also Perham and Thomas 1971). This reagent has been applied to the study of proximity relationships in the ribosome in the following manner. The amino groups of an intact ribosome are reacted with the imidate function of the reagent, in the presence of a reducing agent. After dialysis, the newly introduced SH groups are oxidized with low concentrations of H_2O_2. The resulting disulfide-linked proteins are readily detected on polyacrylamide gel electrophoresis in the presence of sodium dodecyl sulfate, and may be easily converted to their constituent proteins by mild reduction.

A number of studies have been performed with methyl picolinimidate (Benisek and Richards 1968; Plapp et al. 1971) aimed at exploring the usefulness of the metal-chelating properties of such derivatives in the preparation of isomorphous heavy atom derivatives of proteins for X-ray diffraction studies.

A representative amidination procedure is described here. Protein (10 mg/ml) is dissolved in 0.2 M triethanolamine hydrochloride at *p*H 8.5, at room temperature. Immediately before use, ethylacetimidate hydrochloride is dissolved in the same buffer to give a 0.4 M solution, and the *p*H adjusted to 8.5. Equal volumes of protein and reagent solutions are mixed and the reaction allowed to proceed for 2 hr. The derivative is isolated by dialysis and lyophilization. If necessary, reaction may be performed in the presence of 6 M guanidine hydrochloride.

Partial regeneration of amino groups takes place on acid hydrolysis. Hence, residual amino groups in the derivative are most readily determined by titration with trinitrobenzenesulfonate (§ 3.1.2.3), or by measuring incorporation of labeled reagent.

The acetamidino group can be removed by prolonged incubation in concentrated ammonia-glacial acetic acid, 15:1 (v/v), *p*H 11.3. This treatment is harsh and reported to modify the protein (Hunter and Ludwig 1972).

3.1.1.2. Guanidination

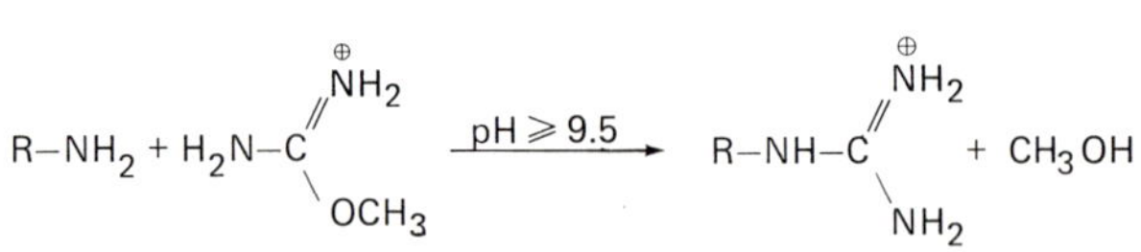

Lysyl residues may be converted to the homoarginine derivative by treatment of proteins with 0-methylisourea at alkaline *p*H. The degree of modification is readily assessed by amino acid analysis, as homoarginine is stable under the usual conditions of acid hydrolysis (§ 2.7.2). α-Amino groups react much more slowly with this reagent than do ε-amino groups. For example, complete guanidination of the lysyl residues of bovine pancreatic deoxyribonuclease A was obtained after 96 hr at 4°C in the presence of 0.5 M 0-methylisourea at *p*H 10.6, with only 20% modification of the α-amino group (Plapp et al. 1971).

In a typical procedure (Kimmel 1967), an aqueous solution of a protein (10 mg/ml) is mixed at 4°C with an equal volume of O-methylisourea, adjusted to *p*H 9.5 with NaOH. The reaction is allowed to proceed for 4–5 days at 4°C, and is then terminated by dialysis against ice-cold deionized water. If lysine modification is found to be incomplete, the reaction may be attempted either at a higher temperature (e.g. 25°C), or at *p*H 10.5–11 at 4°C.

1-Guanyl-3,5-dimethylpyrazole nitrate (Habeeb 1972) has also been employed for the guanidination of proteins. This reagent shows less discrimination between α- and ε-NH_2 groups in proteins than O-methylisourea.

Guanidination of thiol-containing proteins with 0-methylisourea will invariably lead to S-methylation of thiols. Banks and Shafer (1970) have carried out a careful study of the kinetics of this S-methylation.

$$H_2N{-}\overset{\overset{\displaystyle OCH_3}{|}}{C}{=}NH_2^+ + RS^- \longrightarrow RS{-}CH_3 + H_2N{-}\overset{\overset{\displaystyle O}{\|}}{C}{-}NH_2$$

Their study shows that while 0-methylisourea guanidinates primary amino groups at high *p*H values (e.g. *p*H 10.5) more efficiently than it S-methylates thiols, the reverse is true below *p*H 10. Banks and Shafer (1972) exploited this observation in demonstrating that the thiol group at the active site of papain could be selectively S-methylated at *p*H 7 without concomitant guanidination of lysyl residues.

3.1.1.3. Reductive methylation

Selective alkylation of amino groups can be achieved by exposure of proteins, in alkaline solution, to low concentrations of formaldehyde and sodium borohydride. Both α- and ε-amino groups are modified. ε-N-Methyllysine, and ε-N,N-dimethyllysine, may be readily quantitated after acid hydrolysis (see § 2.12.1.2). The physical properties of the alkylated protein derivatives are very similar to those of the un-

$$R{\cdot}NH_2 + HCHO \underset{+H_2O}{\overset{-H_2O}{\rightleftharpoons}} R{-}N{=}CH_2 \xrightarrow{NaBH_4} R{-}NH{-}CH_3$$

$$R{\cdot}NH{-}CH_3 + HCHO \underset{+H_2O}{\overset{-H_2O}{\rightleftharpoons}} R{-}\overset{+}{N}(CH_3){=}CH_2 \xrightarrow{NaBH_4} R{\cdot}N(CH_3)_2$$

modified protein (Means and Feeney 1968). The reductive methylation procedure given below is based on that of Means and Feeney (1968).

Protein (approx. 3 mg/ml) is dissolved in 0.2 M sodium borate buffer *p*H 9.0. To 2.0 ml of this solution, at 0°C, is added a 50 μl aliquot of a freshly prepared solution of $NaBH_4$ (40 mg/ml). Five consecutive increments of 1 μl of 18% (v/v) aqueous formaldehyde solution are then added at 5 min intervals. At the end of 30 min, the reaction mixture is transferred to dialysis tubing and exhaustively dialyzed against ice-cold deionized water at 4°C. The protein derivative is recovered by lyophilization.

If amino acid analysis shows the lysine modification to be incomplete, the derivative is redissolved in the *p*H 9 buffer and the procedure repeated. Several such cycles may be necessary to achieve maximum modification of amino groups in native proteins.

If retention of native structure is not desired, the reaction may be performed in the presence of 6 M guanidine HCl. Complete alkylation of amino groups should then be attainable.

Rice and Means (1971) have employed the following procedure to label a number of proteins and several viruses to specific activities of about 5×10^6 cpm per mg of protein.

Samples of protein (0.1 mg) are adjusted to *p*H 9.0 with 0.1 M NaOH, or 0.2 M sodium borate buffer, *p*H 9.0, and to a volume of 0.1 ml. To the ice-cold solution, 10 μl of 0.04 M ^{14}C-formaldehyde (10 mCi per mmole) are added. This is followed in 30 sec by 4 sequential additions of 2 μl of $NaBH_4$ (5 mg/ml). An additional 10 μl of $NaBH_4$ solution are added after 1 min. The reaction mixture is then dialyzed.

Since either ^{3}H- or ^{14}C-labeled formaldehyde may be used, the reductive methylation procedure lends itself to studies requiring a double label.

It may be noted that reductive alkylation of proteins with acetaldehyde, or acetone, results in the formation of only the corresponding monoalkyl derivatives of lysine.

3.1.2. Modifications of amino groups resulting in conversion to a neutral derivative

3.1.2.1. Carbamylation

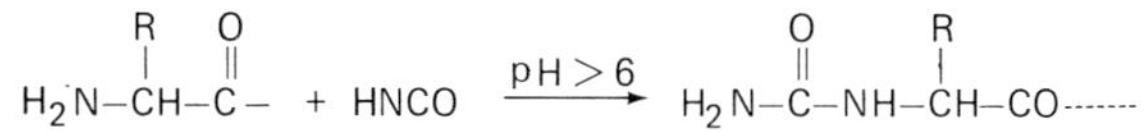

The reaction of proteins with cyanate has been exploited in the development of a method for the quantitative determination of NH_2-terminal residues (Stark 1967a), as well as in a variety of interesting structure-function studies exemplified by those of Smyth (1967) on oxytocin, and Cerami and Manning (1971), as well as Lee and Manning (1973), on sickle cell hemoglobin. Whereas cyanate reacts with α-NH_2, ε-NH_2, thiol, imidazole, and phenolic OH groups of proteins, only the amino group derivatives are stable at alkaline *p*H.

The reaction is performed by dissolving the protein (10 mg/ml) in 0.5 M borate buffer *p*H 8.8, containing 4 M guanidine hydrochloride. Solid KCNO is added to a final concentration of 0.5 M and the reaction mixture is maintained at 30°C for 24 hr. The mixture is then dialyzed against 0.005 M NH_4HCO_3, *p*H 8.2, and the protein derivative lyophilized.

The extent of modification can be assessed either by using ^{14}C-labeled cyanate, or for lysine by determining the homocitrulline content of the protein after acid hydrolysis. Since homocitrulline is slowly hydrolyzed to lysine, the carbamylated protein should be hydrolyzed for 24 and 48 hr, and the values for homocitrulline extrapolated with first order kinetics to zero time (Plapp et al. 1971; § 2.7.4).

A fully carbamylated derivative of rabbit muscle phosphoglucose isomerase was utilized by James and Noltmann (1973), both for a quantitative amino-terminal analysis and for tryptic mapping experiments. Tryptic digestion of the derivative was restricted entirely to the arginyl residues.

It should be noted carbamylation of tyrosyl residues takes place readily (Smyth 1967; Rimon and Perlmann 1968).

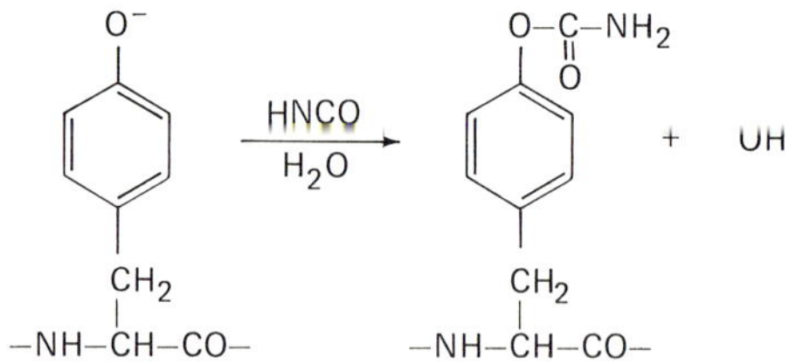

The formation of the carbamyl tyrosine derivative may be monitored spectrophotometrically at 278 nm ($\Delta\varepsilon_M^{278\,nm} = 1145$) (Rimon and Perlmann 1968). Tyrosine is regenerated slowly in aqueous solution, the rate of hydrolysis of the derivative is *p*H-dependent, increasing with increase in *p*H. The derivative is rapidly decomposed at near-neutral *p*H by M hydroxylamine. The possible use of the carbamyl group as a readily removable protecting group for tyrosine has been suggested (Smyth 1967), but not applied to date.

3.1.2.2. *Trifluoroacetylation*

$$R{-}NH_2 + F_3C{-}\overset{\overset{O}{\|}}{C}{-}S{-}C_2H_5 \xrightarrow{\text{pH } 10} R{-}NH{-}\overset{\overset{O}{\|}}{C}{-}CF_3 + C_2H_5SH$$

The reversible blocking of amino groups by trifluoroacetylation provides a means of limiting tryptic digestion to arginyl residues (Goldberger and Anfinsen 1962; Goldberger 1967).

In a typical procedure, protein (25 mg/ml) is dissolved in water and brought to *p*H 10 at 25°C by careful addition of base regulated by a *p*H-stat. Ethylthioltrifluoroacetate (0.25 ml/25 mg of protein) is added, and the *p*H is maintained at 10 by the addition of 1 M KOH. After 1 hr, additional ethylthioltrifluoroacetate (0.1 ml/25 mg of protein) is added and the reaction continued for a further 30 min. The *p*H is then lowered to 5–6 by the cautious addition of 1 M acetic acid. The protein derivative is then precipitated by adding the reaction mixture to 4 volumes of ethanol at $-10°C$ (Goldberger 1967). The precipitate is collected by centrifugation, and washed twice with a mixture of ethanol:0.1 M sodium acetate, *p*H 5.0 (5:1, v/v). The precipitate is resuspended in the ethanol–sodium acetate mixture, dialyzed exhaustively against 0.001 M HCl, and lyophilized.

An alternative isolation procedure may be employed if the protein derivative is partially soluble in the aqueous ethanol. The *p*H of the reaction mixture is lowered to 8 by the careful addition of 1 M acetic acid. The mixture is filtered, and the filtrate, containing the protein derivative, is dialyzed against 0.01 M potassium phosphate buffer *p*H 8, at 4°C, followed by exhaustive dialysis against water, and by lyophilization.

It should be noted that high concentrations of ethanethiol are formed on the hydrolysis of ethylthiotrifluoroacetate at high *p*H. Under alkaline conditions, ethanethiol causes both disruption and rearrangement of disulfide bonds.

A trifluoroacetylation procedure (Levy and Paselk 1973), performed entirely under non-aqueous conditions, appears to eliminate the side-reactions involving disulfide bonds. In this procedure, insulin hydrochloride (24 mg, 4 μmoles) was dissolved in dimethylformamide (5.0 ml) (pre-purified by distillation at 0.2 mm Hg, after refluxing for 2 hr over calcium hydride), and triethylamine (10 μl, 72 μmole), and stirred at 24°C for 5 min. Ethylthioltrifluoroacetate (18.4 mg, 120 μmoles) dissolved in dimethylformamide (1.15 ml) was added to the insulin solution. The reaction was allowed to proceed for 60 min. The product was precipitated by the addition of anhydrous ether (40 ml). The precipitate was isolated by centrifugation, washed with acetone, and ether, and then dried in a dessicator over P_2O_5 under high vacuum.

Two procedures have been utilized for the removal of trifluoroacetyl groups. In the first (Goldberger 1967), the trifluoroacetylated protein (10 mg/ml) is dissolved in 0.5 ml of 1 M piperidine at room temperature, the mixture chilled to 0°C, and allowed to stand for 2 hr. Acetic acid (0.5 M) at 0°C is added to *p*H 6.0, and the regenerated protein is recovered by lyophilization after gel filtration, or dialysis. In the second procedure (e.g. Fanger and Harbury 1965), hydrolysis of the trifluoroacetamide linkage is accomplished by incubation of the protein (10 mg/ml) in 0.15 M K_2CO_3 at 25°C for 30 hr. The first procedure appears less likely to produce side reactions.

3.1.2.3. Trinitrobenzoylation

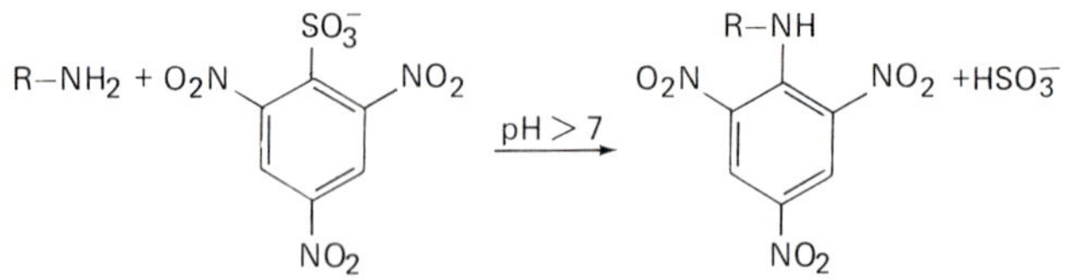

2,4,6-Trinitrobenzenesulfonate (TNBS) was introduced by Okuyama and Satake (1960) as a sensitive colorimetric reagent for the determination of amino groups in proteins and peptides. The absorbance of TNP-amino acids in the visible region of the spectrum is similar to that of DNP-amino acids. The reaction of TNBS with proteins appears to be restricted to α-, and ε-amino groups, and sulfhydryl groups. Under the alkaline reaction conditions the thiol derivative is unstable. In proteins in which sulfhydryl groups are absent or suitably blocked, spectrophotometric determination of the kinetics of the reaction with TNBS provides information both on the content and reactivity of the amino groups. Since the TNP derivatives are stable to acid hydrolysis, the spectrophotometric results can be checked by amino acid analysis.

TNBS readily forms adducts with sulfite, a product of the arylation reaction (see Means et al. 1972).

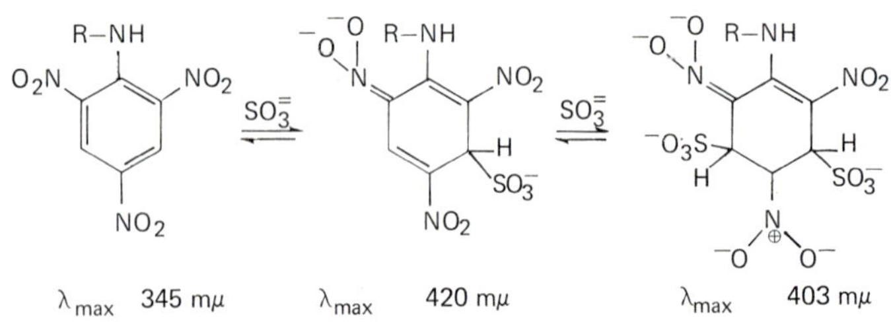

The formation of these complexes profoundly affects the visible spectrum of TNP-amino acids. This complication is resolved in the spectrophotometric procedure of Plapp et al. (1971) by following TNP-amino acid formation at 367 nm, the isobestic point for ε-trinitrophenyl-α-acetyllysine and its sulfite complex. The procedure described by Fields (1971, 1972) exploits the higher extinction coefficient of the sulfite complex at 420 mμ.

Commercially available preparations of TNBS have been reported to be of variable quality. TNBS may be recrystallized by suspending the solid in an equal weight of water and dissolving by heating. HCl is then added to a concentration of 5 M, and the solution is cooled. The resulting white crystals are washed on a filter with cold M HCl and dried over P_2O_5 in a vacuum (water pump), m.p. 189–192°C. The product is believed to be the trihydrate (Fields 1971, 1972; Plapp et al. 1971).

The following method for the spectrophotometric determination of amino groups in proteins with TNBS is based on the procedure of Plapp et al. (1971).

The protein (2 mg/ml) is dissolved in borate buffer (0.05 M $Na_2B_4O_7$ adjusted to *p*H 9.5 with 0.05 M NaOH). A fresh solution of TNBS (7.2 mg/ml of water, approx 0.02 M) is prepared. One ml of borate buffer is placed in a reference cell and 1 ml of protein solution in the sample cell. A 100 μl aliquot of TNBS is added to each cuvette and the change in absorbance at 367 nm followed. Generally 1–4 hr may be required for complete reaction. The extent of trinitrophenylation may be calculated on the basis of an $\varepsilon_{367\text{nm}} = 1.1 \times 10^4\ M^{-1}\,cm^{-1}$. Precise measurement of the kinetics of the reaction requires thermostatting of the cells. (It should be noted that the molar extinction coefficient given above is based on the absorption of a TNP-derivative in an aqueous solution. A proportion of the TNP groups on a native protein may be in environments which perturb the absorption spectrum of the TNP derivative. This may be a source of significant error in the case of proteins containing numerous lysine residues).

Native proteins may contain amino groups which fail to react with TNBS under the above conditions. The number of such groups may be determined from the lysine content of the trinitrophenylated protein, and from the residual α-amino groups which can be detected by end-group methods (§ 2.14).

Where desired, complete trinitrophenylation should be attainable in the presence of high concentrations (4–6 M) of guanidine.

3.1.3. Conversion of amino groups to acidic derivatives

3.1.3.1. Succinylation

The reaction of amino groups with succinic anhydride has been utilized to dissociate multi-subunit proteins, to solubilize proteins, or to limit the action of trypsin to arginine residues. More recently, partial succinylation of multi-subunit proteins has been used to obtain information about the number and type of subunits present (see Klotz 1967; Klapper and Klotz 1972).

In addition to acylating α- and ε-amino groups, succinic anhydride reacts with tyrosyl, histidyl, cysteinyl, seryl and threonyl side-chains. The tyrosyl derivative hydrolyzes spontaneously at alkaline *p*H, and is rapidly decomposed by hydroxylamine at neutral *p*H. The histidyl derivative is presumably very labile. The lability of all of the ester derivatives to hydroxylamine at *p*H 10 permits preparation of a protein modified solely on the α- and ε-amino groups (e.g. Gounaris and Perlmann 1967).

If complete selective modification of amino groups is desired, the reaction should be carried out on a protein derivative in which sulfhydryl and disulfide groups have been converted to a stable derivative. Otherwise, these groups would be exposed to both interchange and oxidation under the conditions required to cleave succinyl esters.

A suitable protein derivative is dissolved in 5.0 M guanidine hydrochloride at *p*H 8.0, and solid succinic anhydride (50 moles/mole of amino group) is added in small portions to a rapidly stirred solution at room temperature. The *p*H is maintained (by means of a *p*H-stat) by the addition of M NaOH. When the addition of succinic anhydride is complete, solid hydroxylamine hydrochloride is added to the reaction mixture to a concentration of 1 M, the *p*H is adjusted to 10 with NaOH and the mixture allowed to stand at room temperature for

60 min. The protein derivative is then isolated either by dialysis or gel filtration and lyophilized.

Determination of the completeness of lysine acylation is performed by dinitrophenylation (Fraenkel-Conrat et al. 1955) of the succinylated protein, followed by acid hydrolysis, and amino acid analysis. Since ε-dinitrophenyllysine is stable to acid hydrolysis, the recovery of lysine reflects the ε-succinyllysine content of the protein.

The presentation by Meighen and Schachman (1970) should be consulted for details of a general method utilizing hybridization of native and partially succinylated subunits of proteins for the study of subunit structure of multimeric enzymes.

3.1.3.2. Reversible modification of amino groups with maleic anhydride and similar reagents

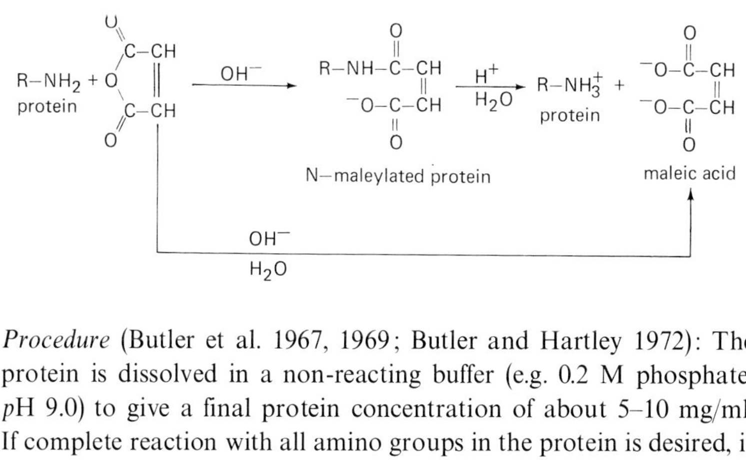

Procedure (Butler et al. 1967, 1969; Butler and Hartley 1972): The protein is dissolved in a non-reacting buffer (e.g. 0.2 M phosphate, *p*H 9.0) to give a final protein concentration of about 5–10 mg/ml. If complete reaction with all amino groups in the protein is desired, it may be necessary to add a denaturing agent, such as 8 M urea or 6 M guanidinium chloride in the buffer. The solution is cooled in ice to 0–2°C and is maintained at this temperature throughout the reaction. This can be done simply by placing a beaker with the protein in it, in a crystallizing dish, containing ice water, which is placed on a magnetic stirrer.

Solid maleic anhydride (preferably purified by sublimation or by recrystallization from chloroform) is added in small aliquots to the protein solution which is stirred and maintained at *p*H 8.5–9.0 by the manual or automatic (*p*H stat) addition of 4 N NaOH (or solid Na_2CO_3 if dilution is undesirable). The maleic anhydride dissolves slowly under these conditions, and the rate of addition of the aliquots is governed by the rate of disappearance of the solid material in the reaction mixture. The final concentration of added reagent (assuming no reaction) should generally be 0.03 to 0.10 M, but preliminary studies should be made to determine the minimum amount of reagent that will give the desired degree of modification; this should minimize the reaction of the reagent with seryl and threonyl residues (see below). When the lack of base uptake indicates the end of the reaction (usually about 5 min after the last addition of reagent), the protein is dialyzed against an alkaline buffer (*p*H 7.0 or higher) that is suitable for the types of studies to be made on the maleylated protein. Acidic buffers will lead to demaleylation (see below).

The total number of maleyl groups incorporated into the protein can best be determined with radiolabeled reagent. Estimates can also be made spectrophotometrically by dissolving the protein in 0.1 N NaOH and using the molar extinction values of 3360 (ε_{250}) and 308 (ε_{280}) for the maleylamino group. However, some maleyl groups may be present as esters of seryl and threonyl residues, and these esters have smaller molar extinction coefficients (see Butler and Hartley 1972). The presence of these esters may be ascertained by observing the loss of radiolabel or a change in electrophoretic migration (see King and Perham 1971) after treating the maleylated protein with 0.5 M hydroxylamine hydrochloride at *p*H 8.3–8.4 for 18 hr at room temperature. Under these conditions N-maleyl groups are stable, but O-maleyl groups are removed. If Asn-Gly bonds are present in the protein, these may also be cleaved by hydroxylamine (see Bornstein and Bollan 1970).

The maleylated protein can be demaleylated at acid *p*H. Near maximal rates are obtained at *p*H 3.0–3.5 but in some studies a higher *p*H and a longer time may be preferable. Any O-maleyl groups must be removed with hydroxylamine (see above). A convenient procedure for carrying out the demaleylation step is to dialyze the protein against a buffer at *p*H 3.0–3.5 (e.g. 0.01 to 0.1 M pyridine, adjusted to *p*H with acetic acid) at 37–40°C for an appropriate time. (The half-time for demaleylation at 37°C and *p*H 3.5 is 11–12 hr.) After the appropriate degree of demaleylation is reached, the protein can be dialyzed under those conditions found to be most favorable for renaturation of the protein. An alternative method for demaleylation (must be used if the protein has been hydrolyzed with trypsin or other proteases) is to lower the *p*H of the reaction mixture to 3.0–3.5 by adding acetic acid (buffer may also be added) and stirring it at 37–40°C for the appropriate time. A few drops of toluene or other agent to inhibit growth of microorganisms may be added. Proteins or peptides may become insoluble during demaleylation, but this has not been found to affect the rate or extent of demaleylation.

Comments: The reversibility of the modification of amino groups in proteins by maleic anhydride makes this an excellent tool for various types of studies including (a) modification of lysyl residues in proteins to limit tryptic cleavage to the COOH side of arginyl residues, (b) studies on the effect of making proteins less positively charged or more negatively charged, (c) dissociation of aggregated systems such as proteins with subunits, (d) study of the reassembly of aggregated systems, (e) solubilization of proteins or peptides with limited solubility, (f) protection of amino groups from modification with other reagents. Succinylation may be preferable if removal of the maleyl groups is not necessary.

The unprotonated amino group is evidently the reactive species in the maleylation reaction. Therefore, it should be possible to obtain some degree of specificity for α-amino groups by utilizing a lower *p*H for the reaction (e.g. *p*H 7.0 to 7.5). The pK_a of α-amino groups is usually lower than the pK_a of ε-amino groups. The *p*H used in the maleylation procedure (*p*H 8.5–9.0) usually gives the maximum rate of modification of ε-amino groups. At higher *p*H the effective rate of maleylation is decreased by the competing reaction in which maleic anhydride is hydrolyzed to maleic acid. The reaction can also be

Subject index p. 201

carried out at higher temperatures, and the reagent can be added as a solution in dioxane (see Butler and Hartley 1972).

Other functional groups are also modified by maleic anhydride, but the products formed with the imidazole nitrogens of histidyl residues and the phenolic groups of tyrosyl residues are unstable and rapidly break down to regenerate these residues. Only the products formed with amino groups, cysteinyl residues (if present) and the hydroxyl groups of seryl and threonyl residues are stable. Although the reaction is obviously non-specific, it can be made operationally specific by converting cysteinyl residues to reversibly-modified derivatives (e.g. disulfide or the S-sulfo derivative, see § 3.8.7, § 3.8.8, § 3.8.10) prior to the reaction, and removing O-maleyl groups after the reaction with hydroxylamine (see above). S-succinylcysteine is the product obtained by *alkylating* cysteinyl residues with maleic anhydride (§ 3.8.9.2). This derivative is stable to acid hydrolysis and can be determined with an analyzer (§ 2.5.7).

In some studies it may be preferable to use a reagent other than maleic anhydride for the reversible modification of amino groups. Table 3.1 lists several of these and compares some of their properties with those of maleic anhydride. All of the derivatives listed in Table 3.1 are less stable at acid *p*H, than those from maleic anhydride and some are significantly unstable at *p*H values below 8.5. In some studies the greater instability of these derivatives may be an advantage, but in any studies where purification of the modified protein (or peptides) is required, the use of maleic anhydride is advised. It should be noted that 2 of the reagents give isomeric products which can sometimes be troublesome. The hexahydrophthalic anhydride reagent may prove useful in modifying proteins with free cysteinyl residues, since this reagent was reported not to alkylate cysteinyl residues.

The removal of added substituents from amino groups, formed with these reagents, depends on the presence of a protonated carboxyl group specifically oriented to participate as an intramolecular catalyst of the hydrolytic reaction. In 3 of the reagents the specific orientation is a result of the *cis*-configuration of the groups about the carbon–carbon double bond, and in the other 2 reagents the specific orientation is

TABLE 3.1

Reversible modification of amino groups in proteins by acid anhydrides*.

Maleic anhydride	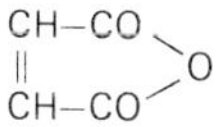	Half-life of ε-N-maleyllysine is 11 hr at *p*H 3.5 and 37°C
2-Methylmaleic (citraconic) anhydride**	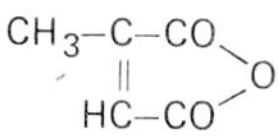	Two isomeric ε-N-acyl derivatives of lysine are produced, differing in pK_a. These have a half-life of approximately 20 min at *p*H 2 and 20°C
2,3-Dimethylmaleic anhydride**	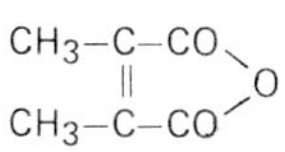	The ε-N-acyl derivative of lysine has a half-life of less than 3 min at *p*H 3.5 and 20°C
Exo cis 3,6-endoxo-Δ^4-tetrahydrophthalic anhydride†	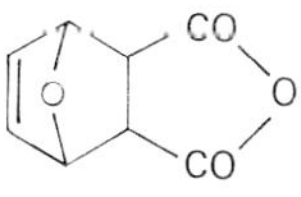	Two isomeric ε-N-acyl derivatives are formed at the same rate. These have a half-life of 4–5 hr at *p*H 3 and 25°C
Exo-cis-3,6-endoxo-Δ^4-hexahydrophthalic anhydride†	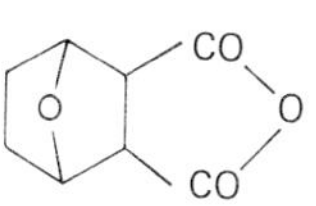	Half-lives of derivatives are the same as for those obtained with the tetrahydrophthalic anhydride. This reagent does not alkylate sulfhydryl groups
Tetrafluorosuccinic anhydride††	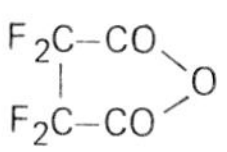	ε-N-acyl derivative is rapidly hydrolyzed at *p*H 9.5 and 0°C

* Both α- and ε-NH_2 groups are modified. Acyl derivatives of tyrosine formed by these reagents hydrolyze spontaneously under mild alkaline conditions. Small amounts of stable acyl derivatives of serine and threonine are formed. These can be quantitatively decomposed by treatment with 1 M NH_2OH at *p*H 8.2 at 25°C for 2 hr. The olefinic reagents alkylate sulfhydryl groups with the formation of stable derivatives.

** Dixon, H. B. F. and R. N. Perham (1968) *Biochem. J. 109*, 312.

† Riley, M. and R. N. Perham (1970) Biochem. J. *118*, 733.

†† Braunitzer, G., K. Beyreuther, H. Fujiki and B. Schrank (1968) *Z. Physiol. Chem. 349*, 265.

produced by the arrangement of the carboxyl groups adjacent to each other on the hydrophthalic ring.

3.2. Modifications of arginine

Several procedures are available for the modification of arginine residues. A partial list of reagents for derivatization of arginine would include butanedione (Yankeelov et al. 1968), phenylglyoxal (Takahashi 1968), malondialdehyde (King 1966) and nitromalondialdehyde (Signor et al. 1971). None of the procedures are ideal since the first two reagents yield products which at present are incompletely characterized while the conditions of derivatization with malondialdehyde and nitromalondialdehyde require strongly alkaline conditions.

Two important motivations exist for the modification of arginine residues. The first would be to restrict the sites of proteolytic digestion by trypsin to lysine residues. The second would be to determine the potential functional importance of an arginine residue in the mode of action of a given protein. The best reagents for the latter purpose are 2,3-butanedione and phenylglyoxal.

3.2.1. Butanedione reaction with arginine

Yankeelov et al. (1968) have reported that the trimer of 2,3-butanedione (I) as well as the dimer (II) are the reactive forms of this reagent. Reaction conditions for the exhaustive modification

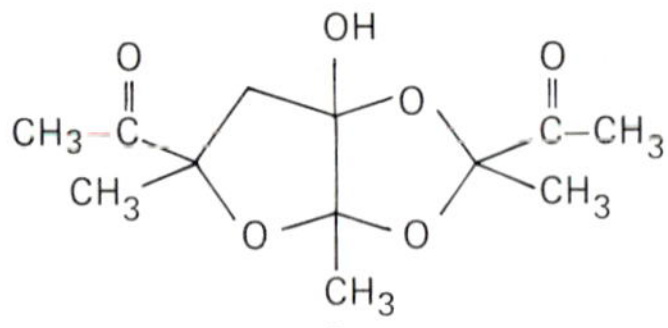

I

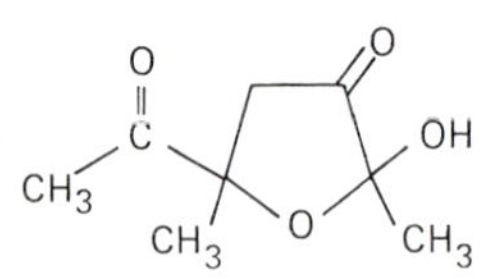

II

of protein arginine with trimeric 2,3-butanedione involve incubation of the 0.4 M reagent I and protein at 25°C in 0.5 M phosphate buffer

(pH 7.0) for 48 hr. The synthesis and structure of the derivative formed have not been reported but whatever its nature, it does not regenerate arginine upon acid hydrolysis.

Since the reagent readily reacts with amino groups at the relatively high concentrations required for complete derivatization of the protein, protection of the ε-amino group is essential if specific cleavage by trypsin at lysine residues is desired. A possible method of protection prior to derivatization with compound I would involve citraconylation of the lysine residues prior to reaction.

Riordan (1973) has reported that the monomer of 2,3-butanedione inactivates carboxypeptidase as effectively as the trimer. One interesting feature of his study is that a 0.05 M borate buffer enhances the rate and possibly affects the distribution of products formed from both monomeric and trimeric butanedione when compared with a 0.05 M veronal buffer at the sample pH. He has attributed this specific buffer effect to the formation of a cyclic borate ester following the initial condensation of the guanidinium group with 2,3-butanedione as indicated in eq. (3.1). The conditions of modification with butanedione used by Riordan (1973) involved incubation of the protein at pH 7.5 at 20°C for 15–60 min at concentrations of butanedione ranging from 2.2×10^{-2} M to 7.5×10^{-2} M.

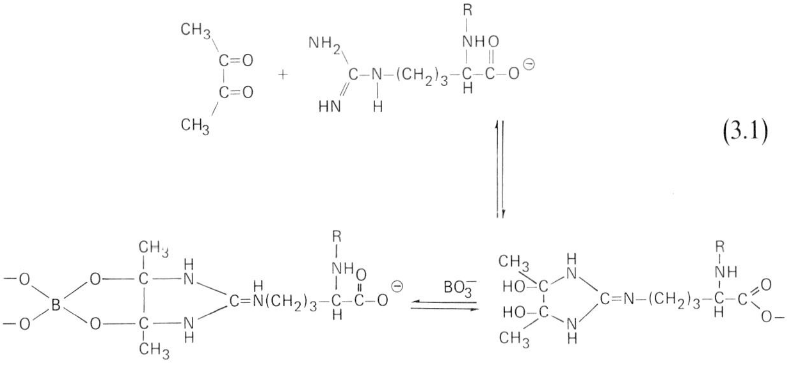

(3.1)

3.2.2. Phenylglyoxal reaction with arginine

Phenylglyoxal was first introduced as a protein modification reagent by Takahashi (1968). The product obtained with either arginine or N-acetyl arginine contains two moles of phenyl glyoxal per mole of amino acid. The precise structure of the derivative formed has not been determined but two suggested structures with N-acetyl arginine are indicated below. Whatever the structure of the product, arginine is not regenerated by acid hydrolysis. Further, the product is unstable even at slightly alkaline *p*H's. For example, 66% of the phenylglyoxal derivative of arginine is regenerated after 48 hr upon incubation at 25°C in 0.1 M N-ethylmorpholine acetate buffer, *p*H 8.0.

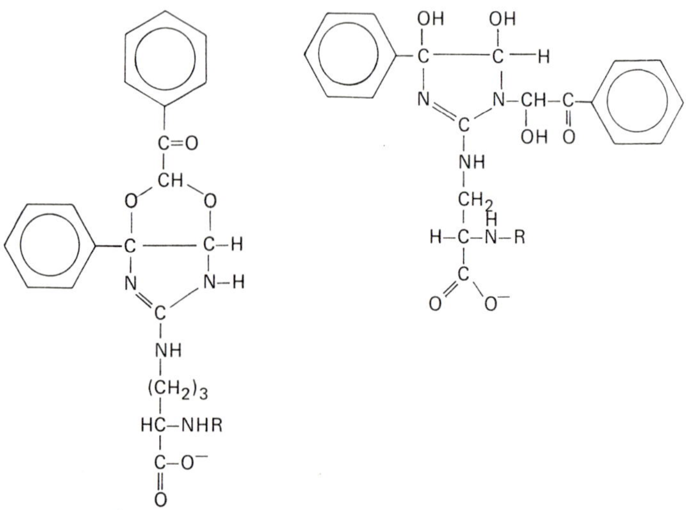

As a general procedure for the modification of proteins by phenylglyoxal, Takahashi (1968) suggested reacting a 0.3 to 3% solution of phenylglyoxal with the protein in 0.2 M N-ethylmorpholine acetate buffer *p*H 8.0 at 25°C. Under these conditions, N-α-dinitrophenyl arginine completely reacts in 20 hr. An important side reaction which limits the usefulness of phenylglyoxal as a modification reagent is its ability to deaminate free amino acids and the N-terminal amino group of peptides. Further, the lability of the phenylglyoxal derivative of arginine in alkaline solution requires mildly acidic conditions to be employed if the isolation of peptide containing the modified arginine residue is desired.

3.2.3. Nitromalondialdehyde reaction with arginine

The products formed by nitromalondialdehyde have been characterized (Signor et al. 1971). Thus N-acetylarginine reacts with nitromalondialdehyde to yield a nitropyrimidine derivative as indicated below in eq. (3.2.).

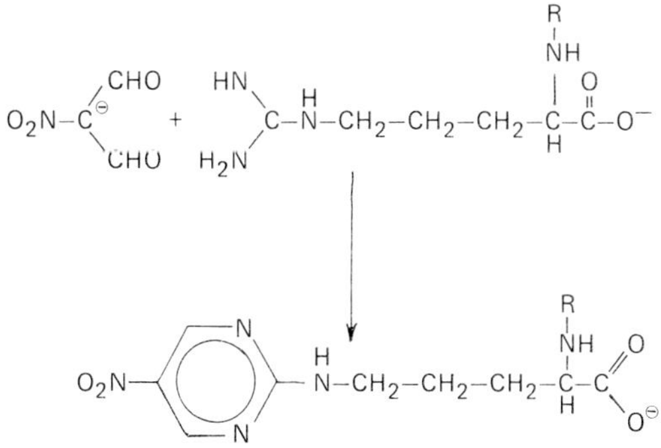

(3.2)

Since the optimum *p*H range for the reaction is between *p*H 12 and 14, the usefulness of nitromalondialdehyde is restricted to denatured proteins.

To modify the S-carboxymethylated B chain of insulin, Signor et al. (1971) added about 3.0 mmoles of the peptide dissolved in 1.0 ml of 1 M NaOH to 1 ml of water containing 10 mg of nitromalondialdehyde (70 mmoles). After 2 hr at 0–5°C excess modification reagent was removed by gel filtration using 50% formic acid as eluent.

Arginine residues modified by nitromalondialdehyde are resistant to tryptic digestion. However, reduction of the derivative by sodium borohydride yields tetrahydropyrimidyl compounds which are susceptible to hydrolysis by trypsin. Modification by nitromalondialdehyde thereby permits the restriction of tryptic digestion to lysine residues but yet would allow the further tryptic cleavage of the resulting peptides after reduction with sodium borohydride.

3.3. Modifications of carboxyl groups

The two reactions most commonly employed for the modification of protein carboxyl groups have been acid-catalyzed esterification (Wilcox 1967), and coupling with nucleophiles mediated by a water-soluble carbodiimide. The latter reaction has been exploited widely in the determination of the carboxyl group content of proteins as well as in studies of carboxyl group function, and would at present appear to be the reaction of choice for these purposes.

The following method has been described by Carraway and Koshland (1972) for the determination of carboxyl group content of proteins. The protein (10 mg/ml) and glycinamide HCl (1 M) are dissolved in guanidine hydrochloride (6 M). The *p*H is adjusted to 4.75 with 1 M HCl using a *p*H stat, and sufficient solid ethyldimethyl-aminopropylcarbodiimide is added as a solid to bring its concentration to 0.1 M. The *p*H is maintained by the automatic addition of M HCl. The reaction is terminated after 1 hr by the addition of an excess of 1 M sodium acetate buffer at *p*H 4.75 which reacts with excess carbodiimide. The residual reagents are removed by exhaustive dialysis. All traces of free glycinamide must be removed. The modified protein is then subjected to amino acid analysis. The difference in glycine content of the protein before and after modification represents the carboxyl group content. This procedure offers considerable flexibility in the choice of nucleophile. For instance, norleucine, or taurine, or ^{14}C-labelled glycinamide or glycine methyl ester may be employed in the place of glycinamide.

It should be noted that the carbodiimide reacts with both sulfhydryl and tyrosyl OH groups as well as with carboxyl groups. Tyrosine can be regenerated by treatment of the derivative with 0.5 M hydroxylamine at *p*H 7 and 25°C for 5 hr. Successful regeneration of thiol groups has not been reported.

The reduction of carboxyl groups and their reaction with diazonium salts, isoxazolium salts, triethyloxonium fluoroborate, have all been exploited to a limited extent. These reactions are discussed in the reviews listed in ch. 1.

3.4. *Modifications of histidine*

Reagents capable of modifying the histidyl residue with complete specificity are not available to date. Reaction with α-haloacids and amides at near neutral *p*H offers the best approach to the modification of histidine in native proteins. In a protein such as insulin, which contains neither methionyl nor cysteinyl residues, reaction with iodoacetate at *p*H 5.6 leads to the formation of a derivative in which the sole modification is the N-carboxymethylation of two histidyl residues (Covelli et al. 1973).

Alkylation of histidyl residues leads to derivatives substituted on either the N-1 or N-3 imidazole nitrogen, as well as to the disubstituted derivative (Crestfield et al. 1963; Heinrikson et al. 1965).

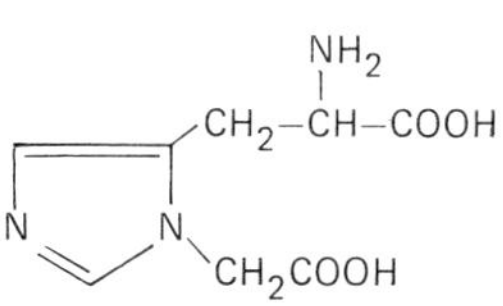

1–carboxymethylhistidine

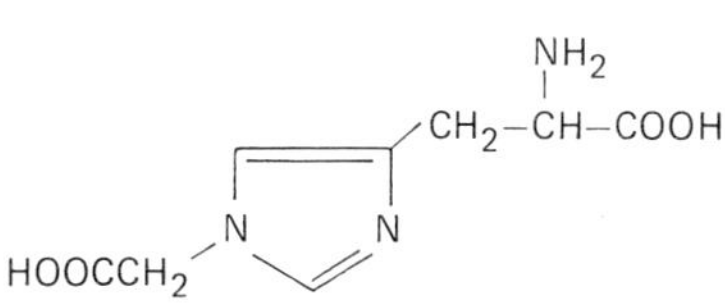

3–carboxymethylhistidine

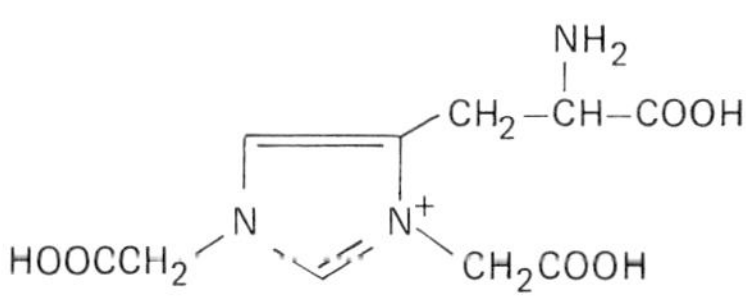

1, 3–dicarboxymethylhistidine

When an unusually reactive histidyl residue, for example at the active site of an enzyme, is alkylated, the reaction tends to be strictly stereospecific, as observed in ribonuclease (Crestfield et al. 1963) or carbonic anhydrase (Bradbury 1969), and only one of the above derivatives is generally formed. However, alkylation of histidyl residues in denatured proteins gives rise to all three products, as does alkylation of native proteins with large excess of reagent (Harris and Hill 1969). In such cases, any histidyl residue may give rise to unequal amounts of derivatives substituted on either of the imidazole nitrogens.

The alkylation of methionine is *p*H-independent, while that of histidyl, cysteinyl and lysyl residues is *p*H-dependent, the rate reflecting the concentration of the unprotonated protein nucleophile.

Dye-sensitized photooxidation (Ray 1967; Westhead 1972) has been employed successfully in a number of cases (e.g. Forman et al. 1973) to obtain selective destruction of histidyl residues.

Other reagents which have been used for the modification of histidyl residues in proteins include 1-fluoro-2,4-dinitrobenzene, diazonium-1H-tetrazole (see Andres and Atassi 1973), iodine (Covelli and Wolff 1966; Wolff and Covelli 1969), N-bromosuccinimide, ethoxyformic anhydride (Melchior and Fahrney 1970), and bromoacetone (Beeley and Neurath 1968). These reagents appear to offer little advantage over alkylation with α-haloacids, or dye-sensitized photo-oxidation. Indeed, some are far less specific.

3.5. Modifications of methionine

Reagents reactive solely toward the methionyl side-chain in *native* proteins have not been described to date. Selective conversion of the thioether to the sulfoxide derivative by photosensitized oxidation has been reported in a protein devoid of free thiol groups. The selective photosensitized oxidation employed methylene blue or hematoporphyrin as sensitizers, and aqueous acetic acid (30–90% v/v), or acidic buffers at *p*H 2–6.5, as solvents (Scoffone et al. 1970). *Anaerobic* photo-oxidation in 4 M aqueous acetone has been reported to lead to the same result (Gennari and Jori 1970). Methionine can be regenerated from the sulfoxide by incubation with thiols (5% aqueous β-mercaptoethanol at *p*H 8.0, for 24 hr under N_2; Jori et al. 1968).

The reaction of iodoacetic acid and iodoacetamide with proteins at

$pH < 4$ is limited to cysteinyl and methionyl residues. Methionine is converted to methionyl sulfonium salts which give a number of products upon acid hydrolysis, thus complicating the quantitation of the extent of derivative formation (§5.3.2.2). The most direct way of estimating methionine sulfonium salt is by performic acid oxidation (§3.2.5.1 and §3.8.1). Methionyl residues are converted to the sulfone, while methionyl sulfonium salts give rise to several decomposition products which do not include methionine sulfone (Goren et al. 1968; Naider and Bohak 1972; §5.3.2.2).

Naider and Bohak (1972) have found that incubation of sulfonium salts with thiols leads to the regeneration of methionine. Complete recovery of methionine was obtained upon incubation of the S-carboxyamidomethylmethionyl sulfonium salt with 0.12 M mercapto-ethanol at pH 8.9 for 24 hr at 30°C. In contrast, the S-carboxymethyl-methionyl sulfonium salt is regenerated to only a minor extent under these conditions.

Parenthetically, it may be noted that the S-carboxyamidomethyl-methionyl residue may be used as a site of cleavage of the polypeptide chain (in a reaction analogous to that obtained with CNBr) by boiling in water for 2 hr (Tang and Hartley 1967, 1970).

3.6. *Modifications of tryptophan*

The reagents employed for the selective modification of tryptophan all react with cysteinyl residues. Hence, either modification or protection of these residues is necessary, and *is assumed in the subsequent discussion.*

Recently, 2-(2-nitrophenylsulfenyl)-3-methyl-3-bromoindolenine (BNPS-skatole) has replaced N-bromosuccinimide, which had been used frequently in earlier studies. At low reagent to protein tryptophan ratios, in 50% aqueous acetic acid, BNPS-skatole reacts selectively with tryptophan residues converting these to the oxindole derivative. Methionine is concommitantly converted to the sulfoxide. At high concentrations of reagent, slow selective cleavage (to the extent of 15–60%) of the peptide bonds involving tryptophanyl residues is obtained. The experimental details concerning the preparation and use of this reagent are discussed by Fontana (1972). Various nitrobenzylhalides have been widely used for the modification of tryptophan as well as for the determination of the content of this amino acid in proteins (Horton and Koshland, 1972). The reaction of these compounds with tryptophan and its derivatives gives rise to complex mixtures of products (Horton and Koshland 1972; Heinrich et al. 1973). Other procedures which have been applied to the modification of tryptophan include ozonolysis in anhydrous formic acid containing resorcinol (Previero et al. 1967a) giving rise to the N-formylkynurenine derivative, and proflavine-sensitized photooxidation in 98–100% acid (Scoffone et al. 1970).

Two apparently highly selective procedures have been developed in recent years: formylation and sulfenylation.

3.6.1. *Formylation of tryptophan*

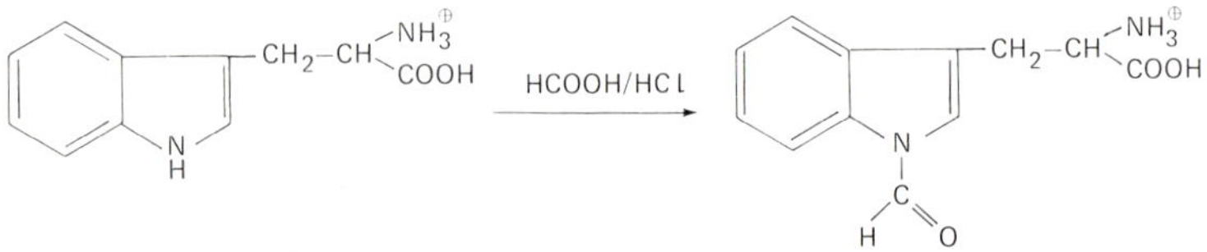

The procedure outlined below, based upon the description of Previero et al. (1967b) has been used successfully, with minor variations for the selective modification of tryptophan residues in lysozyme (Previero et al. 1967b), trypsin (Coletti-Previero et al. 1969), cytochrome *c* (Aviram and Schejter 1971), and thioredoxin (Holmgren 1972).

Protein (10–20 mg) is dissolved in 1 ml of formic acid (98–100%) and 1 ml of formic acid saturated with HCl is added. The mixture is incubated in a glass-stoppered tube at room temperature. At 20 min intervals, 50 μl aliquots of the solution are pipetted into 2.5 ml of 8 M urea-0.05 M sodium acetate, *p*H 4.0, and the absorbance at 298 nm determined. (ε_M for 1-formyltryptophan in 8 M urea at *p*H 4 is 4880.) Hence, the degree of modification can be calculated from the total change in absorbance at 298 nm and the known concentration of protein). When no further change in absorbance at 298 nm is observed, the reaction mixture is diluted 5-fold with ice-cold water, and dialyzed against water at 4°C. The modified protein is then recovered by lyophilization.

1-Formyltryptophan is stable up to *p*H 7 at room temperature. The decomposition of the derivative back to tryptophan at alkaline *p*H forms the basis of the deformylation procedure. The protein derivative (approx. 5 mg/ml) is dissolved in 0.05 M NH_4OH-NH_4Cl, *p*H 9.5, containing 6 M guanidine hydrochloride. After incubation at room temperature for 16 hr, the protein is dialyzed and lyophilized.

3.6.2. Sulfenylation of tryptophan

The reaction of arylsulfenyl halides with proteins at *p*H $\leqslant$ 3.5 is limited to the cysteinyl and tryptophanyl residues (Fontana and Scoffone 1972), as illustrated below for 2-nitrophenylsulfenyl chloride (NPS-Cl).

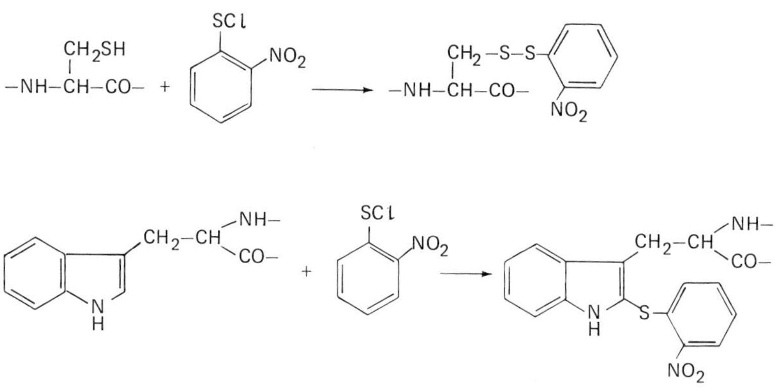

In proteins devoid of –SH groups, or those in which these groups have been alkylated or otherwise modified (§ 3.8), the reaction is restricted to tryptophanyl side-chains.

The protein (10 mg/ml) is dissolved in either water or 5% acetic acid. NBS-Cl (4 moles per mole of tryptophan) dissolved in glacial acetic acid is added, with vigorous stirring, to give a final acetic acid concentration of 25%. After 6 hr in the dark at room temperature the reaction is terminated by passage of the mixture through a column of suitable size of Sephadex G-25 equilibrated with 30% acetic acid. The protein-containing fractions are pooled. Measurement of the absorbance at 365 nm permits the calculation of the concentration of the NPS-tryptophan derivative present ($\varepsilon_{365} = 4000$ L. mole^{-1} cm^{-1}; Scoffone et al. 1968), while the protein concentration is determined on an appropriate aliquot by amino acid analysis. The extent of sulfenylation is then calculated from the relative concentrations of the protein and the NPS-derivative in the fraction.

Site-specific sulfenylation of tryptophan residues in egg-white lysozyme has been attained by either limiting the amount of reagent, or modifying the reaction conditions. Thus, Trp-108 is the major site of modification upon addition of one equivalent of 2-thio-(2-nitro-4-carboxyphenyl)sulfenyl chloride to lysozyme in 25% acetic acid (Veronese et al. 1972). Specific modification of Trp-62 was attained in approximately 8 hr by the addition of 5 consecutive portions of solid NPS-Cl (10 μmole for each ml of reaction mixture) to a solution of lysozyme (0.5 μmole/ml) in 0.1 M sodium acetate at *p*H 3.5 (Shechter et al. 1972). In both cases, the protein derivative was separated from other products, and unreacted enzyme by ion-exchange chromatography.

It may be noted, parenthetically, that a novel reaction of NPS-Cl with the thioether bonds linking the heme to cytochrome *c* leads to quantitative release of the heme (Fontana et al. 1973).

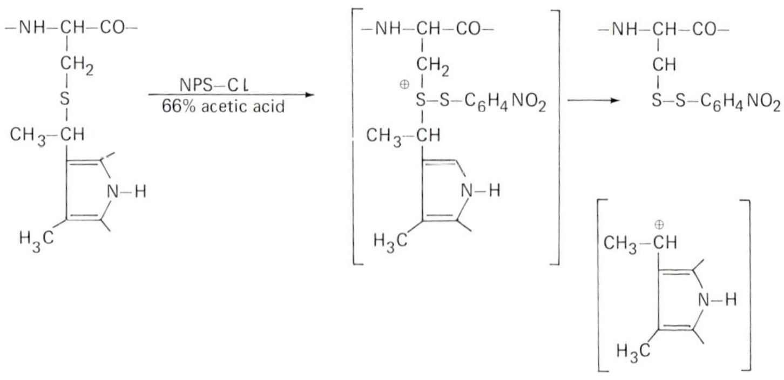

3.7. *Modifications of tyrosine*

Modification of tyrosyl groups in proteins has been performed with acetylimidazole (Riordan and Vallee 1972a), N-bromosuccinimide (Spande et al. 1970), cyanuric fluoride (Gorbunoff 1972), diazonium compounds, such as diazonium-1H-tetrazole (Riordan and Vallee 1972b), tetranitromethane (Riordan and Vallee 1972c), and iodine (or other iodinating reagents). In each case, the specificity of these reagents towards tyrosyl side-chains is far from complete. In native proteins, selective modification may be achieved with any one of these reagents as a consequence of the microenvironment of a given residue. Clearly, this is not predictable in advance.

The two most widely utilized procedures for tyrosine modification, nitration and iodination, are discussed below.

3.7.1. *Nitration of tyrosine*

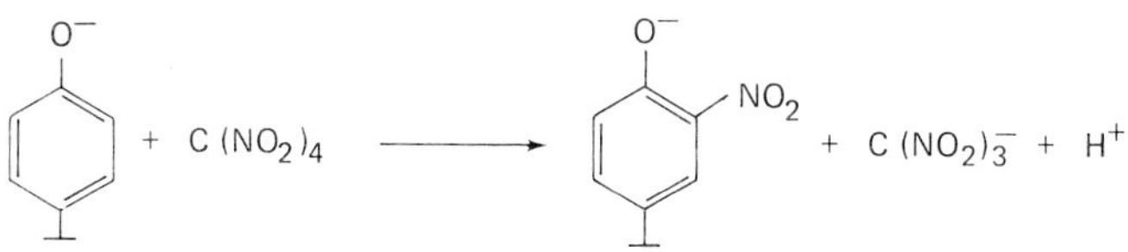

Nitration of tyrosyl residues with tetranitromethane (TNM) is now one of the most frequently attempted modification reactions for native proteins (see Riordan and Sokolovsky 1971 for a review and references). The mechanism of this reaction has been examined by Bruice et al. (1968), who propose the following scheme:

$$XC_6H_4O^- + TNM \rightleftharpoons \text{charge-transfer complex} \xrightleftharpoons[\text{rate-determining step}]{} [XC_6H_4O\cdot + NO_2\cdot] + \underset{\text{nitro-formate anion}}{C(NO_2)_3^-}$$

$$[XC_6H_4O\cdot + NO_2\cdot] \rightarrow O_2NXC_6H_4O^- \qquad [XC_6H_4O\cdot + NO_2\cdot] \rightarrow XC_6H_4O\cdot + NO_2\cdot$$

$$NO_2\cdot + XC_6H_4O^- \rightleftharpoons XC_6H_4O\cdot + NO_2^-$$

$$nXC_6H_4O\cdot \rightarrow \text{coupling products}$$

Awareness of this reaction sequence is of importance to the interpretation of the results of the reaction of TNM with proteins.

The potential advantages of selective nitration of tyrosyl residues in native proteins are numerous. The reaction is performed under mild conditions, giving rise to a 3-nitrotyrosyl derivative ($pK' \sim 7$), which in the acid form absorbs intensely at 350 nm. Hence, the nitrotyrosine content may be readily determined spectrophotometrically, as well as by amino acid analysis (§ 2.2.3). The absorption spectrum of 3-nitrotyrosine is highly sensitive to solvent polarity and exhibits significant optical activity in the long wavelength absorption band. Consequently, nitrotyrosyl residues can be utilized as indicators of conformational change, or of interactions of proteins with other macromolecules or small molecules (e.g. Kirschner and Schachman 1973). Any perturbation in the pK_a of nitrotyrosyl residues is readily determined spectrophotometrically.

3-Nitrotyrosine is readily reduced to 3-aminotyrosine by low concentrations of sodium hydrosulfite ($Na_2S_2O_4$). The pK_a of the phenolic group in the latter derivative ($pK' = 10.1$) is similar to that of tyrosine $-OH$, while the pK_a of the 3-amino group is 4.7. Reduction permits, therefore, a distinction to be made between the effects of the initial nitration reaction, due to the perturbation of the pK_a of the phenolic $-OH$, and those due to steric hindrance or conformational change resulting from the presence of a substituent on the phenolic ring. The 3-aminotyrosyl residue offers opportunities for selective reaction based upon the low pK_a of the aromatic amino group (e.g. Cuatrecasas et al. 1969; Kenner and Neurath 1971), and metal ion chelation.

The awareness of the many advantages of this modification reaction should be matched by the knowledge of the numerous side-reactions observed to result from the reaction of TNM with proteins. In addition to nitration of tyrosine, the following side-reactions have been reported in several (but not all) proteins studied: (1) inter- and intramolecular cross-linking, (2) oxidation of sulfhydryl groups to a variety of products, (3) oxidation of methionine, (4) modification of tryptophan and histidine, (5) modification of prosthetic groups. It is apparent therefore that a successful application of TNM to the selective modification of tyrosine is achieved in those cases where an unusually rapid reaction occurs with specific residues, owing to some factor such as complex formation with the reagent, or, where much effort and care is given to the purification and characterization of a homogeneous component from a complex mixture of products (e.g. Cheng and Pierce 1972).

As expected from the reaction scheme shown above, the rate of nitration is strongly *p*H dependent. Some representative results obtained with carbonic anhydrase are shown in Fig. 3.1. It should be

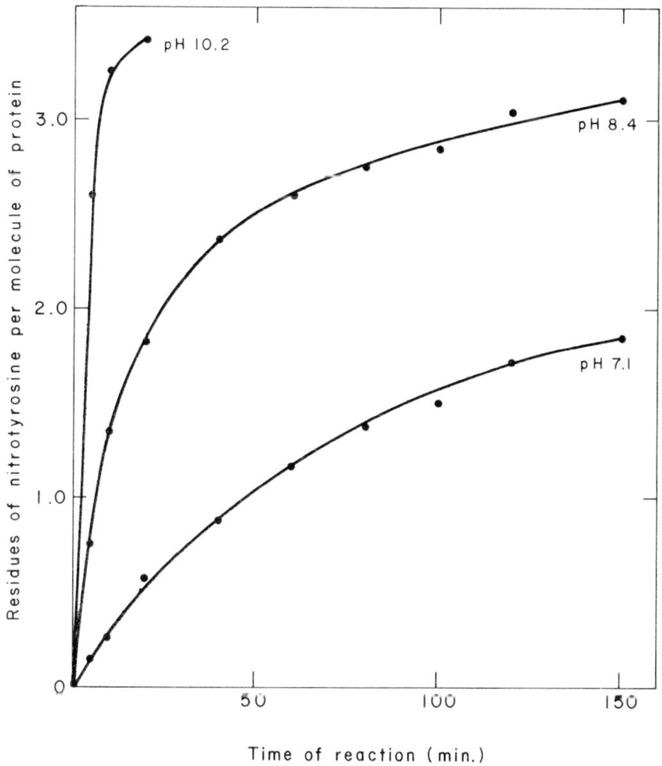

Fig. 3.1. Reaction of human carbonic anhydrase B with tetranitromethane. The reaction mixture contained 5 ml of 0.3% protein and 25 μl of tetranitromethane, buffered at *p*H 7.1 with 0.1 M sodium phosphate, or at *p*H 8.4 and 10.2 with 0.1 M Tris-H_2SO_4. (Data from Dorner 1971).

noted that conformational change in response to alteration in *p*H is commonplace in native proteins and that the *rate and extent* of a chemical modification reaction may well be strongly influenced by this factor.

A procedure applicable to the nitration of a native protein is outlined below.

The protein (2–4 mg/ml) is dissolved in 0.1 M potassium phosphate buffer, *p*H 7.5, containing 10^{-3} M EDTA. A 0.15 M solution of TNM is prepared in 95% ethanol, and 20 μl is added per ml of protein solution (final TNM concentration 0.003 M). After 60 min at room temperature the reaction is terminated by the addition of 50 μl of 1 M mercaptoethanol, followed immediately by exhaustive dialysis against 1% NH_4HCO_3 at 4°C. The dialysis removes excess TNM and the colored nitroformate anion, which is a product both of the nitration reaction and of decomposition of the reagent. The dialyzed protein derivative is lyophilized.

The visible absorption spectrum of a solution containing a known concentration of nitrated protein is measured in a solution buffered at *p*H 9.0, and the absorbance at the maximum (near 428 nm) used to calculate the nitrotyrosine content (ε_{428nm} for the nitrophenoxide ion is 4200). The tyrosine and nitrotyrosine content of the modified protein should also be determined by amino acid analysis. If the sum of these values does not add up to the tyrosine content of the unmodified protein, intra- or intermolecular cross-linking may have occurred. The amino acid analysis may also reveal whether other side-reactions have taken place. Particular attention should be paid to the half-cystine, cysteine, methionine, histidine and tryptophan contents of the modified proteins. Polyacrylamide gel electrophoresis in the presence of sodium dodecyl sulfate offers a rapid and highly sensitive way of detecting products of intermolecular cross-linking. Such products are readily removed by gel filtration.

It should be recognized that variations in *p*H, TNM concentration, or reaction time, from those given above, may be required to produce the desired degree of substitution in a particular case.

Some recent interesting applications of nitration may be found in the work of Piszkiewicz et al. (1971), Dorner (1971), Hugli and Stein (1971), and Cheng and Pierce (1972).

3.7.2. Iodination of tyrosine

The iodination of proteins has long been a very popular modification reaction. This reaction, performed under mild conditions, has been applied to such varied ends as the detection of side-chains at the catalytic sites of proteins, investigation of the relative reactivity of tyrosyl side-chains, and the introduction of heavy atoms in connection with X-ray diffraction studies. The availability of two radioactive iodine isotopes, ^{125}I with a half-life of 56 days, and ^{131}I with a half-life of 8 days, has been very extensively exploited in the preparation of hormone derivatives of high specific activity for radioimmunoassay and receptor studies.

The reaction of proteins with HOI, generated either from triiodide, iodine monochloride, iodine plus chloramine T, etc., may involve a number of side-chains. In native proteins, halogenation of tyrosine takes preferentially, with the formation of the 3-iodo- and 3,5-diiodotyrosyl derivatives – histidine is halogenated less readily to give the 1-iodo- and 3-iodohistidyl derivatives as well as diiodohistidine. In certain cases (see Glazer 1970), reaction with thiol groups leads to the formation of 'stable' sulfenyl iodides (RSI). In addition to these substitution reactions, oxidative reactions involving methionyl, cysteinyl, and tryptophanyl side-chains may also take place. The substitution reactions predominate at alkaline *p*H, the oxidative ones at acid *p*H.

For procedures for non-enzymatic iodination of proteins, most frequently carried out with iodine monochloride, reference should be made to the lucid treatment by Roholt and Pressman (1972).

Recently, application of lactoperoxidase-catalyzed iodination has taken precedence over non-enzymatic procedures. The enzyme-catalyzed reaction is reported to occur through the formation of an enzyme-substrate complex between the protein substrate and lactoperoxidase. No detectable free I_2 is formed by lactoperoxidase, and selectivity in attaining iodination of surface tyrosine residues in proteins without oxidative side-reactions is believed to be high.

The method described by Morrison and Bayse (1970) for the enzymic iodination of tyrosine can be readily adapted to the modification of proteins. The reaction mixture contains, in order of addition, L-tyrosine (8.1×10^{-4} M), KI (1.0×10^{-4} M), lactoperoxidase (7.4×10^{-9} M), in 0.05 M K-phosphate buffer, containing 1×10^{-3} M EDTA, at *p*H 7.4. The iodination is initiated by the addition of H_2O_2 to a concentration of 1.0×10^{-4} M. The specific activity observed for lactoperoxidase under these conditions was 1.05×10^4 moles of L-3-iodotyrosine per min per mole of enzyme at 25°C. At *p*H 7.4, the rate of enzymatic conversion of L-3-iodotyrosine to L-3,5-diiodotyrosine was 0.34 that of monosubstitution (Morrison and Bayse 1970). The desired level of iodination can be attained by successive equimolar additions of KI and H_2O_2 to the reaction mixture. In this manner, only a low concentration of H_2O_2 is maintained, minimizing oxidation reactions. The concentration of lactoperoxidase may be calculated from the millimolar extinction coefficient of 114 at 412 nm, while the concentrations of stock H_2O_2 solutions may be determined from the absorbance at 230 nm and a molar extinction coefficient of 72.4 (Phillips and Morrison 1970).

When radioactive iodine is to be used, it should be purchased as $Na^{125}I$, free of carrier, or reducing agents. Picogram quantities of radio-iodine labelled proteins can be detected readily.

Hormones, iodinated by the lactoperoxidase procedure to high specific activity, show retention of biological activity superior to that observed for preparations labelled by non-enzymatic methods (e.g. Frantz and Turkington 1972).

A micro-scale iodination procedure has been described by Thorell and Johansson (1971). The reaction is performed in an 11×55 mm polystyrene tube at 22°C, and the reactants mixed continuously with a magnetic stirrer. The reagents and polypeptides are dissolved in 0.05 M sodium phosphate buffer, *p*H 7.5. $Na^{125}I$ (carrier-free, without reducing agent) is diluted with the buffer to an activity of ~ 0.1 mCi/μl. The reactants are added in rapid succession in the following order and amounts: 0.5–1.8 mC $Na^{125}I$ (8–15 μl), 5 μg (25 μl) of the polypeptide or protein to be labelled, 4 μg (1.5 μl) lactoperoxidase, 1 μl 0.88 mM H_2O_2. The reactants are mixed for 30 sec, after which the contents of the tube are diluted with 500 μl of 0.05 M sodium phosphate buffer, *p*H 7.5, and immediately transferred to a column of Sephadex G-50 Fine (1 × 15 cm), equilibrated with 0.075 M sodium barbital buffer, *p*H 7.5. (The column is presaturated by the passage of 1 ml of a 1% solution of bovine serum albumin). The first peak of radioactivity is collected and after addition of 0.5 ml of 1% bovine serum albumin per ml it is stored at −20°C.

For the determination of specific activity, an aliquot of the reaction mixture is transferred to a small dialysis tubing and dialyzed for 1 hr at 4°C against two changes of 1000 ml 0.05 M phosphate buffer, *p*H 7.5, containing ~5 g of Amberlite Resin IRA 401. The radioactivity of the reaction mixture is measured before and after dialysis. For a number of proteins, over 80% of the iodine added appears to be covalently bound to the protein.

A water-insoluble lactoperoxidase, linked to CNBr-activated Sepharose beads, capable of iodinating serum albumin, is commercially available (Worthington Biochemical Corp.), and may be useful where avoidance of contamination of the product by the enzyme is important.

The quantitative determination of iodotyrosine and iodohistidine content of proteins can be performed as described in § 2.2.4 and § 2.8.2 after complete enzymic digestion. These derivatives are not stable under the usual conditions of acid hydrolysis.

An alternative procedure for labelling proteins to high specific activities by acylation with a ^{125}I-containing reagent has been described by Bolton and Hunter (1973).

3.8. *Modifications of sulfhydryl and disulfide groups*

The half-cystine residues of many proteins are present in the form of disulfide bridges. Some proteins contain both sulfhydryl and disulfide groups. Since sulfhydryl groups are readily oxidized, and since disulfide interchange complicates the determination of half-cystine pairing in proteins containing several disulfide bonds, it is customary to convert the half-cystine residues to stable derivatives prior to undertaking chemical studies. The most generally accepted approach is the reduction of the disulfide bonds and subsequent modification of the resulting SH groups. Complete reduction of disulfide bonds in proteins, in general requires unfolding of the molecule, and, hence is performed in presence of denaturing agents such as urea, guanidine, or sodium dodecyl sulfate.

The remainder of this chapter deals, in the main, with the preparation of a number of derivatives of the cysteinyl residue; such as the acidic compounds, cysteic acid, S-carboxymethylcysteine, S-sulfocysteine, and the S-sulfenylthiosulfate of cysteine, the basic derivative S-aminoethylcysteine and S-carboxamidomethylcysteine. Procedures are also presented for the application of N-ethylmaleimide, *p*-mercuribenzoate, 5,5′-dithiobis(2-nitrobenzoate), and azobenzene-2-sulfenyl bromide to the spectrophotometric determination of sulfhydryl groups.

3.8.1. Modification by performic acid oxidation

Treatment of proteins with performic acid leads to the oxidation of cysteine and cystine residues to cysteic acid residues (Sanger 1949). Methionine residues are quantitatively converted to the sulfone (Hirs 1956), and tryptophan undergoes oxidative destruction (Toennies and Homiller 1942; Benassi et al. 1965). Other amino acids are not modified, provided that precautions are taken to avoid chlorination (Thompson 1954; Hirs 1956), or bromination (Sanger and Thompson 1963) of tyrosine residues. Cleavage of peptide bonds does not occur on performic acid oxidation at low temperature.

The procedure described by Moore (1963) is the method of choice when performic acid oxidation is employed for the quantitative determination of the half-cystine plus cysteine content of proteins. This procedure is described in detail in §2.5.1. The yield of cysteic acid is $94 \pm 2\%$ and that of methionine sulfone $100 \pm 2\%$.

A widely used procedure for the preparation of oxidized protein derivatives for amino acid sequence analysis has been described by Hirs (1967). A somewhat different procedure, used successfully in our laboratory for a number of years, is as follows: Performic acid is prepared by the addition of 1 ml 30% H_2O_2 to 9 ml of formic acid (98 to 100%) at room temperature. The mixture is allowed to stand for 2 hr and is then cooled to 0°C. The reagent is then added to lyophilized protein in a precooled container, to give a final protein concentration of 1%. After 18–24 hr at 0°C, the reaction mixture is diluted with an equal volume of ice-cold water, and transferred to dialysis tubing. Dialysis is performed against two changes of 100 volumes of water at 0°C, and finally against 100 volumes of 10^{-3} M mercaptoethanol, at 0°C. The protein derivative is then lyophilized.

3.8.2. Reduction and carboxymethylation (or carboxamidomethylation)

The following generally applicable procedure is based on the method of Crestfield et al. (1963), and has been widely used with minor variations for the past ten years.

To 5 to 100 mg of protein in a 10 ml glass-stoppered centrifuge tube, maintained under a nitrogen barrier, is added 3.61 g of deionized crystalline urea, 0.30 ml of EDTA solution (50 mg of disodium EDTA per ml), 3.0 ml of Tris buffer, *p*H 8.6 (5.23 g of Tris and 9 ml of 1.0 N HCl diluted to 30 ml with water), and finally 0.1 ml of mercaptoethanol. The solution is made up to a 7.5 ml mark with water, and deaerated by flushing with nitrogen for several minutes. The tube is then stoppered and allowed to stand at room temperature (22–25°C) for 4 hr, after which a freshly prepared solution of 0.268 g of recrystallized iodoacetic acid in 1.0 ml of 1.0 N NaOH is added. The iodoacetate used is slightly less, on a molar basis, than the amount of mercaptoethanol. The sulfhydryl groups of cysteinyl residues react most rapidly, and since the excess iodoacetate reacts faster with mercaptoethanol above *p*H 8 than with thioether sulfur, alkylation of methionine is kept to a minimum. The three equivalents of Tris per equivalent of iodoacetate keep the solution more alkaline than *p*H 8.3. Both the alkylation reaction, and the subsequent isolation of the protein derivative should be performed in the dark to prevent the formation of iodine. The protein derivative may be recovered by lyophilization, following gel filtration or exhaustive dialysis.

Subject index p. 201

Reduction with dithiothreitol (DTT). The use of DTT, in place of mercaptoethanol, has gained wide acceptance. The reduction proceeds essentially to completion at low levels of DTT, because of the thermodynamically favored formation of a 6-membered ring. The equilibrium constant at *p*H 7 and 25°C for the reduction of cystine by DTT is 10^4, as compared to approximately 1 for mercaptoethanol (Konigsberg 1972).

A representative procedure, patterned upon that employed for the complete reduction and alkylation of a γG immunoglobulin (Waxdal et al. 1968), is given below.

A 10–20 mg/ml solution of protein in 6 M guanidine hydrochloride, 0.5 M in Tris chloride, and 0.002 M in EDTA, at *p*H 8.1, is placed in a glass-stoppered centrifuge tube. The solution is flushed with nitrogen, the tube closed tightly, and placed in a 50°C water-bath for 30 min to denature the protein. Dithiothreitol (50 moles/mole of disulfide in the protein, or if this is not known, 300 moles/mole of protein) is added, the tube flushed briefly with nitrogen and maintained at 50°C for 4 hr. The solution is then cooled to room temperature, and an aqueous iodoacetic acid solution (2-fold molar ratio to the DTT added previously) is added. The *p*H is monitored, and, if necessary maintained at 8.1 by the addition of 1 M NH_4OH. After alkylation for 20 min, in the dark, the reagents are removed (also in the dark) by rapid dialysis against ice-cold water, or by passage through a column of Sephadex G-10, equilibrated with 0.01 M NH_4HCO_3, at *p*H 8.1.

In both of the above procedures, iodoacetamide may be substituted on an equimolar basis for iodoacetic acid with no alteration in reaction conditions.

S-Carboxymethylcysteine is readily determined by amino acid analysis following acid hydrolysis under the usual conditions (§ 2.5.3). The occurrence and extent of any alkylation of lysyl, histidyl, or methionyl residues would be revealed at the same time (§2.5.10, 2.7.1, 2.8.1).

3.8.3. Carboxyethylation of SH

Free S-carboxymethylcysteine, or S-carboxymethylcysteine at the

N-terminus of a peptide, undergoes intramolecular cyclization in acid solution to yield 3-oxo-(2H, 3H, 5H, 6H-1,4-thiazine)-5-carboxylic acid (Bradbury and Smyth 1973), which is ninhydrin-negative.

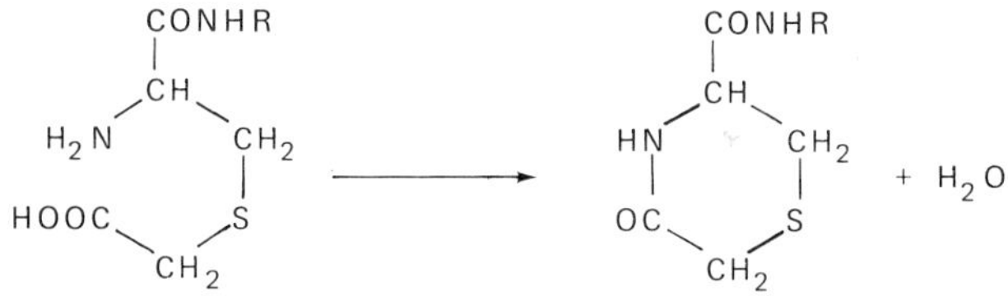

Such cyclization reactions have also been reported for the S-carboxamidomethyl derivative, and for the N-ethylmaleimide adduct of cysteine.

The rate and extent of this reaction depend upon the temperature and *p*H. S-carboxymethylcysteine cyclized most rapidly at *p*H 3.0 only 34% remaining after 16 hr at 110°C in 0.2 M sodium citrate buffer. Under the usual conditions of acid hydrolysis for amino acid analysis, e.g. 6 N HCl, 110°C, 18 hr, S-carboxymethylcysteine was stable (§ 2.5.3).

Bradbury and Smyth (1973) advocate the use of 3-bromopropionic acid in the place of iodoacetic acid, or its amide, in the alkylation reaction. S-carboxyethylcysteine was found to be completely stable at acid *p*H, and could be readily quantitated by amino acid analysis (§ 2.5.3). The half-life of the reaction of the SH-group of cysteine (2 μmoles/ml) with 3-bromopropionate (200 μmoles/ml) at *p*H 8 and 30°C was approximately 10 min. Under the same conditions, the reaction of cysteine and iodoacetate was found to be virtually instantaneous (Bradbury and Smyth 1973).

3.8.4. Aminoethylation of SH

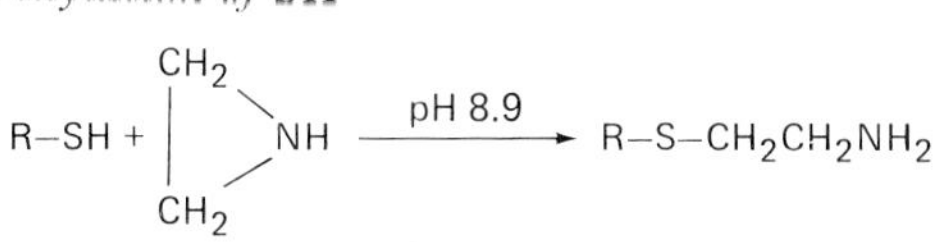

This modification is generally performed to introduce new points for tryptic cleavage within the polypeptide chain (Lindley 1956; Raftery and Cole 1963, 1966). Trypsin cleaves peptide bonds involving residues of S-(β-aminoethyl)cysteine which is an analogue of lysine; cleavage is much slower than for bonds involving lysyl or arginyl residues.

In principle, reduction and aminoethylation of disulfide-containing proteins, after modification of lysyl and arginyl side chains, should lead to a derivative which can be selectively cleaved by trypsin at S-aminoethylcysteinyl residues. Such a sequence of reactions has been applied to a γ-globulin (Slobin and Singer 1968).

Protein (25 mg) is dissolved in 5 ml of fresh 8 M urea (or 6 M guanidine HCl) in M Tris-HCl buffer, *p*H 8.9, containing 75 μl of 2-mercaptoethanol. After 2 hr at room temperature under a N_2 barrier, 150 μl of ethylenimine are added, and the alkylation allowed to proceed for 2 hr under N_2. (The completeness of the alkylation reaction may be assessed by assaying for the absence of free thiol. One drop of the reaction mixture is mixed with a drop each of 10% w/v sodium nitroprusside solution and 1 M NH_3 solution. A negative reaction is indicated by absence of significant purple color.) The completely alkylated reaction mixture is dialyzed, first against 100 volumes of 1% NH_4HCO_3, and then against distilled water. The protein derivative is recovered by lyophilization. Prolonged exposure of the reaction mixture to acidic conditions, prior to the removal of the excess ethylenimine, should be avoided. Significant alkylation of methionine can occur under such conditions (Schroeder et al. 1967). Some alkylation of the α-amino group may be observed (Shotton and Hartley 1973), particularly if the alkylation reaction is allowed to proceed for a prolonged time in the presence of a large excess of ethylenimine.

The S-aminoethylcysteine content of the protein derivative can readily be determined following acid hydrolysis of the protein under the usual conditions, and amino acid analysis (§ 2.5.4).

3.8.5. *Trimethylaminoethylation of cysteine*

The cysteinyl residue may be converted to a strongly basic derivative, 4-thialaminine, by alkylation with (2-bromoethyl) trimethylammonium

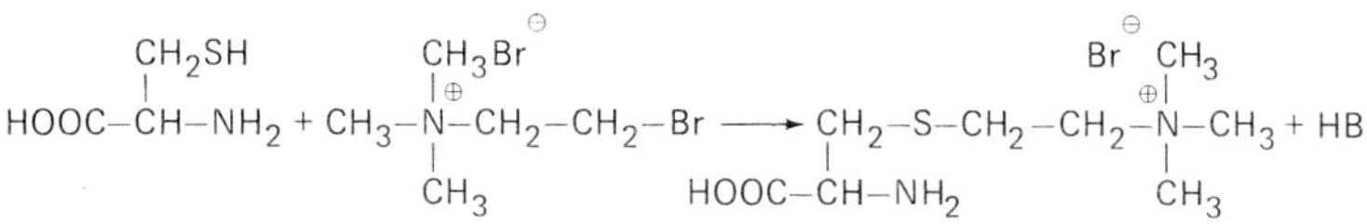

4–thialaminine

bromide (Itano and Robinson 1972).

The virtues of this modification reaction lie in the very high stability of 4-thialaminine under conditions of acid hydrolysis, and the ready solubility of a number of trimethylaminoethylated proteins in aqueous solution.

For complete alkylation of half-cystine residues, after the DTT reduction procedure described in § 3.8.2.1, (2-bromoethyl) trimethylammonium bromide is added in a 3-fold molar excess over the DTT concentration. After reaction for 24 to 48 hr under nitrogen, at room temperature, the protein derivative is desalted either by gel filtration, or exhaustive dialysis, and lyophilized.

The 4-thialaminine content of the protein derivative is determined by amino acid analysis after acid hydrolysis (§ 2.5.6).

3.8.6. Reduction and selective S-methylation

Conversion of half-cystine residues in proteins and peptides to the S-methyl derivatives is advantageous in subsequent studies of amino acid sequence. Under the usual conditions of acid hydrolysis (§ 2.1), S-methylcysteine is recovered in a 90% yield (Heinrikson 1971). The phenylthiohydantoin of S-methylcysteine is readily identified by routine thin layer chromatography procedures (Rochat et al. 1970). With the increasing use of the sequenator, PTH-S-methylcysteine offers a marked advantage over derivatives such as PTH-cysteic acid, or PTH-carboxymethylcysteine, which have to be identified by special techniques (Edman 1960, 1970). S-methylcysteinyl residues provide a new point of cleavage for cyanogen bromide (5).

The procedure described below is taken from a detailed publication of Heinrikson (1971).

Lyophilized or crystalline protein (10 to 50 mg) is dissolved in 5 ml of a solution at *p*H 8.6 containing 6 M guanidine hydrochloride, 0.25 M

Tris, 3.3 mM disodium EDTA, and 25% (v/v) of acetonitrile. (The organic solvent must be included to ensure solubility of the reagent, methyl-*p*-nitrobenzenesulfonate.) The solution is flushed with nitrogen, and a 50-fold molar excess of *β*-mercaptoethanol over the half-cystine content of the protein is added under a nitrogen barrier. The tightly closed vessel is then incubated at 50°C. After 1 hr, the reduction mixture is cooled to 37°C, and 0.5 ml of a solution of methyl-*p*-nitrobenzene-sulfonate in acetonitrile is added under a nitrogen barrier. The amount of methylating agent added is in a 2-fold molar excess with respect to the mercaptoethanol. After incubation for 2 hr at 37°C, the clear yellow solution is treated with 5 *μ*l of mercaptoethanol and dialyzed exhaustively against distilled water. The protein derivative tends to precipitate during dialysis and is recovered by lyophilization.

Under the above conditions, the modification is totally restricted to sulfhydryl groups (Heinrikson 1971). S-methylcysteine is quantitated by amino acid analysis after acid hydrolysis (§ 2.5.5).

3.8.7. *S-Sulfonation*

In the presence of catalytic amounts of cysteine, or *β*-mercapto-ethylamine, and oxygen, sodium sulfite converts the half-cystine and cysteine residues of proteins to the S-sulfonate derivatives.

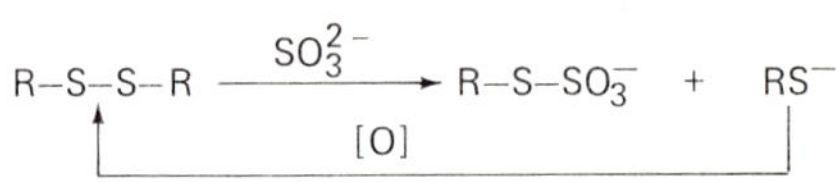

The S-sulfo derivative is stable at neutral and acidic *p*H. Sulfitolysis has been employed as a mild procedure for the cleavage of disulfide bonds in multi-chain proteins, as a preliminary to polypeptide fractionation, and also to provide a protective blocking group for the cysteinyl residue. The S-sulfo derivative is readily reduced back to the thiol by the addition of sulfhydryl compounds, e.g. *β*-mercaptoethanol.

The following sulfitolysis procedure is based upon the work of Chan (1968).

Protein (2–5 mg/ml) is dissolved in 0.1 M Tris chloride buffer, *p*H 8.0, containing 8 M urea (or 6 M guanidinium chloride), 2×10^{-4} M β-mercaptoethylamine, and 0.05 M Na_2SO_3. The mixture is stirred gently at room temperature for 1 hr, and then dialyzed exhaustively against distilled water. The derivative is then lyophilized.

The completeness of the reaction is best assessed by employing $Na_2{}^{35}SO_3$, of known specific activity, and determining the incorporation of radioactivity into the protein (Chan 1968).

Chan (1968) describes the following procedure for the regeneration of free thiol groups.

The S-sulfonated protein (1 mg/ml) is dissolved in 1 M Tris chloride buffer (pH 7.5) containing 4 M urea, and β-mercaptoethanol is added to a final concentration of 0.7 M. The mixture is incubated for 2 hr at 25°C, and then dialyzed against a buffer solution, appropriate to those further manipulations to which the protein is to be subjected.

3.8.8. Conversion to the S-sulfenylsulfonate derivative

The high reactivity of sulfhydryl groups imposes serious limitations on attempts to modify selectively other amino acid residues in proteins containing cysteinyl residues. The reversible blocking of free sulfhydryl groups in native proteins with tetrathionate offers one solution to this problem:

$$\text{protein–SH} + S_4O_6^{=} \rightleftharpoons \text{R–S–S–}SO_3^{-} + S_2O_3^{=} + H^{+}$$

An illustration of this approach may be seen in the studies on streptococcal proteinase (Liu 1967). The activity of this enzyme is dependent upon the presence of a free sulfhydryl group. The active form of the enzyme was first converted to the inactive S-sulfenylsulfonate derivative. Treatment of this derivative with a chemically-reactive substrate analogue, α-N-bromoacetylarginine methyl ester, resulted in the alkylation of a single histidine residue. The sulfhydryl group of the modified enzyme was regenerated by reduction, however, this did not restore enzymatic activity, thus providing presumptive evidence for the involvement of both a cysteinyl and a histidyl residue in the active site of this enzyme.

This method of reversible modification of sulfhydryl groups has also

Subject index p. 201

proved very useful in minimizing autolysis and proteolysis during purification of sulfhydryl proteases and, also, of other proteins from extracts containing high concentrations of sulfhydryl dependent proteolytic enzymes.

Protein (1 μmole) is dissolved in 5 ml of 0.02 M sodium phosphate buffer at *p*H 7.0, 0.001 M in EDTA, and 35 mg of sodium tetrathionate ($Na_2S_4O_6 \cdot 2H_2O$). After 60 min at room temperature, the reaction mixture is passed through a Sephadex G-25 column (approx. 1.5×40 cm) equilibrated with 0.02 M phosphate, 0.001 M in EDTA at *p*H 7, to remove excess reagent. The thiol groups may be regenerated by adjusting the *p*H to 7.6, adding β-mercaptoethanol to a concentration of 0.1 M and incubating at 37°C for 15 min. If prolonged storage of the S-sulfenylthiosulfate protein derivative is desired, this should be done in the presence of 0.001 M sodium tetrathionate.

It should be noted that the formation of a stable sulfenylthiosulfate is a phenomenon observed with *native* proteins (Pihl and Lange 1962). When simple thiols such as cysteine are reacted with an excess of tetrathionate, S-sulfocysteine is formed (Inglis and Liu 1970). If thiol is in excess, the sulfenylsulfonate can react with a second molecule of thiol to form a disulfide.

Inglis and Liu (1970) have developed a procedure for the quantitative determination of cystine and cysteine in acid hydrolyzates of proteins, dependent upon the quantitative conversion of cysteinyl residues to S-sulfocysteine, and subsequent quantitation of this derivative by amino acid analysis (§ 2.5).

3.8.9. Addition of thiols to activated double bonds

3.8.9.1. Spectrophotometric titration with N-ethylmaleimide (NEM)

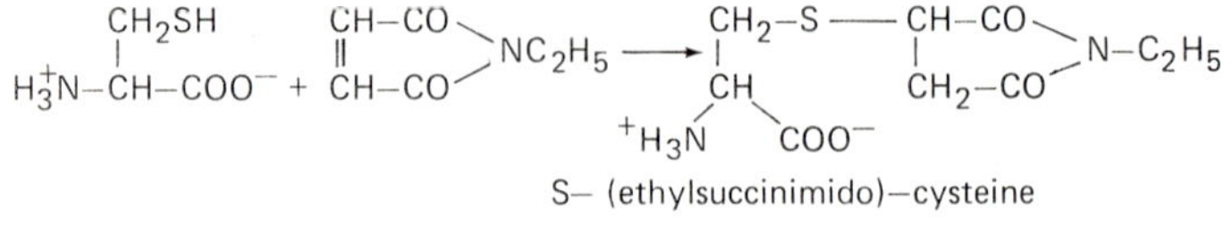

S– (ethylsuccinimido)–cysteine

The spectrophotometric procedure requires freshly prepared stock solutions of NEM (1.25×10^{-3} M) in either 5 M guanidine hydrochloride, or in 2% sodium dodecyl sulfate, in 0.1 M sodium phosphate buffer at *p*H 7.0, and a stock protein solution (approximately 5×10^{-4} M) in the same solvent as the NEM. The following solutions are then prepared.

A: 2.0 ml NEM solution +0.5 ml solvent
B: 2.5 ml solvent
C: 2.0 ml NEM solution +0.5 ml protein solution
D: 2.0 ml solvent +0.5 ml protein solution

The absorbancy (A_1) of solution A (sample cell) *versus* solution B (reference cell), and the absorbancy (A_2) of solution C *versus* solution D, are then determined in 1 cm pathlength spectrophotometer cells. The reaction with denatured proteins is generally rapid and complete within 10 min under the conditions specified here. Lack of further change in absorbance over an additional period of 10 min indicates that the reaction is indeed complete.

The ε_M at 305 nm for NEM is 620 whereas S-(ethylsuccinimido)-cysteine does not absorb at this wavelength. Hence, the sulfhydryl titer is given by the following relationship.

$$\text{sulfhydryl concentration} = \frac{A_1 - A_2}{620} \text{ moles/liter}$$

3.8.9.2. Other applications of N-ethylmaleimide and related compounds

Although NEM has been largely superceded as a spectrophotometric titrant for thiol groups, the reagent offers other useful features. Upon acid hydrolysis, S-(ethylsuccinimido)-cysteine gives rise to S-succinyl-cysteine (more precisely, 2-amino-2-carboxyethyl-mercaptosuccinic acid), which is stable to acid hydrolysis and can be quantitated by amino acid analysis (§2.5.7). Ethylamine, the other product of the hydrolytic cleavage of the derivative, can likewise be quantitated by amino acid analysis (§2.5.7). Since this product arises also from the hydrolytic cleavage of NEM itself, such quantitation is useful only after complete removal of excess reagent by exhaustive dialysis, or gel filtration, before subjecting the derivatized protein to acid hydrolysis. It should be noted that complete conversion of S-(ethylsuccinimido)-cysteine to S-succinylcysteine requires 72 hr of hydrolysis in 6 N HCl at 110°C *in vacuo* (Smyth et al. 1971; Guidotti and Koningsberg 1964).

Parenthetically, it should be noted that the reaction of maleic anhydride with sulfhydryl-containing proteins also leads to the formation of S-succinylcysteine derivatives, by the reaction sequence

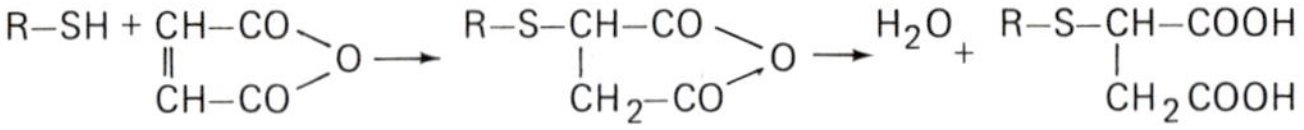

NEM is not completely specific for sulfhydryl groups. Reaction with amino groups occurs readily in native proteins. Formation of such derivatives would be detected by a comparison of the yield of S-succinylcysteine and ethylamine, or by the appearance of N-ε-succin-2-yl-lysine, or N-succin-2-yl-histidine (Holbrook and Jeckel 1969) upon acid hydrolysis of the modified protein (cf. ch. 2).

Radioactive reagents, such as ^{14}C-ring labeled NEM (see, for example, Klee and Gladner 1972), or N(N′-acetyl-4[^{35}S]-sulfamoyl-phenyl)maleimide (Holbrook and Pfleiderer 1965; Holbrook and Jeckel 1969) have been employed to tag specific residues in proteins and facilitate purification of peptides containing these residues.

The colored derivative, N-(dimethylamino-3,5-dinitrophenyl)-maleimide (DDPM) (Witter and Tuppy 1960) has been used to label cysteinyl residues in several proteins. Purification of peptides incorporating this derivative has been facilitated in several instances by their strong adsorption to talc (Witter and Tuppy 1960; Gold and Segal 1964, 1965). It should be noted that the DDPM derivative of N-acetylcysteine exhibits an $\varepsilon_{440\text{nm}}$ of only 3000 (Gold and Segal 1964), i.e. it is a relatively weak chromophore in the visible region of the spectrum.

Derivatives formed by the nucleophilic addition of sulfhydryl groups to the activated double bonds of acrylonitrile (Plummer and Hirs 1964), and 4-vinylpyridine (Cavins and Friedman 1970) have also been exploited in sequence and analytical studies.

3.8.10. Titration of thiols with 5,5′-dithiobis(2-nitrobenzoate) (DTNB; Ellman's reagent)

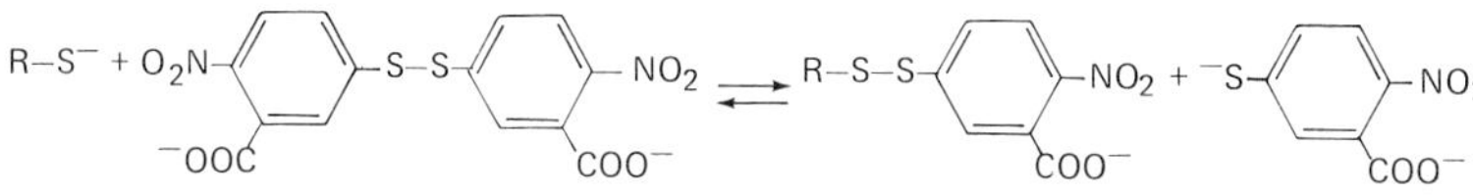

Following its introduction in 1959 (Ellman), this sensitive spectrophotometric procedure for the determination of thiols has gained wide acceptance. The mixed disulfide product can be exploited as an intermediate in the preparation of other useful derivatives of the cysteinyl residue.

For the determination of total sulfhydryl group content, protein (0.02 to 0.05 μmole) is dissolved in 2.5 ml of 0.1 M Tris chloride buffer at *p*H 8.0, containing 0.01 M EDTA, and either 6 M guanidinium chloride, 8 M urea, or 1% sodium dodecyl sulfate. A fresh solution of DTNB (0.01 M in 0.05 M sodium phosphate buffer, *p*H 7.0) is prepared. The solvent (2.50 ml), in which the protein is to be dissolved, is placed in the reference cell of a spectrophotometer, and 2.5 ml of the protein solution in the sample cell. DTNB solution (100 μl) is added to each cell, and the absorbance at 412 nm is recorded with time. After the development of the maximum color the downward sloping line (a consequence of the spontaneous hydrolysis of DTNB) is extrapolated to zero time to determine the concentration of thiol. Where conjugated proteins, absorbing in the visible region, are under study, or where the protein contributes significant light scattering, the absorbance of the protein solution at 412 nm should be determined against a water blank, and the appropriate correction made.

The values quoted for ε_{412} of 3-carboxylato-4-nitrothiophenolate in aqueous solution have ranged from 13 600 (Ellman 1959, Janatova et al. 1968) to 14 140 M^{-1} cm^{-1} (Gething and Davidson 1972). The value of 13 600 is that generally used. In 6 M guanidinium chloride, $\varepsilon_{412} = 13\,880$ M^{-1} cm^{-1}, and in 8 M urea, $\varepsilon_{412} = 14\,290$ M^{-1} cm^{-1} (Gething and Davidson 1972).

Where a determination of total half-cystine plus cysteine content of proteins is desired, the protein may be reduced by any of the procedures described in § 3.8.2, and freed of reducing agent by gel filtration on a column of Sephadex G-25, equilibrated and eluted with the solvent used for the titration.

The paper by Janatova et al. (1968) should be consulted for a careful study of the optimum conditions for the determination of the sulfhydryl content of native proteins by titration with DTNB.

It should be noted that incomplete conversion of protein sulfhydryl groups to the mixed disulfide leaves open the possibility of intramolecular reactions leading to the formation of disulfide bonds.

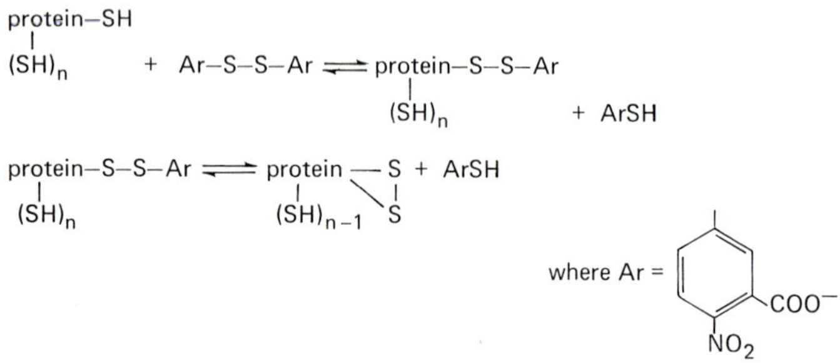

Such interchange reactions have been observed with a number of proteins, and are particularly likely to occur where initial reaction of the most rapidly reacting sulfhydryl groups on a protein molecule is followed by removal of excess DTNB, and a denaturing treatment which leads to the exposure of previously unavailable thiol groups.

3.8.11 Cyanylation of SH

Degani et al. (1970) and Degani and Patchornik (1974) demonstrated that quantitative cyanylation of sulfhydryl groups in proteins may be achieved by reaction with 2-nitro-5-thiocyanobenzoate (NTCB).

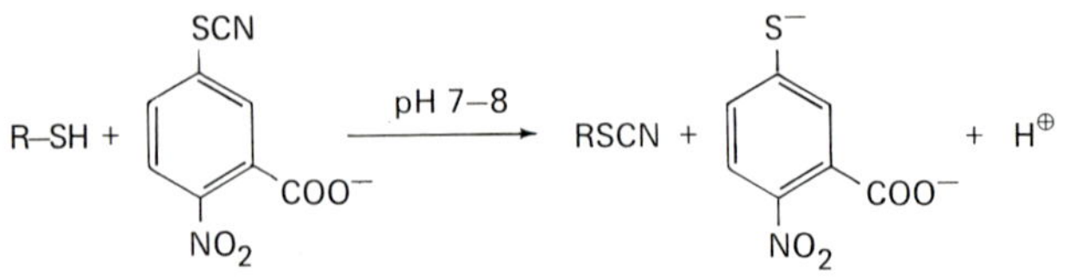

The preparation of NTCB has been described by Degani and Patchornik (1971). To a 150 ml aqueous solution containing 7.5 g of $KHCO_3$ and 2.0 g (31 mmol) of KCN, 3.0 g (7.5 mmol) of 5,5′-dithiobis-(2-nitrobenzoic acid) were added with stirring. After 30 min, a freshly prepared 3% solution of CNBr in water was added slowly (10 min) to the stirred deep orange solution until the color was completely discharged. This required 27 ml. The *p*H was then decreased to 5 by the dropwise addition of glacial acetic acid, excess cyanide was removed by bubbling a stream of N_2 through the solution for 12 hr. Upon acidification to *p*H 2.3 with 6 N HCl a white solid crystallized out. After cooling the mixture with ice, the solid was filtered, washed with cold water and air-dried, yield 3.42 g (94%) of chromatographically and electrophoretically pure NTCB, mp 248°C.

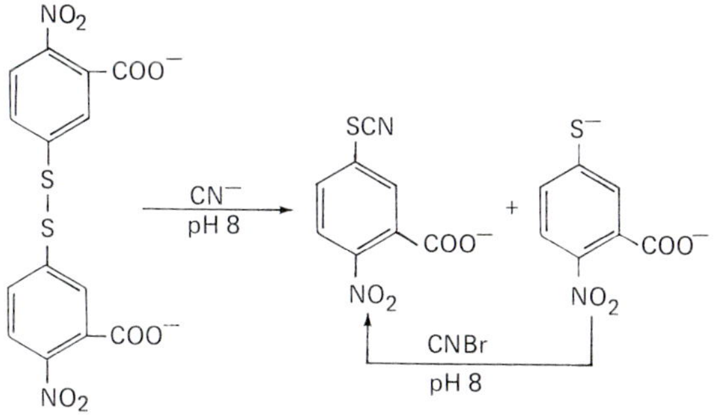

For complete cyanylation of sulfhydryl groups, protein (1×10^{-4} M, or less than 10 mg per ml; concentrations higher than this should be avoided) is dissolved at room temperature in 0.1 M phosphate, *p*H 7.4, containing 6 M guanidine HCl and 1 mM EDTA, and the solution freed of oxygen by flushing with N_2. A 5-fold molar excess of NTCB in the same buffer is then added and the rate of reaction followed by monitoring the absorbance at 412 nm, due to the 2-nitro-5-thiobenzoate anion ($\varepsilon_M = 13\,600$). When the reaction is complete, the protein is separated from the reagents by either dialysis or gel filtration at near-neutral *p*H.

If conversion of both sulfhydryl and disulfide groups to the thiocyanate derivative is desired, the protein should first be reduced with dithiothreitol in 6 M guanidine HCl (§ 3.8.2.1) and the reduced protein separated from the reducing agent either by gel filtration or dialysis prior to being subjected to the above cyanylation procedure.

NTCB will undoubtedly prove to be a very popular reagent for the modification of sulfhydryl groups. The reagent appears to be totally specific. The –CN substituent on the –SH group is small in comparison with that introduced by reaction with 5,5′-dithiobis(2-nitrobenzoate), *p*-mercuribenzoate, N-ethylmaleimide or indeed any of the other commonly used –SH reagents. Hence, this reagent may permit clarification of situations where loss of biological activity due to reaction with sulfhydryl groups results from steric hindrance due to the substituent rather than to the substitution of a functionally vital thiol group. Another advantage is that labeled reagent is readily synthesized by using $Na^{14}CN$.

Selective cleavage of the polypeptide chain at the thiocyanatoalanine residues may be achieved by incubation at alkaline *p*H, e.g. *p*H 9.0 for 24 hr at 37°C. Under these conditions some conversion to an uncleaved dehydroalanine peptide also occurs.

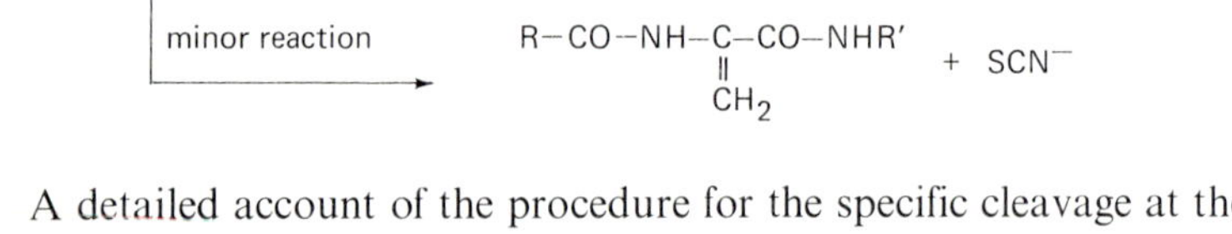

A detailed account of the procedure for the specific cleavage at the amino peptide bonds of cysteine and cystine residues of several proteins, utilizing NTCB, has been presented by Jacobson et al. (1973).

3.8.12. Reaction of thiols with organomercurials

3.8.12.1. Titration with p-mercuribenzoate (PMB)

Reagent grade sodium *p*-chloromercuribenzoate (9 mg) is dissolved in

1 ml of 0.04 M NaOH, the solution is made up to 25 ml with water, and centrifuged to remove particulate material. This solution (approximately 8×10^{-4} M PMB) should be stored at room temperature in the dark. Prior to use, the exact concentration of the reagent is determined by measuring the absorbance of diluted solutions obtained by adding 0.5 ml of the stock solution of PMB to 9.5 ml of 0.33 M sodium acetate buffer at *p*H 4.6 ($\varepsilon = 1.74 \times 10^4$ M^{-1} cm^{-1} at 234 nm).

For an initial determination on a protein of unknown thiol content, it is appropriate to use a stock solution of protein at a concentration of 1 mg per ml in 0.33 M sodium acetate at *p*H 4.6, containing either 8 M deionized urea, or 2% sodium dodecyl sulfate. This solution should be centrifuged prior to use. (At this protein concentration, a ΔA at 255 nm of approximately 0.2 would be observed upon titration of a macromolecule of molecular weight of 30 000 containing a single cysteinyl residue). Precisely measured aliquots (10 μl) of stock PMB solution are then delivered to a reference 1 cm light path silica cell containing 3.0 ml of solvent and to a matching cell containing 3.0 ml of protein solution. The contents of the cells are mixed after each addition (very small Teflon coated magnetic stirring bars are very useful for spectrophotometric titrations), and the change in absorbance at 255 nm is recorded. The titration is continued until no further change in absorbance is observed. The equivalence point is determined graphically (see Fig. 3.2), and the thiol content computed from the known concentrations of the reagent and the protein.

The $\Delta\varepsilon_M$ at 255 nm for PMB-cysteinyl residues is in the range of 6000–8000 M^{-1} cm^{-1} at *p*H 4.6, depending on the solvent.

An excellent detailed discussion of the application of PMB to the determination of sulfhydryl groups in native proteins has been presented by Benesch and Benesch (1962).

3.8.12.2. Reaction with mercurated nitrophenols

McMurray and Trentham (1969) and Stefanini et al. (1972) have described the synthesis of several mercurated nitrophenols (Table 3.2). The spectra of these organomercurials show large changes in the visible region when thiols displace more weakly bound ligands from

Subject index p. 201

TABLE 3.2

Spectral properties of mercurated nitrophenols*

Compound	Structure	λ_{max} $m\mu$	ε(in 0.1 M KOH) $M^{-1}cm^{-1}$
2-chloromercuri-4-nitrophenol	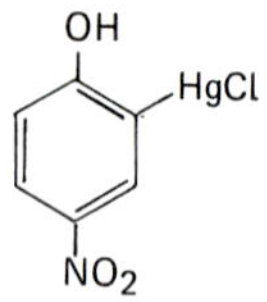	405	1.74×10^4
2-chloromercuri-4,6-dinitrophenol	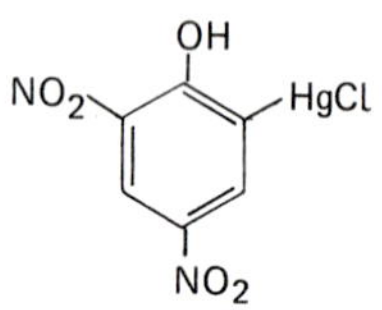	371	1.57×10^4
4-chloromercuri-2-nitrophenol	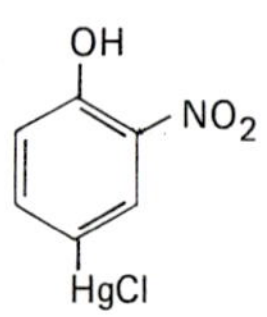	416	4.1×10^3
2,6-dichloromercuri-4-nitrophenol	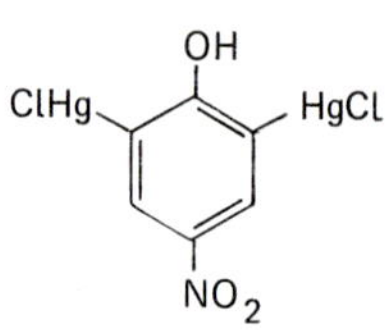	410	1.74×10^4
2-acetoxymercuri-3-nitrophenol	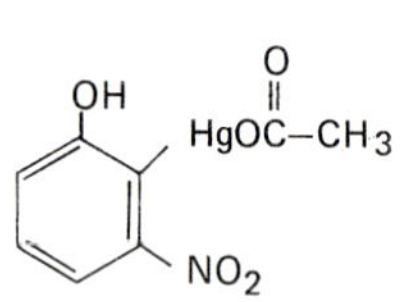	410	1.7×10^3**

* Data from McMurray and Trentham (1969), and Stefanini et al. (1972).
** In 0.1 M NaOH.

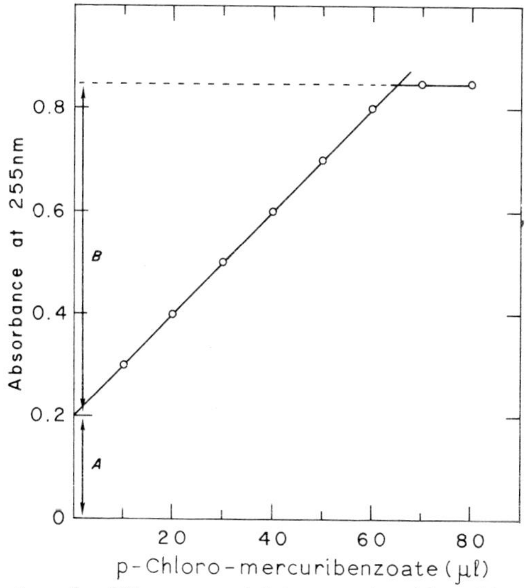

Fig. 3.2. Titration of a SH-group containing protein with *p*-chloromercuribenzoate (PMB). A, is the absorbance of the protein solution prior to the addition of PMB. The *increment* in absorbance, B, due to mercaptide formation, observed upon titration with PMB (as described in the text), is a measure of thiol concentration in the solution.

the mercury atom. These spectral changes are very largely a consequence of the perturbation of the p*K* of the nitrophenols. These compounds have been used as probes of the environment of sulfhydryl groups in native proteins, as well as in the preparation of crystalline mercurial derivatives of proteins for X-ray diffraction analysis. Aside from these applications, the mercurated nitrophenol derivatives may be used for the spectrophotometric titration of sulfhydryl groups in the same manner as PMB, with the added advantage that the spectral shifts associated with mercaptide formation may be followed in the visible region of the spectrum where interference from protein absorbance is minimal.

3.8.13. Reaction of cysteinyl residues with azobenzene-2-sulfenyl bromide

Azobenzene-2-sulfenyl bromide is reported to react selectively with cysteinyl residues in proteins. The reagent is soluble in water and reacts readily with thiols in acid solution (*p*H 1–5).

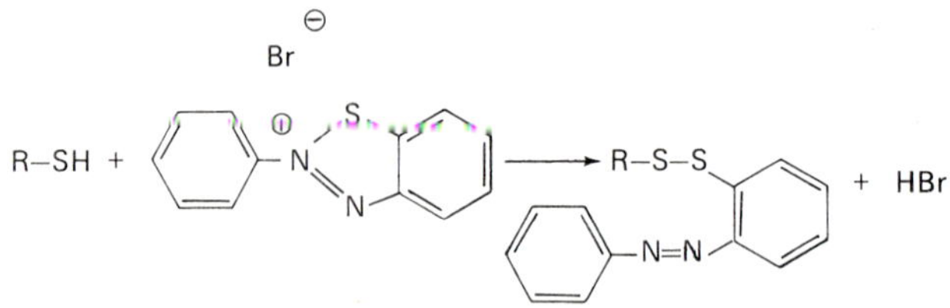

The following procedure, applied to egg-white lysozyme, was described by Fontana et al. (1968).

Protein (40 mg) was dissolved in 2 ml 8 M urea solution, adjusted to *p*H 8.6 by the addition of 5% methylamine, and β-mercaptoethanol (20 μl) added. After 1 hr at room temperature, the protein was precipitated with acetone: 1 N HCl (39:1, v/v) at −5°C, separated by centrifugation, and washed with acetone. The protein was dissolved in 2 ml of 25% (v/v) aqueous acetic acid. Azobenzene-2-sulfenyl bromide (35 mg) was dissolved in 50% aqueous acetic acid (1 ml), and added to the solution of the reduced protein. After 30 min at 22–24°C, the protein derivative was freed of excess reagent by passage through a column of Sephadex G-25 (90 × 1 cm), equilibrated and developed with 0.2 M acetic acid, and lyophilized.

The modified protein was dissolved in 0.1 N HCl (2 mg/ml) and an aliquot (0.3 ml) added to 2.7 ml of 8 M urea adjusted with HCl to *p*H 1. The concentration of azobenzene-2-sulfenyl residues ($\varepsilon = 16\,700$ at 353 nm) was determined spectrophotometrically, and extent of modification calculated by comparing this concentration with the concentration of protein in the 0.1 N HCl solution, determined by amino acid analysis on an appropriate aliquot.

The mixed disulfide is readily reduced by thiols, such as β-mercaptoethanol, or DTT, or by sodium borohydride.

Site-specific modification of native proteins with group-specific reagents

The general objectives for the site-specific modification of native proteins include: (1) the identification of amino acid residues at the catalytic site of enzymes and the ligand-binding sites of regulatory proteins, and of immunoglobulins as well as enzymes; (2) the introduction of physico-chemical reporter groups such as fluorescent, spectrophotometric or spin-label probes; and (3) the labelling of a specific protein in order to isolate it from a multicomponent system such as a ribosome or mitochondrion. The potential use of irreversible inhibitors as pharmacological agents provides another motivation for their study. As the term will be used here, site-specific modification implies either the exclusive derivatization of a single amino acid residue or the incorporation of a single mole of modification reagent per mole of protein subunit.

The site-specific modification of native proteins is not one of the routine procedures in protein chemistry. It cannot be placed in the same category as end-group labelling or determination of amino acid composition and sequence. The specific chemical modification of a native protein can never be guaranteed because the reactivity of amino acids in a native protein is rarely predictable even if the three-dimensional structure of the protein is known. Unusual pK_a's of side chains, steric and solvent effects and the proximity of the amino acid residue to a ligand-binding site all influence its reactivity, frequently in opposite directions. However certain well-defined avenues of in-

Subject index p. 201

vestigation are available which the skillful experimenter may follow to answer his specific question.

In general, there are two approaches to the site-specific modification of a protein: side chain specific modification reagents such as those discussed in ch. 3 and affinity labels or active site-directed irreversible inhibitors. The latter type of compound shares important structural similarities to ligands known to have affinity for a particular binding site but is distinguished from reversible inhibitors by the possession of reactive groups capable of forming covalent bonds with amino acid side chains. Most commonly, the reactive groups are alkylating agents such as haloketones or haloacids although acylating and arylating groups have been employed. New types of reactive substituents currently receiving active attention are photoactivatable or capable of being transformed into a reactive group by the catalytic site of an enzyme.

Many side-chain specific reagents have been successfully used for the stoichiometric modification of native proteins. This approach accounts for most of the papers published in this area. Although the likelihood of a successful site specific modification with these reagents is significantly less than that with a well designed affinity label, many more experiments with these compounds are probably attempted because minimal commitment of resources is necessary to initiate such studies. Most of the site-specific reagents are readily available, whereas affinity labels usually must be synthesized, often by difficult routes.

The unexpected specificity which can be achieved with functional group modification reagents is an apparent consequence of the native protein's ability to impose a unique chemical environment on a given amino acid under a given set of experimental conditions. It is important to emphasize that the site-specific modification of a protein is a kinetic phenomenon and selective modifications result from the ability of the protein to alter the reaction rate of a single residue under one clearly defined condition of *p*H, ionic strength and temperature. For example, it is entirely possible that if, at *p*H 7.0, one lysine residue is substantially more reactive than either free lysine or other lysine residues in the protein it may well be less reactive than these at *p*H 9.0.

4.1. Effect of complex formation

Two factors are chiefly, but not exclusively, responsible for the fact that, under certain conditions, amino acids in native proteins react more rapidly than free amino acids in solution. The first and most general is the capacity of proteins to bind modification reagents at or near the functional groups of amino acid residues in orientations favorable to reaction. The reversible binary complexes formed between proteins and modification reagents prior to reaction are analogous to enzyme-substrate complexes. As a result, most site-specific modifications of native proteins probably proceed by the scheme summarized in eq. (4.1) rather than by the strictly bimolecular scheme summarized in eq. (4.2) where P' designates the derivatized protein and R is the modification reagent.

$$P + R \underset{k_{-1}}{\overset{k_1}{\rightleftharpoons}} P-R \xrightarrow{k_2} P' \tag{4.1}$$

$$P + R \xrightarrow{k_R} P' \tag{4.2}$$

These two mechanistic alternatives can often be distinguished kinetically. The pseudo first-order rate constant for the modification of the protein (k_{obs}) for the schemes summarized in eqs. (4.1), (4.2) are given in eqs. (4.3), (4.4), respectively, where the

$$k_{obs} = \frac{k_2(R)}{(R)+K_R} \tag{4.3}$$

$$k_{obs} = k_R(R) \tag{4.4}$$

modification is carried out under conditions in which the reagent is present in large excess relative to the protein and where in eq. (4.1) k_2 is assumed to be small relative to k_{-1}. If the scheme involving the formation of the binary complex (eq. 4.1) is valid, then the first order rate constant for modification will not always be linearly dependent on the concentration of the modification reagent. The simplest procedure to determine if intermediate complexes form during a modification reaction is to measure the pseudo first-order rate constant as a function of reagent concentration and then plot the reciprocal of this rate constant *versus* the reciprocal of the modification reagent concentration. Since eqs. (4.5), (4.6) are the reciprocal forms of eqs. (4.3), (4.4) respectively, a finite intercept in these double reciprocal plots indicates that an intermediate complex is probably formed. The ratio of the slope to the intercept in the double reciprocal plots yields $K_{R'}$ the dissociation constant of the protein-modification reagent binary complex.

$$\frac{1}{k_{\mathrm{obs}}} = \frac{1}{k_2} + \frac{K_R}{k_2}\left(\frac{1}{R}\right) \tag{4.5}$$

$$\frac{1}{k_{\mathrm{obs}}} = \frac{1}{K_R} \cdot (R) \tag{4.6}$$

Failure to detect a complex by this kinetic procedure is not proof that it does not form. If the concentration of the modification reagent is substantially less than K_R, then eq. (4.3) reduces to eq. (4.7) – an expression which is indistinguishable from a strictly bimolecular mechanism.

$$k_{\mathrm{obs}} = \frac{k_2(R)}{K_R} \tag{4.7}$$

One alternative approach for demonstrating the existence of a complex during the course of a modification reaction is stereochemical in nature. For example, if enantiomers of a modification reagent give either different rates of modification or different products, the importance of multiple sites of interaction between the reagent and the protein, and hence intermediate complex formation is indicated. Examples of studies of this type include the alkylation of bovine pancreatic ribonuclease and papain by a variety of haloacids (Heinrikson et al. 1965; Eisele and Wallenfels 1968).

The simple numerical analysis below indicates the significant rate acceleration which can be achieved if a modification proceeds through the formation of a reversible complex (eq. 4.1) rather than through a strictly bimolecular reaction (eq. 4.2) as would be the case for a free amino acid in solution. Rates of intramolecular reactions are usually compared to those of intermolecular reactions by determining the ratio of the first-order rate constants to the second order rate constants. The units of this ratio are concentration and the ratio is at least 5 M for simple organic reactions if no specific orientation effects are involved. Ratios of this size are generally interpreted in terms of the increased local concentration of one reactive group relative to another in the intramolecular reaction.

If one considers that the ratio of k_2, the first order rate constant of eq. (4.1), to k_R, the second order rate constant of eq. (4.2), is 5 M, the expression in eq. (4.8) permits the comparison of the observed pseudo first-order rate constant for modification according to eq. (4.1) (k^1_{obs}) and eq. (4.2) (k^2_{obs}). The reaction which proceeds according to eq. (4.2) can be considered the rate of modification of the free amino acid.

$$\frac{k^1_{\text{obs}}}{k^2_{\text{obs}}} = \frac{\dfrac{k_2 R}{R+K_R}}{k_R(R)} = \frac{\dfrac{5\,k_R(R)}{R+K_R}}{k_R(R)} = \frac{\dfrac{5\,k_R(10^{-2}\,\text{M})}{10^{-2}\,\text{M}+0.5\,\text{M}}}{k_R(10^{-2}\,\text{M})} = 10 \qquad (4.8)$$

Assuming that the affinity of the modification reagent for the protein is slight so that K_R is 0.5 M and that the modification reagent concentration is 10^{-2} M, it is readily apparent that the rate of modification of an amino acid in a native protein is ten times greater than that for a free amino acid in solution. This conclusion is remarkable for it shows that, without assuming highly specific geometric constraints or a marked affinity of the reagent for the protein, it is still possible to achieve a significant rate enhancement if a complex is formed. Since site-specific modification with a side-chain specific reagent is exclusively a kinetic phenomenon this analysis shows one reason why amino acids of the same type on a given protein can have widely disparate reactivities.

Related to the ability of the protein to interact with modification reagents and thus form binary complexes, is its probable role of providing a reaction matrix which can preferentially stabilize the

Subject index p. 201

transition state of a particular modification reaction. The effect is roughly equivalent to the capacity of an enzyme to coordinate or chelate the transition state of the particular reaction that it catalyzes. Clearly, a number of specific interactions between protein, modification reagent and reactive amino acids are responsible for the stabilization of the transition state. They would include electrostatic effects, hydrogen-bonding interactions and unique microenvironments of varying dielectric constants. If the transition state of the modification reaction is stabilized by additional interactions with the protein, then the selectivity of the modification reaction will be considerably enhanced. The unusual rate enhancements observed for the reaction of some functional group reagents with specific amino acids undoubtedly are explicable in these terms. Perhaps the most outstanding example is the reaction of serine esterases with diisopropyl fluorophosphate (Sanger, 1963).

4.2. *Effects of pK_a perturbations*

The perturbation of the acid dissociation constant of an amino acid residue as a consequence of its environment within a protein represents another mechanism for enhancing its reactivity relative to a free amino acid in solution. Most amino acid residues react with their respective modification reagents in their unprotonated form instead of in their conjugate acid form. Eq. (4.10) describes the *p*H dependence of the simple bimolecular reaction (eq. 4.9) of the free base form of nucleophilic amino acid side chain with a non-ionizable modification reagent where K_a is the acid dissociation constant and A_T is the total concentration of amino acid.

$$A + R \xrightarrow{k_R} A - R \tag{4.9}$$

$$\frac{d(A-R)}{dt} = K_R \left(\frac{K_a}{H^+ + K_a} \right) (A_T)(R) \tag{4.10}$$

If a *p*H-dependent rate constant (k_R') is defined by eq. (4.11),

$$k_R' = k_R \left(\frac{K_a}{H^+ + K_a} \right) = k_R \alpha_A \tag{4.11}$$

it is apparent that the observed rate constant at any *p*H will be a function of the reactivity of the nucleophile (the magnitude of k_R) and the fraction of the nucleophile in its deprotonated form $[\alpha_A = K_a/(H^+ + K_a)]$. At any given *p*H, k_R' will increase with increase in K_a. In effect, by increasing the acid dissociation constant (or decreasing the pK_a) the protein generates a larger concentration of the nucleophilic form of the amino acid residue.

However, the bimolecular rate constant changes as a function of the pK_a of the nucleophilic group according to the Bronsted relation (eq. 4.12) where γ is a reaction constant which depends on the nature of the modification reaction and β describes the sensitivity of a series of nucleophiles on the pK_a.

$$\log k_R = \beta \mathrm{p}K_a + \gamma \qquad (4.12)$$

This standard free energy relation indicates that the rate acceleration gained as consequence of increasing the reactive form of the nucleophile is partially offset by the decrease of k_R. But since the values of β are often close to 0.5, a net rate acceleration usually results especially if the *p*H of the reaction mixture is near the pK_a of the ionizing nucleophile. The exceptional reactivities of lysine residues in glutamate dehydrogenase and acetoacetate decarboxylase with pyridoxal and 2,4-dinitrophenyl acetate respectively are almost certainly due to the greatly perturbed pK_a's of the modified residues (Piszkiewicz and Smith 1971; O'Leary and Westheimer 1968; Kokesh and Westheimer 1971). The pK_a of the ε-NH_2 group of reactive lysine in glutamate dehydrogenase is 7.9 while that in acetoacetate decarboxylase is 6. The normal pK_a of lysine is 10.2

Recently, Kaplan et al. (1971) devised a new procedure for determining the ionization constants and reactivities of individual amino group of proteins with a competitive labelling technique. This method represents the first comprehensive attempt to relate the reactivity of amino acid side chains to their pK_a's and nucleophilicities. The method consists of reacting the protein and a free amino acid standard with a limiting amount of a radioactive group-specific reagent such as acetic anhydride. The protein, which is initially heterogeneously labelled with the radioactive modification reagent, is then exhaustively modified with non-radioactive reagent to yield a chemically homogeneous but radiochemically heterogeneous final product. The internal standard (phenylalanine was used in the published studies with elastase) is present when the acetylation is performed with the non-radioactive as well as with the radioactive acetic anhydride.

After digestion of the modified protein and isolation of the radioactive peptides, the specific activities of these peptides and of the acetylated amino acid standard are determined. This procedure is repeated at several *p*H's

$$\alpha_A r = \alpha_S \, X \, \frac{\text{specific radioactivity of acetylated peptide}}{\text{specific radioactivity of acetylated internal standard}} \tag{4.13}$$

Since the pK_a of the internal standard is known, the product $\alpha_A r$ in eq. (4.13) can be determined at any *p*H where α_A and α_S are fractions of a particular lysine residue and internal standard present in the deprotonated form, respectively, (i.e. α_A is defined as in eq. 4.11); and r is the quotient $k_R^{\text{lys-X}}/k_R^{S}$ where $k_R^{\text{lys-X}}$ is the second order rate constant for the reaction of acetic anhydride with the unprotonated form of lysine residue X on the protein and k_R^{S} is the comparable constant for the reaction of the internal standard with acetic anhydride. Experiments at varying *p*H values permit the determination of the acid dissociation constant of the particular lysine residue under study.

The results obtained for porcine elastase have revealed that the ε-amino groups of both lysines 224 and 87 have normal pK_a's (about 10.3) and nucleophilicities anticipated for primary amines of this pK_a. That is, the second order rate constants for the reaction of the unprotonated ε-amino groups of these lysine residues with acetic anhydride fit approximately on the Bronsted plot for the reaction of acetic anhydride with a variety of amines. The results for valine-16, which is known to be in a salt linkage in the interior of the enzyme, indicate that this α-amino group has an apparent pK_a of 9.7 but a nucleophilicity of only 4% of that anticipated from the Bronsted plot for an amine of this pK_a. The unusually low reactivity of this valine is consistent with the significant steric hindrance that would be expected from a residue involved in a salt linkage and shielded from the solvent. Although no highly reactive lysine residues were present in porcine elastase, the competitive labelling techniques of Kaplan et al. (1971), in principle, provide a method to determine if a site-specific modification reaction at a given *p*H is unusually rapid due to the unusual nucleophilicity of this residue or to its unusually low pK_a. Exceptional nucleophilicity or reactivity of the residue is likely to be the consequence of the formation of preliminary binary complex of reagent and protein or of the stabilization by the native protein of the transition state for the modification reaction.

In summary, the ability of the protein to bind modification reagents both prior to reaction and/or in the transition state, coupled with its capacity to increase the reaction rate by perturbing the pK_a's of the nucleophiles can account for the selectivity of a modification reagent with no apparent affinity for the protein modified. Clearly, in certain reactions, only one of these sources of rate enhancement is operative. The ability to rationalize the selectivity which can be achieved with modification reagents specific for amino acid side-chains should not be confused with the capacity to predict the results of the modification of any given protein with a particular modification reagent. For this reason, this experimental approach remains highly empirical and the ease of attempting experiments of this type should be weighed against the low probability of their success and their low information content. Clearly in the absence of sequence information and a precise understanding of the protein's functional role and properties, an isolated specific modification of a protein has very little intrinsic importance. Since the experimenter possesses very few means of controlling the course of a modification reaction with functional group-specific reagents, the use of affinity labels constitutes the most rational approach for the site-specific modification of a protein. It is the only method which can be used with any hope of success in a complex protein mixture.

4.3. Widely employed site-specific reagents

Several reagents which do not bear a strong structural homology to natural ligands have proved generally useful in either classifying enzymes as to basic mechanism or modifying specific types of binding sites. For example, diisopropyl fluorophosphate has played an historically important role in defining the class of serine esterases and proteases (Sanger 1963). Pyridoxal phosphate has been extremely useful in the modification of lysine residues at or near the binding site for inorganic phosphate or phosphate esters in various enzymes. Procedures involving these two generally useful site-specific reagents are now presented.

4.3.1. Diisopropyl fluorophosphate

Clearly all experiments performed with the nerve gas, diisopropyl fluorophosphate (DFP), must be done in a fume hood with the utmost care. DFP rapidly hydrolyzes in 1 N NaOH, so that all glassware which comes in contact with the nerve gas should be soaked in this alkaline solution for at least 1 hr as a precaution prior to its reuse. (*Warning*: DFP is a potent poison. Atropine is an effective antagonist. For details of treatment, see Goodman, L. S. and Gilman, A., 1965, 'The Pharmacological Basis of Therapeutics,' The Macmillan Co., New York, 3rd Ed., p. 454).

Stock solutions of DFP can be conveniently prepared in isopropanol in concentrations from 0.1 M to 0.001 M. These solutions are stable for a month in the refrigerator (Jansen et al. 1949). Moon et al. (1965), in their studies of the reaction of chymotrypsin with DFP, have determined the normality of stock solution of DFP in the following manner. Roughly 0.03 moles of DFP were added to an aqueous solution of 0.17 moles of KOH in a volumetric flask. The solution was allowed to stand for 12 hr at 25°C to permit complete hydrolysis, and was titrated to *p*H 7.0 with 0.1 N HCl. Identical titrimetric results were obtained after 43 hr standing in alkali indicating that complete hydrolysis had taken place after 12 hr. To determine the amount of free acid, if any, in the DFP, the same amount of DFP that was used in the basic hydrolysis is added to water and then titrated with KOH to *p*H 7.0. The amount of DFP in the stock solution can then be readily calculated from the two sets of titrimetric data.

The derivatization of an enzyme by DFP is accomplished simply by incubating DFP with the protein. Aliquots of the incubation mixture can then be assayed for activity in the presence of DFP or after its removal by either gel filtration or dialysis. The second-order rate constant at neutral *p*H for the inactivation of chymotrypsin by DFP is roughly 3×10^6 M^{-1} sec^{-1} (Main 1964). This is the most rapid rate of inactivation by DFP so far observed. The rate of inactivation of acetylcholinesterase is an order of magnitude slower (Froede and Wilson 1971).

Although DFP has been and still is widely used to test if an enzyme possesses an unusually reactive serine, it should be noted that phenylmethane sulfonyl fluoride can also be used for the same purpose (§ 5.7). This reagent is in some ways preferable as it is non-volatile and relatively non-toxic. Therefore, it can be employed with fewer precautions.

4.3.2. Pyridoxal-5-phosphate

Several proteins are readily derivatized by pyridoxal-5-phosphate but react only slowly with pyridoxal. They include fructose-1,6-diphosphatase (Marcus and Herbert 1968), glutamate dehydrogenase (Piszkiewicz et al. 1970), glyceraldehyde-3-phosphate dehydrogenase (Ronchi et al. 1969), hemoglobin (Benesch et al. 1972), phosphofructokinase (Uyeda 1969), 6-phosphogluconate dehydrogenase (Rippa et al. 1967), and phosphoglucose isomerase (Schnackerz and Noltmann 1971). Since most, if not all, these proteins possess specific phosphate binding sites, the best explanation for the effectiveness of pyridoxal phosphate as opposed to pyridoxal as a modification reagent is that it preferentially binds to these sites. Generally, pyridoxal-5-phosphate inhibits these enzymes by the formation of Schiff base with a reactive lysine residue. However, since this type of linkage is readily hydrolyzed, irreversible inhibition usually can be obtained only if the Schiff base is reduced by sodium borohydride.

In their studies with 6-phosphogluconate dehydrogenase, Rippa et al. (1967) incubated the enzyme with concentrations of pyridoxal phosphate ranging from 10^{-5} to 10^{-4} M for 15 min at *p*H 7.5 in 0.01 M phosphate buffer. After 5-fold dilution the mixture was incubated a further 5 min. Aliquots were then assayed for activity in standard substrate solutions which contained a concentration of pyridoxal phosphate equal to that in the second incubation mixture. The additional pyridoxal phosphate was added to prevent reversal of the reaction. Piszkiewicz and Smith (1971) obtained significant amounts of inhibition simply by withdrawing aliquots of enzyme from its incubation mixture with pyridoxal-5-phosphate without including any additional pyridoxal phosphate in the assay mixture. Clearly, the ease of reversibility of the pyridoxal phosphate inhibition will vary from enzyme to enzyme and both procedures should be employed in exploratory studies. The site of attack of pyridoxal-5-phosphate can be conveniently explored by determining which substrate and/or coenzyme protects the protein from derivatization by pyridoxal-5-phosphate. For example, Rippa et al. (1967) have shown that 6-phosphogluconate and inorganic phosphate protected 6-phosphogluconate dehydrogenase from inhibition while $NADP^+$ had no effect. The latter finding indicates that phosphate buffers may not be ideal for use in studies with pyridoxal-5-phosphate. At the very least, the rate of inactivation by pyridoxal-5-phosphate should be measured as a function of phosphate concentration to determine if phosphate inhibits the modification reaction.

The borohydride reduction of Schiff base formed between a protein and pyridoxal phosphate should be carried out at a mildly acidic *p*H. Although sodium borohydride is more unstable in acidic solution, this disadvantage is offset by the exceptional reactivity of the Schiff base salts which are formed in mildly acidic solution (*p*H 4.5–6.5) (Schellenberg 1963). Reductions have been carried out after the protein and pyridoxal-5-phosphate have been incubated at a *p*H of 7.5 which is then changed to 4.5 or 6.5 with acetic acid (Rippa et al. 1967; Dempsey and Christensen 1962; Piszkiewicz et al. 1970) or after initial incubation at *p*H 6.0 (Schnackerz and Noltmann 1971). The relative merit of either procedure depends on whether or not the Schiff base formed with the given protein is freely reversible.

Prior to reduction with sodium borohydride, octyl alcohol can be added to avoid foaming. Then a solution of 0.05–0.06 M sodium borohydride in either water or 0.001 N sodium hydroxide is added in equal aliquots until roughly a 100-fold molar excess has been added. After each addition, the *p*H of the reaction mixture should be readjusted to the initial acidic *p*H by the addition of either acetic acid or hydrochloric acid. The temperatures of the reaction mixture have ranged from 4–25°C. The modified protein can then be isolated either by precipitation, dialysis or gel filtration under conditions where the native protein is normally stable.

Proof that a lysine residue has been modified can be readily obtained because pyridoxyl derivatives of lysine possess characteristic white-blue fluorescence (Ronchi et al. 1969). In addition, they have a distinctive absorption maximum at 325 nm with ε_M of 9710 M^{-1} cm^{-1} (Fisher et al. 1963). Finally, a radiochemical label can be introduced by reducing the pyridoxal-5-phosphate protein complex with tritium-labelled sodium borohydride. The peptide containing the derivatized lysine can therefore be detected either by fluorimetry, spectrophotometry or radiochemical techniques following routine procedures of proteolytic digestion and fractionation. Acid hydrolysis in 6 N HCl for 24 hr of peptides containing pyridoxal-5-phosphate lysine yields pyridoxyl-lysine since phosphate esters are readily hydrolyzed under these conditions. Pyridoxyl-lysine is eluted between lysine and histidine from a 55 cm column of Beckman 50 resin with 0.15 M citrate buffer *p*H 5.28.

Authentic pyridoxyl-lysine has been prepared by Schnackerz and Noltmann (1971) by borohydride reduction of a mixture of poly-L-lysine hydrochloride (20 mg) and 0.38 moles of pyridoxal, which had been allowed to stand for 10 min at 0°C in 50 mM sodium phosphate (*p*H 6.0). Low molecular weight impurities were removed by dialysis against 50 mM sodium acetate buffer (*p*H 6.0). After dialysis the resulting product can be hydrolyzed in 6 N HCl to yield pyridoxyl-lysine and some lysine. The latter contaminant can be minimized by

Subject index p. 201

reacting the partially pyridoxylated-polylysine for a second time prior to acid hydrolysis.

An alternative procedure which can provide analytically pure pyridoxyl-lysine involves the prior synthesis of ε-pyridoxyl-N-acetyl lysine (Dempsey and Snell, 1963). A mixture of 1.20 g of α-N-acetyl lysine and 470 mg of potassium hydroxide was dissolved in 20 ml of absolute methanol. Then 1.37 g of pyridoxal is added and the resulting mixture is stirred for 15 min at 25°C and filtered. 50 mg of PtO_2 is added and the solution is hydrogenated at room temperature at 1 atmosphere for 1 hr. After removal of catalyst by filtration, the *p*H of the filtrate is reduced to 6.0 (as measured by moist indicator paper) by the addition of methanolic HCl. Concentration of the reaction mixture to roughly one-third of its original volume causes precipitation of KCl which is then removed by filtration. When the apparent *p*H is decreased to about *p*H 4.4 by the addition of more methanolic HCl, the product precipitates and it can be collected and washed extensively with methanol. The yellow product, ε-pyridoxyl-α-N-acetyl lysine, melts at 174–174.5°C (Dempsey and Christensen, 1962).

Deacetylation was accomplished by treating 258 mg of the above product for 40 min with 5 ml of 6 N HCl at 121°C. The resulting was dried under reduced pressure and dissolved in water. After adjusting the *p*H to 7.0 with aqueous ammonia, the solution was evaporated to dryness again. The residue was dissolved in a little water and applied to a 0.9 × 30 cm column of resin XE-64 which had been previously equilibrated with 1 M ammonium formate *p*H 4.0 and washed with 250 ml of water. The column was washed with 850 ml of water after application of the sample followed by 70 ml of 0.72 M acetic acid to remove unhydrolyzed material. The ε-pyridoxyl lysine was eluted with 0.81 M acetic acid, and fractions containing the product were evaporated to dryness. On recrystallization of pyridoxyl-lysine from ethanol the yield was 110 mg of pale yellow crystals, m.p. 214–214.5°C. On paper chromatography in butanol:pyridine:acetic acid-H_2O (30:20:6:24 v/v) $R_f = 0.28$ (Ronchi et al. 1969).

Affinity labels

Affinity labels or active-site directed inhibitors represent a deliberate attempt to exploit the rate enhancements possible when a modification reagent forms a binary complex with the protein prior to covalent attachment. Because they are designed to be structurally similar to known substrates, inhibitors or ligands, affinity labels have a high probability of interacting tightly with the ligand-binding sites of a protein. In §4.1, we have presented a simple numerical analysis which demonstrated that the formation of even a weak binary complex prior to reaction led to a significantly enhanced rate of modification. Here we will demonstrate that if a very stable binary complex forms, the rate enhancement will be even more significant even if no pronounced orientation effects influence the magnitude of the first-order rate constant for covalent modification. For example, if the dissociation constant for the protein-modification reagent complex is 10^{-3} M in eq. (4.8) and the concentration of the modification reagent is equal to this dissociation constant, then this affinity labelling reagent, with only a modest affinity for the protein, would react 2500 times faster with an amino acid near its binding site than with the same amino acid in free solution, by a strict bimolecular mechanism.

This calculated rate acceleration is conservative since the ratio of 5 M presented in eq. (4.8) assumes no significant orientation effects. Rate ratios as high as 10^5 M have been found for a variety of intramolecular reactions. A careful study of a series of affinity labels for trypsin has revealed that the first order rate constants for reagents with comparable reactive groups vary by at least a factor of 5. The differences in these first order rate constants must reflect the difference in the

Subject index p. 201

orientation of the alkylating agent relative to the nucleophilic amino acid (Shaw 1970a).

5.1. Affinity labels versus group-specific reagents for site-specific modification

The significant advantages of affinity labels as opposed to functional group modification reagents for the site-specific modification of proteins are several. Although the syntheses required for all affinity labels are time-consuming, the likelihood that the compound will accomplish the chemical modification of its particular protein is reasonable. Even if the reagent is unsuccessful, it will provide a basis for the design of other labels. The failure to achieve site-specific modification with functional group-specific reagents is not very informative and does not suggest any new experiments.

The results of chemical modification experiments with affinity labels are far easier to interpret than those with functional group-specific reagents, even if a stoichiometric modification is achieved by both approaches. For example, the amino acid modified by an affinity-labelling reagent must be at or near the active site or ligand-binding site. An examination of the structure of the affinity label used should suggest whether the amino acid is involved in ligand binding or catalysis. By systematically varying the structure of the affinity label, additional amino acids may be modified and the relative orientation of the various derivatized residues can be inferred.

In this regard, implicit in the use of affinity labels for the modification of proteins is that all experiments should be attempted under conditions where the protein is biologically active and binds its specific ligands and/or substrates. Incubation of the affinity label with the protein under any other conditions may provide misleading information that will undermine the inherent information content of the technique. In all cases of affinity and photoaffinity labels which have been cited in this monograph, the protein has been incubated with the modification reagent under conditions of temperature, *p*H and ionic strength where the macromolecule was stable and active.

In contrast to affinity labelling, it is frequently difficult to prove if a side chain of an enzyme modified by a functional group-specific reagent is at the active site. One standard technique for demonstrating this is to show that substrates or known competitive inhibitors block the modification reaction. If they do, it is often concluded that the active site is modified. But this conclusion must be regarded as inferential and not conclusive. Designating the role of the amino acid in the active site, even assuming its location in this region of the enzyme, is even more tenuous. Possible roles, if any, of the modified residue may include binding the substrate or serving as one of the catalytic residues. No potential for the systematic variation of the structure of the group specific modification reagent exists to probe these questions.

All site-specific modifications provide valuable information for correlating the three-dimensional structure of a protein in the crystalline state and in solution. However, modifications by affinity labels are of greater potential value than group-specific reagents. In addition to unambiguously localizing the active site of an enzyme, affinity labels yield derivatized proteins which are uniquely useful materials for X-ray crystallographic analysis. Difference Fourier maps of subtilisin BPN′ (derived from *Bacillus subtilis* strain BPN′) derivatized with affinity labels have permitted a detailed analysis of the enzyme-substrate interactions not only near the active site serine but also in the entire substrate-binding groove (Robertus et al. 1972). Group specific reagents have no similar potential.

In addition, two important future directions of research in the chemical modification of proteins will include 1) labelling a specific protein in a multicomponent system in order to facilitate its isolation and/or localization within a membrane system; and 2) the use of irreversible inhibitors for pharmacological purposes. For each of these goals, affinity labelling is the only reasonable approach because of its high inherent specificity. Clearly the modification of the desired protein must proceed significantly more rapidly than the reaction with the free amino acid to avoid the generation of undesirable side products. The achievement of the necessary degree of kinetic differentiation with group specific reagents seems exceedingly improbable.

Subject index p. 201

5.2. *Reactive groups for affinity labels*

The design of affinity labels possesses two clearly defined components. The first is the choice of the basic structure with affinity for the protein of interest. The second is the selection of the reactive grouping that will be used for the covalent attachment to the enzyme. In the sections which follow, some common reactive groups will be discussed in terms of their reactivity, synthesis, and the nature of the possible products formed. Since the choice of the basic structural skeleton depends on the individual protein to be studied, this aspect of the design of affinity labels will not be considered here.

5.3. *Haloketones*

5.3.1 Haloketone derivatives of amino acids

The striking successes achieved by Shaw (1970a) and his coworkers with haloketone derivatives of N-tosyl-phenylalanine and α-N-tosyl-lysine as affinity labels for chymotrypsin and trypsin, respectively, have stimulated their use in a large number of affinity labels. Haloketones are potentially reactive with all the nucleophilic amino acid residues in proteins. Examples of residues modified by haloketones include methionine (Sigman et al. 1970), glutamate (Visser et al. 1971), cysteine (Porter et al. 1971), histidine (Schoellman and Shaw 1963) and serine (Schroeder and Shaw 1971).

Two synthetic approaches for the preparation of haloketones include halogenation and the acidification of the corresponding diazoketone with the appropriate halo acid. Direct halogenation is most appropriately performed only with bromine.

5.3.1.1. Synthesis of haloketones by bromination

An example of the synthesis of a bromoketone, *p*-guanido-phenacyl bromide hydrobromide, is provided by Schroeder and Shaw (1971). Various other phenacyl bromides are readily synthesized in an analogous fashion. For the synthesis, *p*-guanidinoacetophenone hydrochloride (2.6 g, 10 mmole) was suspended in 20 ml of glacial acetic acid containing 13% HBr and a solution of bromine in acetic acid (0.75 ml in 2.5 ml) was added to the vigorously stirred suspension. Within 10 min, the bromine color was discharged and solution was complete. After 2 hr, water was added and the mixture was taken to dryness; recrystallization of the residue from acetonitrile-ether gave 3.2 g (9.6 mmole) of *p*-guanidinophenacyl bromide hydrobromide, m.p. 181–183°C.

5.3.1.2. Synthesis of haloketones by acidification of diazoketones with haloacids

The synthesis of haloketones via their corresponding diazoketones is probably a more useful route for three reasons. They include 1) the fact that chloroketones as well as bromoketones can be readily prepared; 2) the potential for oxidation of the affinity label by bromine is eliminated; and 3) the radioactive form of the reagents can be readily synthesized using ^{14}C-diazomethane. The relevant synthetic route for the procedure is indicated in eq. (5.1).

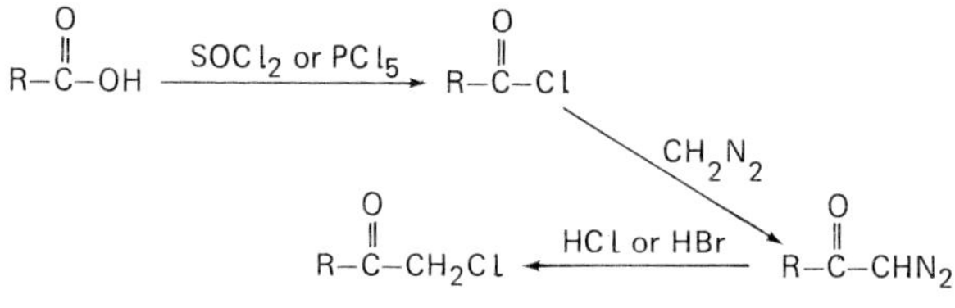

(5.1)

Various routes exist for the synthesis of the acid chlorides of amino acid derivatives. The following procedure for α-N-tosyl phenylalanyl chloride originated by Popenoe and Du Vignaud (1954) has been repeated by Schoellman and Shaw (1963) and also used by Visser et al. (1971) for the synthesis of N-tosyl-L-alanyl chloride. Phosphorus pentachloride (3.90 g) was added to 5.4 g of tosyl-L-phenylalanine suspended in 75 ml of anhydrous ether at 0°C. The mixture was shaken for 10 min at 0°C, then for 10 min at room temperature and finally stored at 0°C for 1 hr. The crystalline product was filtered off, washed on the funnel quickly with a little ether and then with ice-water and dried for 2 hr in a vacuum desiccator. The yield was 5.07 g (88 %) of a product which melted with decomposition at 128–129°C.

One general synthetic difficulty in the preparation of acid chlorides of amino acids, particularly those in which the α-NH_2 is protected by acylation, is the formation of azlactones. Tosyl derivatives partially avoid this difficulty.

Synthesis of diazoketones: The synthesis of diazoketones of α-N-tosyl alanine by Visser et al. (1971) was performed using ethereal diazomethane generated by the method of Arndt (1943). It proceeded as follows. A solution of tosyl-L-alanyl chloride (3.9 g, 15 mmoles) in 100 ml of anhydrous ether was added dropwise to a gently stirred (Teflon bar) anhydrous ether solution at 0°C containing 30 mmoles of diazomethane*. The resulting solution was stirred for about 45 min, then left at room temperature overnight. The ether was removed under a stream of dry nitrogen; the residue redissolved in ether and evaporated. The infrared spectrum of the yellow syrup has a strong band at 2100 cm^{-1} which is diagnostic of the diazo (C=N=N) stretching frequency (Bellamy 1956). Attempts to crystallize it were unsuccessful, but elution from a silica gel column with chloroform followed by ethyl acetate gave two 360-nm absorbing fractions. The first fraction eluted with $CHCl_3$ had infrared characteristics compatible with an N-methyl derivative of I

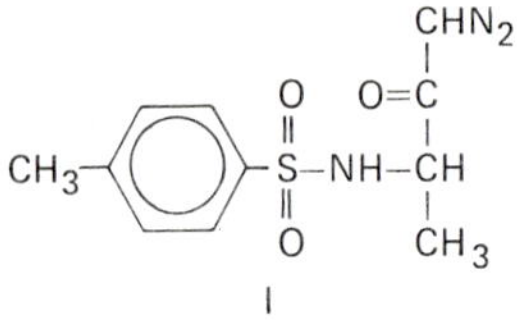

I

while the second fraction had an infrared spectrum consistent with the diazoketone. This procedure underscores the fact that one hazard of the synthetic approach using diazomethane is the prevalence of insertion reactions, especially into N-H bonds. It further stresses the

* Diazomethane is both poisonous and explosive.

importance of the infrared band in the region of 2100 cm^{-1} to prove the structure of diazoketones.

Preparation of diazomethane: The ethereal solution of diazomethane used in the above synthesis was prepared in the following way (Arndt 1943). The virtue of this procedure is that it is rapid and easy. However, it does not provide a fully anhydrous solution.

To 100 cc of ether is added 30 cc of 40% potassium hydroxide, and the mixture is cooled to 5°C. To this two-phase system with continued cooling and shaking is added 10 g of finely powdered nitrosomethylurea in small portions over a period of 1–2 min. The deep yellow ether layer can be decanted readily; it contains about 2.8 g of diazomethane, together with some dissolved impurities and water. The water may be removed by drying for 3 hr over pellets of pure potassium hydroxide. Solutions of diazomethane in benzene and other water-immiscible organic solvents may be prepared in the same way.

The following procedure has been used by Hartmann (1963) to prepare alcohol-free ^{14}C-diazomethane in about 60–65% yield. N-Methyl-C^{14}-N-nitroso-*p*-toluenesulfonamide (22 mg, 0.103 mmole, 0.1 mC of C^{14}) was dissolved in 1 ml of anhydrous, peroxide-free diethyl ether in a 5-ml distilling flask fitted with a gas inlet tube. The side arm was bent vertically downward near the top and connected through a two-holed rubber stopper to a 10-ml Erlenmeyer flask. A tube from the second hole led to the back of the hood. The latter flask was cooled in a Dry-Ice-Cellosolve bath. With the reaction flask at room temperature, 1 ml of a solution of 10 mg of sodium metal in dry *n*-octyl alcohol was added all at once. The gas inlet tube was immediately connected and a slow stream of dry nitrogen was passed through the system. The temperature of the mixture was then raised to 70°C in an oil bath and the ^{14}C-diazomethane was flushed into the cooled collection flask for about 15 min. A further 1 ml of ether was then added through the gas inlet tube and collection was continued until the distillation of the ether was complete. Use of ^{14}C-diazomethane represents the most general method for the introduction of radioactivity into a haloketone.

Acidification of diazoketones: The conversion of the diazoketone into a chloroketone is usually routine. Schoellman and Shaw (1963), in their synthesis of the chloromethyl ketone derived from phenylalanine, prepared an ethereal solution of the corresponding diazoketone and then treated it with dry HCl for 2 hr. The chloroketone could then be isolated following the removal of solvent. Visser et al. (1971) added concentrated HCl to an ethyl acetate solution of the diazoketone derivative of N-tosyl alanine until the evolution of nitrogen ceased. Removal of solvent, followed by crystallization from chloroform-heptane yielded an analytically pure product. A carbonyl absorption in the region of 1720 cm^{-1} is diagnostic of haloketones.

5.3.2. *Amino acid derivatives formed by haloketones*

The identification of the amino acid residue modified by haloketones often represents a challenging problem. In fact, one inherent limitation in the use of most affinity labels is that authentic samples of the various amino acid derivatives formed are not readily available since the syntheses from the free amino acids and the affinity label are not simple.

5.3.2.1. *Histidine*

The derivatives of histidine formed by haloketones are probably generally stable to acid hydrolysis. At the very least, histidine is not regenerated following hydrolysis in 6 N HCl for 20 hr. Stevenson and Smillie (1965) in their studies of the modification of chymotrypsin by the chloromethyl ketone of N-tosyl phenylalanine or compound II have shown that oxidation by vapors of performic acid for 2 hr of peptides derivatized by the above reagents yields 3-carboxymethyl

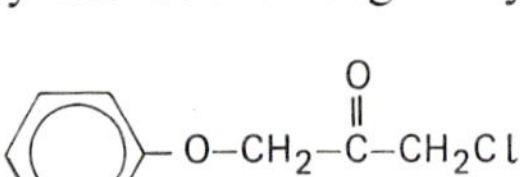

II

histidine. Since this amino acid derivative can be readily identified chromatographically (§ 2.8.1), this procedure might be generally useful in the analysis of chemical modifications by haloketones. It is capable of distinguishing alkylation at N-1 or N-3 of the imidazole side chain of histidine.

5.3.2.2. *Methionine*

The derivatives of methionine formed by haloketones are not stable to the usual conditions of acid hydrolysis. These sulfonium salts are degraded in three different ways. Some methionine is regenerated, some homoserine and homoserine lactone is formed and possibly the homocysteine derivative of the general structure indicated below is produced where X represents the rest of the affinity label.

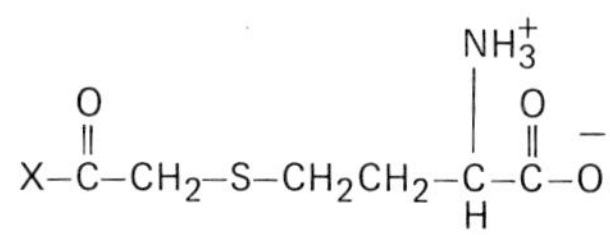

The degradation product of the sulfonium salt formed in the greatest yield after acid hydrolysis is undoubtedly a function of the structure of the affinity label. Generally, if the total amino acid composition of the modified protein was determined, low yields of methionine and increased yield of homoserine would be indicative, but certainly not proof of, the modification of a methionine residue. Sulfonium salts of methionine are generally not oxidized by hydrogen peroxide (Sigman and Blout 1967).

5.3.2.3. *Serine*

The derivatives of serine formed by haloketones are stable to acid hydrolysis. The resulting ether linkage is apparently not cleaved by the usual hydrolytic conditions so that the loss of a serine residue, if it can be accurately determined, can be used as evidence for the modification of a serine residue (Schroeder and Shaw 1971).

5.3.2.4. *Aspartate and glutamate*

The esters formed when haloketones react with glutamate or aspartate residue are not stable to acid hydrolysis. The glutamate or aspartate residues are quantitatively regenerated. An elegant procedure which both proves that an aspartate or glutamate has been modified and can determine which of these amino acids has been derivatized involves treatment of a protein containing a side-chain aspartate or glutamate ester successively with hydroxylamine, dinitrofluorobenzene and alkali. This sequence of steps leads to the conversion of a glutamate or aspartate residue into diaminobutyric or diaminopropionic acid, respectively. These two basic amino acids can be readily identified on the amino acid analyzer after acid hydrolysis. The Lossen rearrangement forms the basis of this procedure.

Such a procedure adapted from Gross and Morell (1966) and Blumenfeld and Gallop (1962) is as follows. Visser et al. (1971) treated 2.5 to 10 mg of a modified elastase with 1 N NH_2OH–HCl, adjusted to *p*H 9 by addition of sodium hydroxide, for 2 hr at 25°C. The excess hydroxylamine was removed either by dialysis or by precipitation of the protein at *p*H 3.0. The protein was then dissolved, brought to *p*H 8.0 by addition of NaOH and treated with an equal volume of a 1% solution of 1-fluoro-2,4-dinitrobenzene in ethanol. The *p*H of the solution was maintained at 8 by the continuous addition of NaOH. The reaction is complete when no additional alkali must be added for 5 min. The mixture is then extracted three times with ether and the aqueous phase subjected to the conditions of the Lossen rearrangement (i.e. heating to 100°C under alkaline condition (0.1 N NaOH) for 10 min). Acid hydrolysis followed by amino acid analysis permits the identification of either diaminopropionic or diaminobutyric acid which would result from either aspartate or glutamate modification, respectively. Diaminopropionic and diaminobutyric acids may be estimated on the short column of the amino acid analyzer. Diaminopropionic acid emerges with histidine. (Color values do not seem to be available.)

5.3.2.5. *Cysteine*

Several sulfhydryl enzymes have been modified specifically by haloketones. They include clostripain, papain, ficin, and bromelain (Porter et al. 1971; Whitaker and Perez-Villaseñor 1968; Stein and Liener 1967; Murachi and Kato 1967). For these enzymes, the chloromethylketone of N-tosyl-phenylalanine and N-tosyl-lysine were used as the site-specific modification reagents. The derivatives formed by the alkylation of cysteine by haloketones do not regenerate cysteine upon acid hydrolysis. Therefore, the evidence for cysteine modification primarily rests on the loss of cysteine subsequent to protein hydrolysis. At present, the isolation of a cysteine derivatized by a haloketone has not yet been accomplished. All the present evidence for cysteine as the site of modification by these alkylating agents has been based on the loss of the cysteine residue as determined by amino acid analysis or by one of the several spectrophotometric titrimetric methods discussed in ch. 3.

5.4. Amides and esters of haloacids

Amides and esters of haloacids have been frequently used in the synthesis of affinity labels. Like haloketones, these derivatives react with all the nucleophilic amino acids. Their advantages as modification reagents are two-fold. First, they are relatively more easy to synthetize than haloketones. Any substrate or reversible inhibitor with a free amino or hydroxyl group can be potentially converted into an affinity labelling reagent. Second upon acid hydrolysis, the modified protein yields carboxymethylated derivatives which are known and therefore readily identifiable and quantifiable.

5.4.1. Synthesis of amides of haloacids

Several routes exist for the synthesis of amides of halo acids. Cuatrecasas et al. (1969) used two different bromoacetylating reagents in the synthesis of water soluble inhibitors of staphylococcal nuclease. The N-hydroxysuccinimide ester of bromoacetate was one of the reagents used. It is particularly useful for the synthesis of radioactive derivatives since ^{14}C-bromoacetic acid is commercially available. Synthesis of the hydroxysuccininimide ester is accomplished by dissolving 87 mg (630 μmoles) of bromoacetic acid and 86 mg of N-hydroxysuccinimide in 3 ml of dioxane. To this solution, 132 mg (700 μmoles) of dicyclohexylcarbodiimide is added. Urea precipitates immediately and after 1 hr, is removed. The solution of bromoacetyl N-hydroxysuccinimide ester is brought to 5 ml. It can then be used without any further purification.

The synthesis of the water-soluble irreversible inhibitor deoxythymidine bromoacetyl-5-*p*-aminophenylphosphate (III) from the

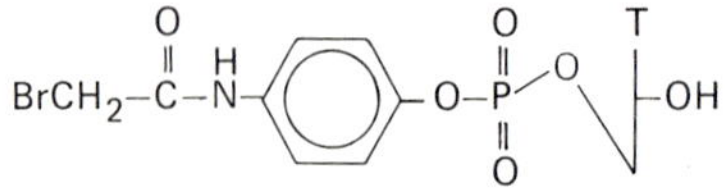

III

corresponding aminophenyl phosphate derivative was accomplished as follows: 50 μmoles of the aminophenyl ester were dissolved in 0.3 ml of water and 0.7 ml of dioxane, and 1 ml (125 μmoles) of the stock solution of O-^{14}C-bromoacetyl-N-hydroxysuccinimide ester was added. After 3 hr, 1 volume of water was added, and the solution was extracted 5 times with ether and concentrated to dryness. The product was dissolved in methanol and precipitated with ether. Yields were 90% and the compound was chromatographically pure on thin layer chromatography using 2-propanol:NH_4OH:H_2O (7:1:2) and 1-butanol:acetic acid:water (5:2:4).

Bromoacetic anhydride was the second bromoacetylating reagent used by Cuatrecasas et al. (1969). In order to synthesize bromoacetyl *p*-aminophenylphosphate, they dissolved 100 μmoles of the corresponding aminophenyl derivative in 1 ml of water and then added 2 ml of dioxane containing 420 μmoles of bromoacetic anhydride. One volume of water was added after 1 hr and the mixture was then extracted several times with ether. The aqueous solution was concentrated to dryness, dissolved in methanol and precipitated with ether. Yields were reported to be quantitative and the compounds were chromatographically pure.

An alternative method for preparing derivatives of bromoacetate involves using bromoacetyl bromide or bromoacetyl chloride. The synthesis of the N-bromoacetyl derivative of L-arginine methyl ester with bromoacetyl bromide was carried out by Liu (1967). The product N-bromoacetyl-L-arginine methyl ester was a successful affinity label for streptococcal proteinase. L-Arginine methyl ester dihydrochloride (780 mg 3 mmoles) was dissolved in 6 ml of ice-cold 1 N $NaHCO_3$. Over a period of 20 min, freshly distilled bromoacetylbromide, 3 mmoles, was added. During the course of the addition and for 30 min thereafter, the solution was stirred and maintained between *p*H 8.4 and 8.6 by the addition of N $NaHCO_3$. At this point, the entire reaction mixture was placed on a Sephadex G-10 column and eluted with 0.1 N acetic acid at 4°C. A fraction was obtained which was Sakaguchi positive and ninhydrin negative. It was lyophilized and shown to be homogeneous by paper electrophoresis at *p*H 6.15. Elemental analysis demonstrated that it was N-bromoacetyl-L-arginine methyl ester.

Bromoacetyl derivatives of free amino acids can be prepared in a comparable manner. Product in this case can be readily precipitated by acidification of the reaction mixture to *p*H 2.0 with 1 N HCl.

5.4.2. Synthesis of esters of haloacids

Chase and Tubbs (1969) prepared the bromoacetate ester of carnitine by taking the appropriate enantiomer of carnitine chloride, dissolving it in bromoacetic acid at 53°C and heating it with an excess of bromoacetyl bromide for 4 hr. Excess bromoacetic acid and bromoacetyl bromide was removed by distillation *in vacuo*. The residue was dissolved in absolute ethanol and precipitated by ether. The derivatives can be recrystallized from butanol.

The following procedure is useful for preparing ^{14}C-bromoacetyl chloride. (1-^{14}C)Bromoacetyl chloride was prepared by Hass and Neurath (1971a) by dissolving 693 mg of bromoacetic acid in 20 ml of anhydrous ether and then adding 1.0 gram of phosphorus pentachloride. After all the PCl_5 had dissolved (about 1 hr) the solution was evaporated on a rotatory evaporator at 30°C.

5.4.3. Analysis of acid hydrolysis products

As already pointed out, the chief advantage of using derivatives of haloacetates as modification reagents is that the carboxymethyl derivatives of most of the nucleophilic amino acids have been described. The chromatographic behavior of the carboxymethylated derivatives of lysine, cysteine and histidine have been described in ch. 2. O-Carboxymethyl tyrosine appears as a single peak in the long column of the amino acid analyzer, located between valine and the breakthrough of the second buffer.

An additional product of acid hydrolysis with affinity labels containing haloacid groups is glycolic acid. This product would be expected from the esterification of either glutamate or aspartate. Takahashi et al. (1967) have found that the hydrolysis of the carboxymethyl ester of glutamate in 6 N HCl at 110°C for 23 hr yields 1.0 eq. of glutamic acid and 0.6 eq. of glycolic acid. Since glycolic acid itself is only recovered to the extent of 60 % after its incubation under identical conditions, hot 6 N HCl must transform glycolic acid into some other product, possibly chloroacetic acid. Glycolic acid emerges at 25–26 ml from the 50 cm column of the amino acid analyzer from which cysteic acid emerges at 14 ml (Hass and Neurath 1971b). Therefore if a radioactive haloacetate derivative is used initially, the production of glycolic acid can be readily monitored.

A chemical method for the determination of glycolic acid has been reported by Takahashi et al. (1967). It is carried out as follows. Glycolic acid (1–50 nmoles) is added to a test tube and if the volume of the solution exceeds 50 μl it is evaporated to dryness. This step is essential since water interferes with color development. One ml of a freshly prepared solution of 2,7-dihydroxynaphthalene (0.01 % in concentrated sulfuric acid) is then added. The color development is accomplished by heating the test tube in boiling water for 20 min. The absorption at 540 nm, which is stable for several hours, is then read against a reagent blank. The color produced is linear up to 50 nmoles of glycolic acid and 10 nmoles of the standard gave an absorbance of 0.226 per cm.

5.5. *Epoxides*

Epoxide (3-member cyclic ether) groups are effective broad-spectrum alkylating agents which have not as yet received a great deal of attention in the design of affinity labels. Their reactions with proteins were first studied by Fraenkel-Conrat (1944) who found that they reacted with the basic forms of most nucleophiles in proteins. Their chief advantage relative to haloketones and haloacid derivatives is that they are smaller so that steric hindrance may not be as significant a problem in their reactions with proteins.

One of the chief drawbacks of epoxides is that it is difficult to predict the structure of the derivative which might be formed with the various nucleophilic amino acid residues. All epoxides incorporated into affinity labels will have the general structure (IV). Nucleophiles can therefore react at either of the carbon atoms and since it is generally unlikely that the *R′* and *R″* will be identical, the formation of at least two types of derivatives might be expected.

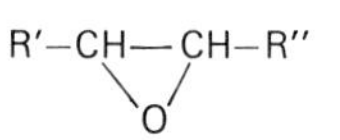

IV

Since epoxides are very sensitive to acid-catalyzed nucleophilic attack, whichever carbon will yield the most stable carbonium ion will be the most likely target for nucleophilic attack if an acidic group on the protein facilitates the modification reaction by hydrogen bonding to the epoxide. On the other hand, epoxides are also subject to S_N-2 displacement reactions. In this case the carbon which will be attacked will be the least sterically hindered of the two. Unfortunately, there is no *a priori* way to know the mechanism of the modification reaction so that if an affinity label containing an epoxide group derivatizes a protein at least two possible products must be anticipated.

Examples of epoxides which have been used as affinity labels include compounds V–VIII.

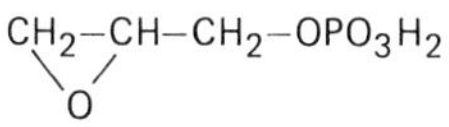

V

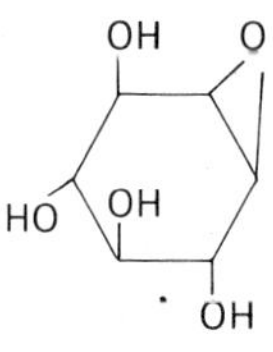

VI

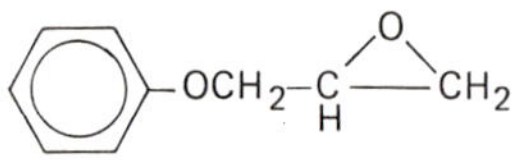

VII

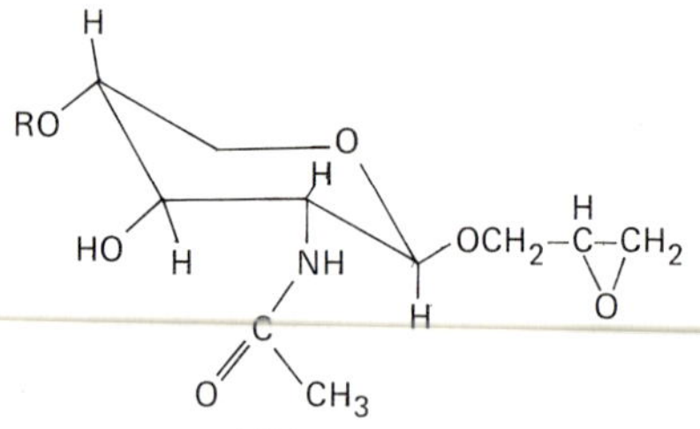

VIII

Compound V or glycidol phosphate was used by Rose and O'Connell (1969) to study muscle triosephosphate isomerase because it closely resembles the presumed ene-diol intermediate in this enzyme's reaction mechanism. Coincidentally, it also proved to be an effective inhibitor of enolase even though it is not closely analogous to substrates of this enzyme. The structure of glycidol phosphate is similar to phosphononomycin (IX), an antibiotic isolated from fermentation broths of *Streptomyces fradiae* (Christensen et al. 1969).

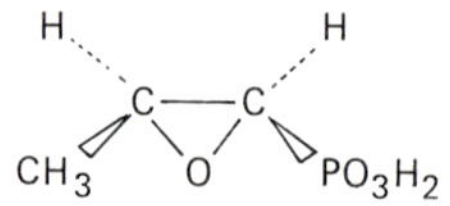

IX

5.5.1. Synthesis

5.5.1.1. Synthesis of glycidol phosphate from glycidol

Glycidol phosphate was synthesized by phosphorylation of commercially available glycidol with $POCl_3$ in trimethylphosphate with added N, N-dimethylaniline to prevent ring opening which occurs with Cl^- at acid *p*H. A solution of 1 mmole of DL-glycidol in 0.5 ml of trimethylphosphate was added to a solution of 0.5 ml trimethylphosphate, 0.25 ml of dimethylaniline and 1 mmole of $POCl_3$ which had previously been cooled to 0°C. The mixture was kept for 1 hr at 0°C, and then added dropwise to 10 ml of cold water; NaOH (2 N) was used to maintain the *p*H range 5–9 during this addition. The final *p*H was adjusted to 7 and then dimethylaniline was extracted twice with ether

(6 ml). Barium acetate (1 M, 2 ml) was added to the aqueous solution and the precipitate which formed was discarded. Ethanol (2.5 vols) was added and the precipitated barium salt of glycidol phosphate was collected after 30 min at 0°C. The material could be recrystallized by dissolving in 10 ml of water, removing any precipitate, and then adding ethanol at 30°C until crystals began to form. The crystals were harvested after standing in the cold overnight. The resulting glycidol phosphate had the strong characteristic I.R. adsorption peaks of an epoxide at 830, 915 and 1255 cm^{-1}.

5.5.1.2. Synthesis of epoxides from alkenes

The 2′,3′-epoxypropyl β-glycoside of di(N-acetyl-D-glucosamine) where *R* is N-acetyl glucosamine specifically inactivates hen lysozyme and several other bird lysozymes (Maron et al. 1972). The residue of hen lysozyme specifically modified by VIII is asp. 52 (Eshdat et al. 1973). X-ray analysis reveals that the two glucosamine residues of the affinity label occupy subsites B and C of the substrate binding cleft (Moult et al. 1973). The synthesis of the affinity label was accomplished by the most general procedure for the synthesis of epoxides, namely oxidation of alkenes with peroxyacids.

The starting materials for the synthesis of the various derivatives used in these studies were the appropriate allyl glycosides which have the general structure indicated in (X). Allyl derivatives may be the most general precursor for the synthesis of epoxides. The various allyl glycosides were synthesized by the following procedure of Thomas (1970) for allyl-2-acetamido-3,4-6-tri-0-acetyl-2-deoxy-β-D-glycopyra-

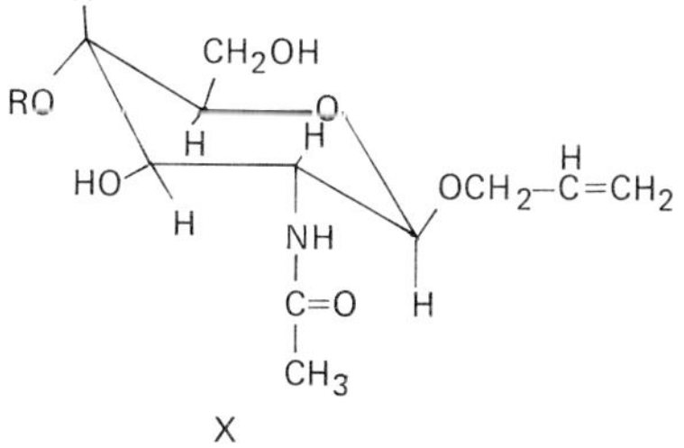

X

noside. Dry allyl alcohol (150 ml), silver carbonate (4.25 g), and powdered anhydrous calcium sulphate (15 g) were stirred with exclusion of light and moisture for 2 hr. 2-Acetamido-3,4,6-tri-0-acetyl-2-deoxy-α-D-glucosyl chloride (5.6 g) and silver perchlorate (200 mg) were added, and stirring was continued for 6 hr. The mixture was then filtered through Celite, the filtrate evaporated to dryness, and the residue dissolved in methylene chloride. After washing with N HCl, 10% aqueous $KHCO_3$, and water, the organic layer was dried ($MgSO_4$) and evaporated to a colorless syrup which crystallized on triturating with propan-2-ol. Recrystallization from methanol-ether gave material (3.5 g, 52%) having m.p. 160°C, $[\alpha]_D^{23}$ −15.1°C (*c* 2.06, chloroform).

The appropriate allyl glycoside (1 mmole) for the various affinity labels was dissolved in methylene chloride (10 ml) containing peroxyphthalic acid (*ca.* 2 mmoles), and the solution was refluxed gently for 3 hr. After cooling to 0°C, phthalic acid was filtered off, and the filtrate was extracted twice with cold 0.5 M $KHCO_3$ and twice with water. After drying ($MgSO_4$) and evaporation, the corresponding epoxide (essentially one component as shown by thin-layer chromatography) was crystallized from methanol-ether.

As a guide to the stability of epoxides, the procedure used for the deacetylation of the above glycosides is presented. The appropriate epoxypropyl glycoside was suspended in dry methanol (10% w/v) with rapid magnetic stirring, and treated with methanolic barium methoxide to give a final concentration of 0.02 M. After dissolution, precipitation of the O-deacetylated products began within 5 min. After 12 hr at 3°C, the solids were collected, and crystallized from aqueous acetone.

Ross (1950) has provided a simple procedure to determine the reactivity of epoxides which may be useful in monitoring their stability if they are to be used in affinity labels. Addition of an epoxide to a neutralized solution of 0.2 M sodium thiosulfate in 50% acetone containing phenolphtalein followed by heating causes the generation of a pink color which can be reversed by addition of 0.2 N acetic acid from a burette. When no further OH^- is produced upon heating, the volume of acetic acid used is a measure of the titer of epoxide present.

According to Ross (1950), the half-life of epoxides in water is about 100 hr. Acid catalyzed decomposition reactions do not take place rapidly until the *p*H is below 4.2.

5.5.2. *Analysis of products*

Since epoxides potentially will react with a variety of amino acids, many products may be formed if they are incorporated into affinity labels. However at present affinity labels containing epoxides have been shown to modify either glutamate or aspartate residues in pepsin, lysozyme, triose phosphate isomerase and β-glucosidase. The only other residue which has as yet been modified by epoxides is methionine 192 of chymotrypsin. In general, the other possible products should be similar in stability to derivatives formed by haloketones. Therefore the methods for identification of the amino acid derivatives formed by reaction with epoxides closely parallel those described in connection with haloketones (§ 5.3.2).

5.6. *Sulfonyl fluorides*

Sulfonyl fluorides have been used extensively in the design of affinity labels for two types of enzyme systems – serine esterases and proteases and dihydrofolate reductase. Sulfonyl fluorides are significantly less reactive than sulfonyl chlorides in general base catalyzed reactions and in non-specific sulfonylations of nucleophilic amino acid residues. Yet they still are sufficiently good sulfonylating reagents to be attractive groups to incorporate into affinity labels. The initial important work calling attention to their potential value was that of Fahrney and Gold (1963) who demonstrated that sulfonyl fluorides were potent specific modification reagents for chymotrypsin.

5.6.1. *Synthesis of phenylmethylsulfonyl fluoride*

The following procedure was used by Gold and Fahrney (1964) to prepare ^{14}C-phenylmethanesulfonyl fluoride. It illustrates both a route for the preparation of sulfonyl chlorides as well as a method of converting sulfonyl chlorides into sulfonyl fluorides. To 105 mg of (7-^{14}C)benzyl chloride (0.83 mmoles) (specific activity, 1.20 mc/mmole),

Subject index p. 201

1 ml of methanol and 70 mg of thiourea (0.92 mmoles) were added. Following a reflux period of 30 min, the methanol was evaporated in a stream of nitrogen. Water (4 ml) was added to the residue, the mixture was magnetically stirred, and then cooled to 5°C. Chlorine gas was then passed through the stirred aqueous solution. The resulting phenylmethanesulfonyl chloride was collected after 5 min on a sintered glass funnel, washed with ice water and dried overnight *in vacuo* over NaOH pellets.

The conversion of the sulfonyl chloride to the sulfonyl fluoride was carried out as follows. The sulfonyl chloride was removed from the filter by washing it with alcohol-free chloroform into a 5-ml round-bottom flask. The chloroform was then removed and 0.5 ml of aceto-nitrile and 167 mg of dry powdered sodium fluoride was added. The resulting mixture was magnetically stirred at 90°C for 6 hr, 2 ml of alcohol-free chloroform was then added and the mixture was filtered into a sublimation apparatus and the solvent was removed in a stream of nitrogen. The product sublimed readily at 45°C (0.3 mm) and could then be recrystallized from benzene-cyclohexane to yield crystals with m.p. 90–92°C.

An alternate procedure for preparing sulfonyl chlorides is to stir the corresponding free sulfonic acid or hydrated sodium salt with thionyl chloride for 2–4 hr at 50°C. Conversion to the corresponding sulfonyl fluoride can be accomplished as indicated above in the synthesis of phenylmethylsulfonyl fluoride.

An alternate method of converting sulfonyl chlorides to sulfonyl fluorides has been reported by Sigler et al. (1966) in the synthesis of benzene sulfonylfluoride. Benzenesulfonyl chloride (18 g, 0.1 mole) was dissolved in 100 ml of acetone and then mixed vigorously at room temperature for 4 hr with 100 ml of aqueous 4 M potassium fluoride. On evaporation of the acetone, the pale yellow liquid product separates. It can be dried after dissolution in methylene chloride over anhydrous $MgSO_4$ and then distilled as a colorless oil (b.p. 63–67°C/6–7 mm).

5.6.2. Synthesis of sulfanilyl fluorides

Baker and his colleagues have prepared a series of sulfonyl fluorides as affinity labels for dihydrofolate reductase. The sulfonyl fluoride was attached to an aromatic nucleus with high affinity for the active site of this enzyme. The goal of these studies was to achieve modification of an amino acid residue which was remote from the active site (Baker 1969).

One group of compounds prepared had the general structure of XIV which could be synthesized by the indicated route. As presented in the synthetic scheme, the sulfonyl fluoride moiety was introduced as

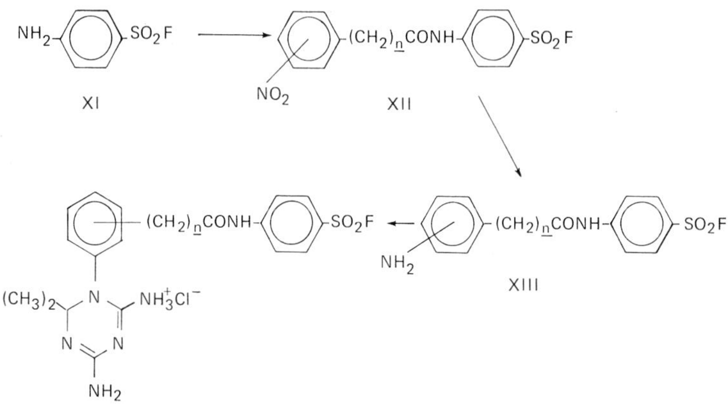

sulfanilyl fluoride which is commercially available or can be readily prepared (DeCat and Von Pouche 1963). The steps for the synthesis of N-(m-(4,6 diamino-1,2-dihydro-2,2 dimethyl-s-triazinyl)-benzoyl) sulfanilyl fluoride hydrochloride (XIV) where $n=0$ are indicated mostly to illustrate the stability of the sulfonyl fluoride group with respect to acid hydrolysis and to reduction by hydrogen using Raney nickel as catalyst.

The synthesis of N-(m-nitrobenzoyl)sulfanilyl fluoride (XII, $n=0$) by Baker and Lourens (1967) was performed as follows. A mixture of 1.75 g (10 mmoles) of sulfanilyl fluoride (XI), 1.86 g (10 mmoles) of *m*-nitrobenzoyl chloride, and 50 ml of xylene was refluxed for 2 hr during which time about 15 ml of the xylene was allowed to distill and HCl was evolved. The mixture was cooled, the product was collected by filtration, then washed with xylene. Recrystallization from EtOAc-petroleum ether (b.p. 30–60°C) gave 2.32 g (72%) of buff crystals, m.p. 216–217°C.

The same authors synthesized N-(*m*-aminobenzoyl)sulfanilyl fluoride (XIII, $n=0$) in the following manner. A suspension of 1.95 g (6 mmoles) of (XII, $n=0$) and 1 g of Raney nickel (Grace Co.) in 100 ml of EtOH was shaken with H_2 at 2–3 atm until 18 mmoles of H_2 was absorbed (20 min). The solution was filtered through a celite pad and the filter cake was washed (EtOH). The combined filtrate and washings were concentrated to about 10 ml on the rotary evaporator and then diluted (H_2O) and cooled. The solid product was collected and recrystallized from aqueous EtOH; yield, 1.00 g (57%) of buff crystals, m.p. 200–204°C dec.

The last step in the synthesis of the affinity label XIV involved the following steps. A mixture of 589 mg (2 mmoles) of XIII, 185 mg (2.2 mmoles) of cyanoguanidine, 15 ml of reagent acetone, and 0.18 ml of 12 N HCl was refluxed with stirring for 24 hr, during which time the product crystallized from the solution. The cooled mixture was filtered and the product was washed with acetone. Recrystallization from ethanol gave 380 mg (42%) of white crystals, m.p. 231–233°C dec.

5.6.3. *Analysis of products*

Sulfonyl fluorides have so far been reported to react at only two amino acid residues, cysteine and serine. The chemical evidence for the reaction of phenylmethylsulfonyl fluoride at the reactive cysteine of papain is indirect (Whitaker and Perez-Villaseñor 1968). However, the strong chemical evidence for the attack of phenylmethane sulfonyl fluoride at the serine of chymotrypsin (Gold and Fahrney 1964) has been confirmed by the X-ray crystallographic structure of tosyl-chymotrypsin (Matthews et al. 1967) which had been prepared from tosyl fluoride (Sigler et al. 1966).

Generally sulfonyl esters of serine are relatively stable with respect to reactivation by a nucleophile such as hydroxylamine (Alexander et al. 1963). However, treatment of the sulfonyl derivatives of chymotrypsin with 0.1 N NaOH at 0°C yields a dehydroalanine residue in place of a serine and the anhydrochymotrypsin residue thus formed is completely inactive (Strumeyer et al., 1963). Baker (1969) has assumed that the sulfonyl fluorides used as inhibitors of dihydrofolate reductase react at a serine residue, but this contention has not yet been proved.

5.7. *Diazo compound–aryl diazonium salts*

Various types of diazo linkages have been used as the reactive group for affinity labels. At present, only the light-independent reactions of diazo derivatives will be discussed. The recent application of diazo derivatives as photoreactive affinity labels is discussed in § 6.1.1. The reactive diazo cation (XV) can only be isolated when attached to a benzene ring. Alkyl systems are too unstable to be isolated. However, the same group appears as the charged resonance form of certain

$$\mathrm{R{-}\overset{+}{N}{\equiv}N{:}}$$

XV

neutral diazo compounds such as α-diazoketones or diazoacetyl derivatives. For example, resonance structures of diazoketones can be written as indicated in eq. (5.2).

$$\mathrm{R{-}\overset{\overset{\displaystyle O}{\|}}{C}{-}CH{=}\overset{+}{N}{=}\overline{N}{:}} \longleftrightarrow \mathrm{R{-}\overset{\overset{\ominus}{\overset{\displaystyle O}{|}}}{C}{=}CH{-}\overset{+}{N}{\equiv}N} \qquad (5.2)$$

5.7.1. *Reactive properties of aryl diazonium salts*

Aryl diazonium cations are electrophilic reagents and appear to react predominantly with four types of amino acids – lysine, tyrosine, histidine and cysteine. Although the precise structure of the cysteine derivatives is unclear, aryl diazonium salts can react with lysine, histidine and tyrosine as indicated in eq. (5.3) below to give the various substituted derivatives.

Each of the monosubstituted amino acids can react with a second mole of diazonium salt to give the derivatives XVI, XVII and XVIII. However, if the diazonium salt is incorporated into an affinity label,

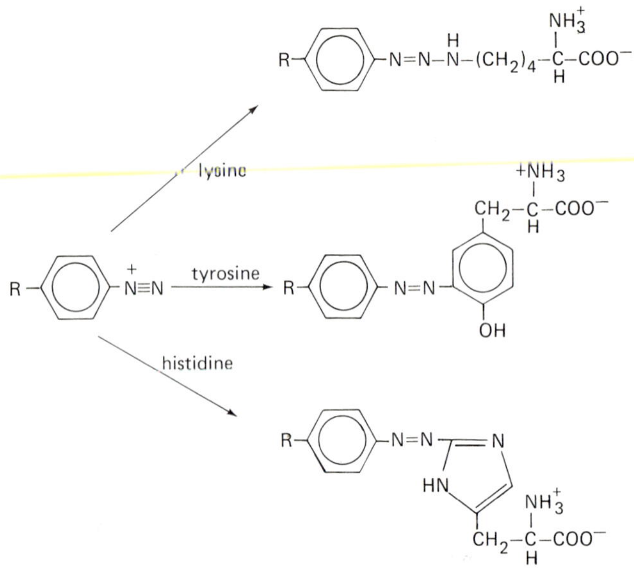

(5.3)

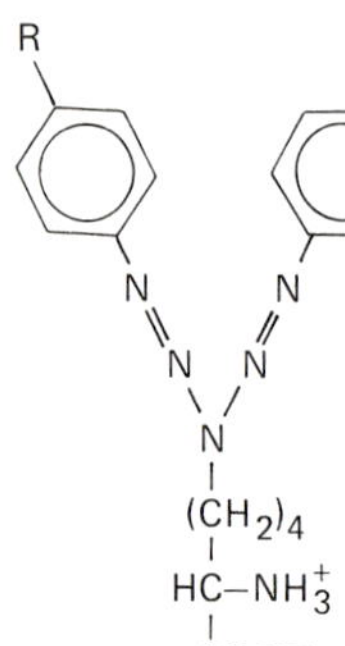

XVI

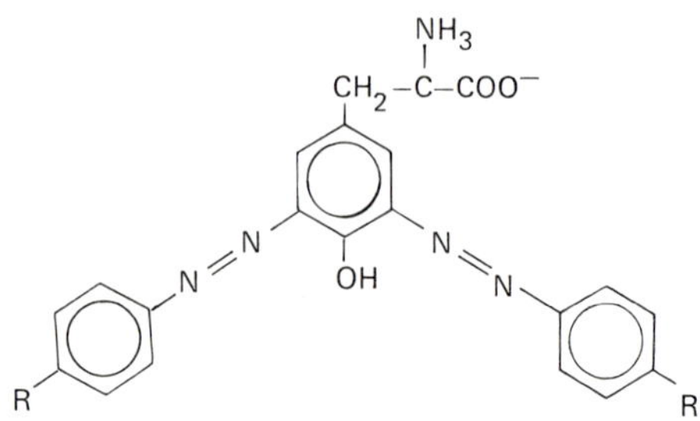

XVII

steric constraints may inhibit, to a large extent, the second substitution reaction.

The monazo and bisazo derivatives of lysine, tyrosine, and histidine are unstable to acid hydrolysis and the native amino acids are not regenerated. Therefore, the best method to quantitate the extent of derivatization is with radioactive reagent. The characteristic absorp-

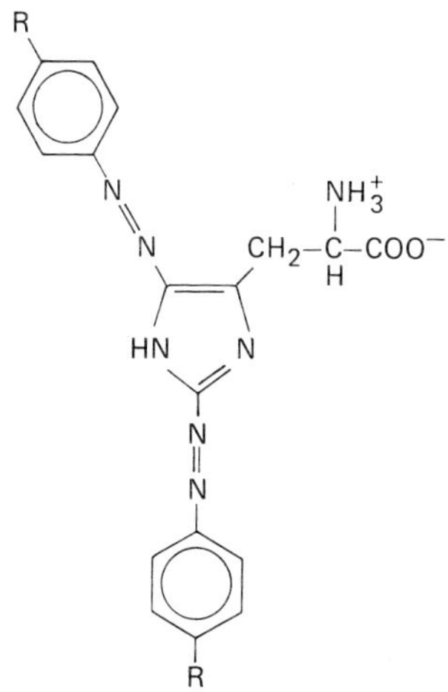

XVIII

tion spectra of the histidine and tyrosine derivatives can be used to determine which of these two residues have been modified if appropriate model compounds comprising each of the amino acids and the various diazonium salts used as affinity labels are prepared. On the other hand, it is probably risky to use the absorption spectrum of the modified protein to determine the extent of reaction, since it is not necessarily a valid assumption that the extinction coefficient of the modified residue in the native protein is identical to that of the model compound.

The relative lability of diazonium salts dictates that the modification reaction be carried out between 0–5°C and that whenever possible the counterion of the diazonium salt be an inert anion such as tetrafluoroborate. Diazonium salts readily undergo solvolytic reactions when exposed to ambient temperatures in hydroxylic solvents. They easily lose molecular nitrogen and will react with any available nucleophilic anion. For example, in an aqueous solution of potassium iodide the following reaction will take place (eq. 5.4).

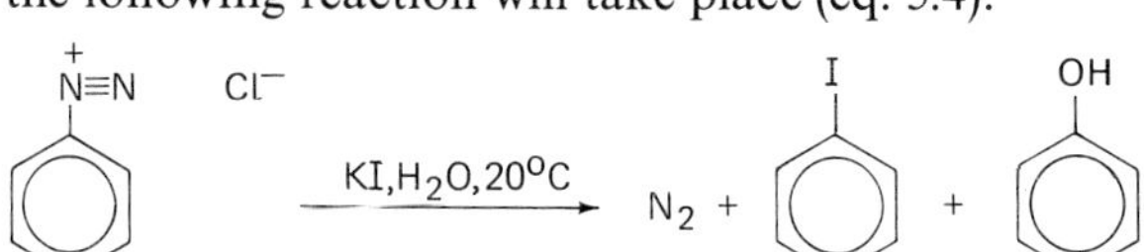

(5.4)

Attempted coupling with the protein at an elevated temperature will cause an excessive consumption of reagent and a large degree of non-specific reaction with the protein. In addition, a great deal of background absorbance will be generated since the product phenols or other biphenyl derivatives will combine with unreacted diazonium salt to yield highly colored products.

Frequently if the diazonium salt is isolated in dry crystalline form, with a nucleophilic anion such as chloride, an explosive reaction will ensue (eq. 5.5). However, the diazonium salts with a non-nucleophilic anion such as tetrafluoroborate are relatively stable. These salts are therefore of particular value if the synthesis of a stable radioactive reagent is desired.

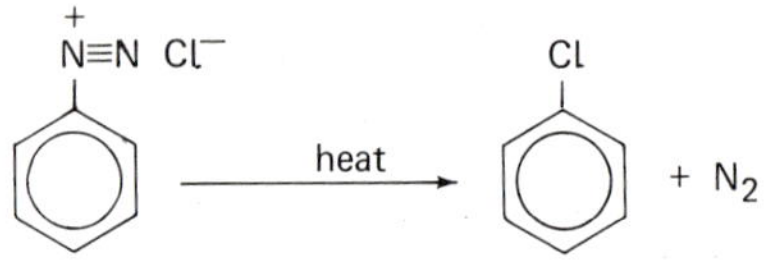

(5.5)

5.7.2. Synthesis of typical diazonium salts

Traylor and Singer (1967) have provided a detailed synthesis of the diazonium salts XIX and XX. Compound XIX has been used as an affinity label for acetylcholinesterase on erythrocyte membrane (Wofsy and Michaeli 1967) and for the cholinergic receptor from eel electroplax (Changeux et al. 1967). XX has been used for the modifica-

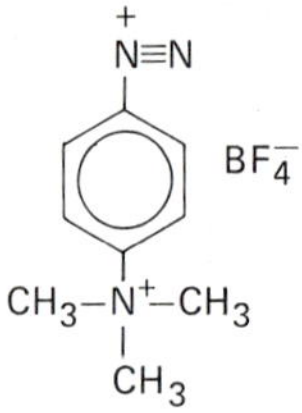

XIX

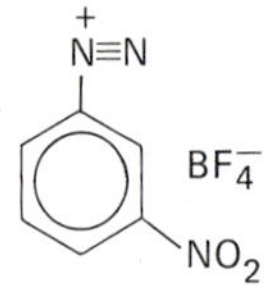

XX

tion of rabbit antibodies to the 2,4 dinitrophenyl determinant (Good et al. 1967).

The synthesis of nonradioactive XIX (Traylor and Singer 1967) is as follows. An aqueous solution of sodium nitrite (35.5 mg, 0.515 mmole, in 0.25 ml) was added drop-wise to a stirred cooled suspension (0–5°C) of 100 mg (0.448 mmole) of trimethyl (*p*-aminophenyl)ammonium chloride hydrochloride in 1.2 ml of 50% (w/v) fluoroboric acid. Stirring was continued for 15 min after the addition was complete. The reaction mixture was then kept at −20°C for 3 hr after which the product had precipitated. It was collected by filtration and washed successively with ice-cold 50% fluoroboric acid, anhydrous ethanol, 2,2-dimethoxypropane and anhydrous ether. The white crystals obtained (110 mg) could be recrystallized by dissolving in a minimum volume of 25% fluoroboric acid followed by addition of methanol to yield fluffy white crystals which decomposed at 170–171°C. Elemental analysis revealed the product ($C_9H_{13}B_2F_8N_3 \cdot NaBF_4$) cocrystallized with 1 mole of sodium tetrafluoroborate per mole of diazonium compound.

These same workers accomplished the synthesis of the radioactive XX as follows. Sodium nitrite (38.2 mg, 0.553 mmole) in 0.17 ml of water was added dropwise to a solution of 34.4 mg of (^{3}H)-*m*-nitroaniline and 30.9 mg of carrier *m*-nitroaniline in 0.5 ml of 50% fluoroboric acid and 0.25 ml of water. The reaction mixture was stirred magnetically during the addition and for an additional 1 hr. After the product precipitated as a cream solid, it was filtered and washed successively with ice cold 25% fluoroboric acid, anhydrous ethanol and anhydrous ether. The product could be recrystallized as white needles from acetone-ether if the temperature did not exceed 50°C. The yield was 39.3 mg; specific activity was 7.72×10^7 dpm/μmole. The product can be stored at −20°C in 0.01 M hydrochloric acid at a concentration of 2×10^{-3} M.

As standards for spectrophotometric measurements, Traylor and Singer (1967) prepared the monoazo derivatives of histidine and tyrosine with the various diazonium salts. The spectra of the products of reaction of N-acetyl histidine with the diazonium salt were obtained after reaction of a 100-fold excess of N-acetyl histidine with the diazonium salt in 0.1 M borate at *p*H 9.0. The spectral constants for the histidine and tyrosine derivatives are recorded in Table 5.1.

TABLE 5.1

Spectral properties of monoazo coupling products with histidine and tyrosine*

Compounds coupled		*p*H 5.6–6.2		*p*H 12.7–13.2	
Diazonium salt**	Aromatic compound	λ_{max} (mμ)	ε	λ_{max} (mμ)	ε
XIX	N-chloroacetyl tyrosine	320	19 530	325	12 710
				490	10 020
	N-acetylhistidine	367	20 000	415	22 000
XX	N-chloroacetyl tyrosine	340	20 700	345	13 400
				520	12 800
	N-acetylhistidine	392	23 000	472	27 500

* Traylor and Singer, 1967.
** See text for formulae

The monoazo derivative of tyrosine formed with XX was prepared in the following way. A solution of 237 mg (1.0 mmole) of XX in 30 ml of 0.01 N HCl was added dropwise to N-chloroacetyltyrosine (309 mg, 1.2 mmoles) in 25 ml of 0.2 M sodium phosphate buffer, pH 6.2, with continuous stirring at 0°C. Aqueous sodium hydroxide was added constantly to maintain the reaction mixture at *p*H 6.2. Three hr after the completion of the addition of N-chloroacetyl tyrosine, the stirring was discontinued and the reaction mixture was left at room temperature overnight. The reaction mixture formed a gel and then was acidified to *p*H 2 with 12 N HCl. The product precipitated out and could be recrystallized from methanol and then aqueous acetone. The crystals thus obtained melted at 214–215° with decomposition.

5.8. *Diazo compounds – diazoketones and diazoacetates*

5.8.1. *Reactive properties*

Neutral diazo compounds such as diazoketones, diazoacetates and diazomethane are efficient alkylating agents with weakly acidic nucleophiles. Consistent with the instability of the alkyl diazonium salt, alkylation by diazocompounds, including diazomethane, probably proceeds by an acid-catalyzed mechanism. For example, the generally useful esterification reaction of carboxylic acids by diazomethane probably proceeds via eq. (5.6). Likewise the esterification of acetic

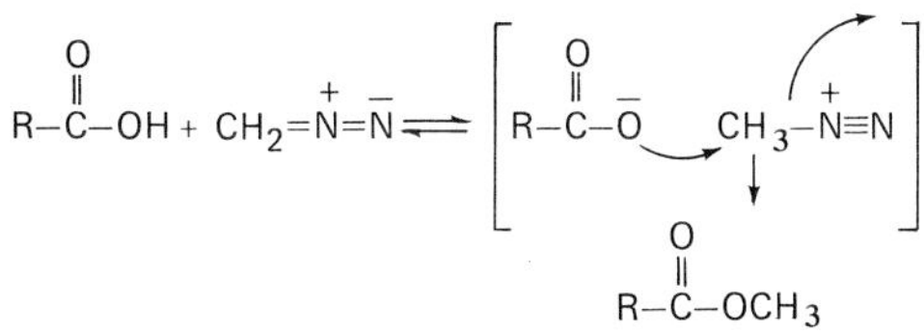

(5.6)

acid by α-diazoacetophenone probably proceeds by eq. (5.7). The decomposition of the intermediate indicated in both schemes likely takes place by a two step Sn-1 type mechanism where molecular nitrogen is readily lost, followed by nucleophilic attack of the carboxylate group on the resulting carbonium ion.

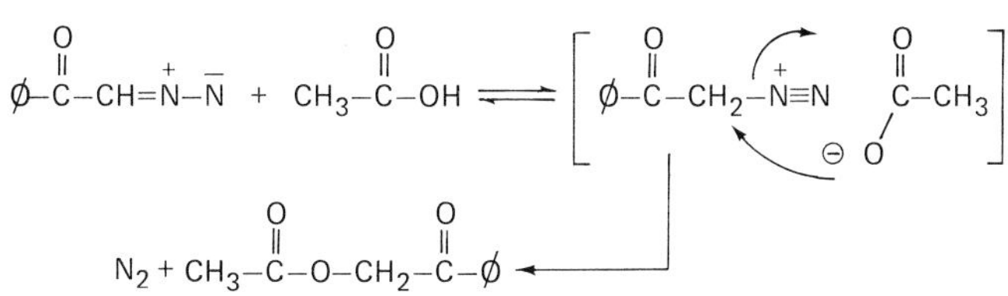

(5.7)

Neutral diazocompounds, in their light-independent reaction, do not react exclusively via acid-catalyzed pathways. For example, diazomethane in its dipolar form XXI adds to carbonyl groups.

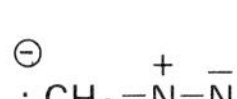

XXI

Indeed in the synthesis of diazoketones described in the synthesis of haloketones, this very process takes place. Diazoacetyl and diazoketone derivatives can also decompose via carbenes instead of carbonium ions even in the absence of irradiation. For example diazoketones lose nitrogen and rearrange to ketene in the presence of silver oxide via the following reaction pathway known as the Wolff rearrangement.

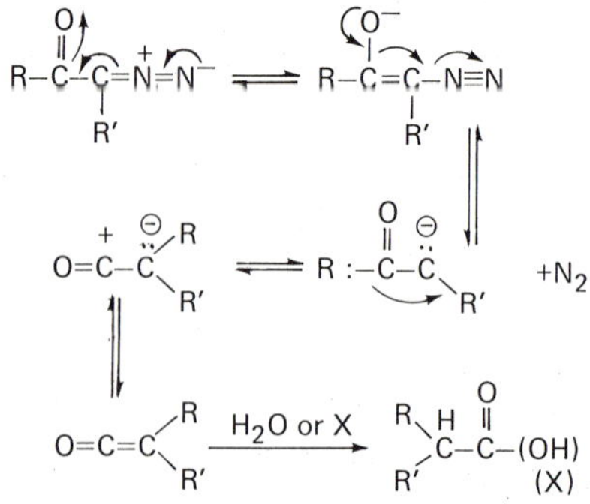

Reactions involving diazo groups are also affected by heavy metals such as cuprous ion. For example, in the well known Sandemeyer reaction, cuprous ion can catalyze the decomposition of aryl diazonium salts. Although the exact mechanism is unknown and may involve free radical processes, the anion of the cuprous salt replaces the nitrogen of the diazonium salt.

5.8.2. Synthesis of diazoacetyl derivatives

The general procedures for the synthesis of diazoketones have been described in § 5.3.1 on haloketones. Two other possible routes for the synthesis of diazoacetyl groups are indicated below. Bayliss et al. (1969) have synthesized N-diazoacetyl-L-phenylalanine methyl ester by the following procedure. A solution of 8.2 g of glycyl-L-phenylalanine methyl ester hydrobromide in 40 ml of 2 M sodium acetate with 2.0 ml of glacial acetic acid was cooled in an ice bath. Then 3.0 g of solid sodium nitrite was added over 1 hr. Some yellow solid formed after the solution was left for 3 hr. The resulting mixture was then extracted with three 50 ml aliquots of ice cold chloroform. The combined chloroform extracts were dried over $MgSO_4$ and then petroleum ether was added to the cloud point. After the solution was left overnight, yellow needles formed which melted between 126–128°C.

An alternate procedure was used by Shafer et al. (1966) in their synthesis of *p*-nitrophenyl diazoacetate. The key to this synthesis was the use of a chloroformate intermediate. To a 16-fold excess of diazomethane in ether (10 ml) was added dropwise a solution of 48.4 mg of *p*-nitrophenyl chloroformate. After the solution stood overnight at 4°C, the excess diazomethane was removed under a stream of N_2 and the ether evaporated under reduced pressure. The residual yellow oil was dissolved in 2 ml of benzene and chromatographed on an alumina column using benzene as the eluant. The first fraction contained 48 mg of product which could be recrystallized from chloroform-hexane (m.p. 92–94°C). These authors reported that several other diazoacetates can be prepared by this procedure.

5.8.3. *Analysis of products*

The light-independent reactions of diazoketones and diazoacetates can involve modification of any of the nucleophilic amino acid residues. The same amino acid derivatives that might be formed with haloketone and haloacid derivatives will be formed with these two types of diazo derivatives. At present, glutamate and aspartate appear to be the residues most usually modified by neutral diazo derivatives. For example, Bayliss et al. (1969) have shown that N-diazoacetyl-L-phenylalanine methyl ester reacts readily with pepsin causing loss of all proteolytic and peptidolytic activity. The residue modified in this case was an aspartate. One interesting feature of this study is that cupric ion catalyzes the esterification of the enzyme. Rajagopalan et al. (1966) had reported a similar phenomenon with pepsin when they used diazoacetyl norleucine methyl ester as the modification reagent. The precise function of the cupric ion in this reaction is not yet clear but the reactive species appears to be the metal ion complexed carbene. The observation by Lundblad and Stein (1969) that silver ion, which catalyzes the Wolff rearrangement, facilitates the modification of pepsin with diazoacetyl compounds, strengthens this suggestion.

Two other residues which have been modified by affinity labels containing diazo linkages are sulfhydryl groups and histidine. Hartmann (1963) has shown that 6-diazo-5-oxo-L-norleucine (XXII),

Subject index p. 201

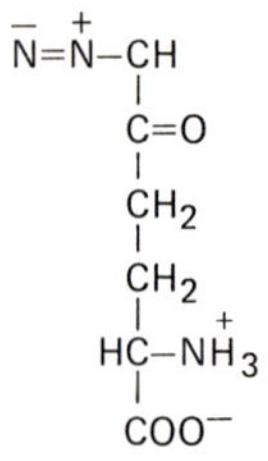

XXII

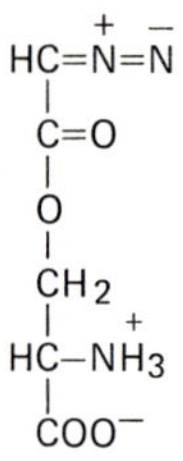

XXIII

a structural analog of L-glutamine, modified a cysteinyl sulfhydryl group of phosphoribosyl pyrophosphate amido transferase. Azaserine (XXIII), another structural analog of glutamine reacts with a sulfhydryl group of 2-formamido-N-ribosylacetamine-5′-phosphate : L-glutamine amido-ligase (adenosine diphosphate) (French et al. 1963; Dawid et al. 1963). Shafer et al. (1966) have shown that diazoacetyl chymotrypsin generates 1-carboxymethyl histidine in an apparently light independent reaction. Clearly, a properly oriented diazoacetyl group at the active site of an enzyme is capable of modification of a histidine residue.

Photoaffinity labels

The various reactive groups for affinity labels which have been described in ch. 5 are unable to modify all the amino acids in proteins. Although most of the reactive groups have broad specificity with respect to the various nucleophilic amino acid residues, their potential site of derivatization is limited to this class of amino acid residues. Generally, the formation of a covalent bond with the protein would be anticipated if a nucleophilic amino acid residue was vicinal to the modification reagent. Rapid reactions could be rationalized in terms of very favorable orientations between the electrophilic center of the affinity label and the target nucleophilic residue. However, if no nucleophilic center was close to the affinity label, no matter how perfect a substrate analog the modification reagent was, no reaction would take place.

Generally, catalytically important nucleophilic amino acid residues will be present near the substrate binding sites at the active sites of enzyme. However, there is a much lower probability that such a residue will be present at the ligand binding site of immunoglobulins, receptor proteins, or modifier (non-catalytic) sites of enzymes. In short, the type of functional group one might want to incorporate into an affinity label for a receptor site is very different from that for an affinity label for the active site of enzyme. Affinity labels for receptor proteins should possess highly reactive functional groups capable of reacting with both hydrophobic and polar residues. Indeed the research objectives are very different in the two types of experiments. One goal in the design of affinity labels for enzymes is to determine the catalytically important residues. In this case, the modification of a single amino acid residue is desirable. Local concentration and orientation effects hopefully will control the modification of an uniquely essential amino acid residue. On the other hand, the goal of the modification of a receptor protein is to tag it specifically in order to facilitate its isolation or localization within a complex membrane system. The identification of the amino acid residue modified is not as important as the specific labelling of the desired protein.

However since hydrophobic and some polar residues are relatively unreactive, highly activated reagents would be necessary to accomplish their derivatization. Yet even if such reactive reagents could be designed so that they would not react nonspecifically with proteins, they would likely react immediately with water and none would remain for the derivatization of the amino acid residue in the region of the ligand-binding site. An approach to the solution of this dilemma is to incorporate a relatively unreactive group into the affinity label and activate it when it is bound to the ligand-binding site of interest. One way to accomplish this goal is to use photoactivatable functional groups which are unreactive in the absence of light but which upon photolysis yield a highly reactive intermediate which can rapidly react with the protein.

Two types of photoactivatable reagents have been employed. The first involves prior covalent attachment of a photoactivatable group to the protein followed by photolysis of the derivatized enzyme. This approach was used in the pioneering studies of Westheimer and his colleagues in which they attached a diazoacetyl group to the reactive serine of chymotrypsin (Singh et al. 1962).

The second and more generally applicable approach involves the use of reversibly bound ligands containing groups capable of photoactivation. These reagents have been termed photoaffinity labels (Kiefer et al. 1970) and have been designed for a series of proteins including yeast alcohol dehydrogenase (Browne et al. 1971), acetylcholinesterase (Kiefer et al. 1970), antibodies (Fleet et al. 1969; Converse and Richards 1969), and phosphofructokinase (Brunswick and Cooperman 1971). In principle, these reagents can be expected to have great specificity if the ligand is light-activated when bound to the site and reacts with the protein before it dissociates.

6.1. Types of photoactivatable groups

6.1.1. Carbenes

Westheimer and his associates have used carbenes in their studies (Singh et al. 1962; Shafer et al. 1966; Vaughan and Westheimer 1969; Browne et al. 1971; Hexter and Westheimer 1971). Carbenes are capable of reacting not only with polar residues but also with hydrophobic residues. Carbenes have been generated from diazoacetates and diazomalonate derivatives. Diazoacetates were initially employed since they may be photolyzed at 370 nm. This minimizes the potential for photochemical decomposition of the protein – one of the important limitations of photoaffinity labels.

The analysis of the results of the photolysis of diazoacetylchymotrypsin represented a significant experimental challenge which illustrates both the strengths and weaknesses of the use of carbenes. After formation of the diazoacetyl enzyme with *p*-nitrophenyl diazoacetate (synthesis described in §5.8.2) in quantitative yield and the removal of the excess ester by extraction with a mixture of acetone and ether, the diazoacetyl enzyme was photolyzed. Depending on the *p*H of the photolysis solution and the concentration of the diazoacetylated enzyme, seven products were identified. The radioactive components that were isolated using nitrophenyl-^{14}C diazoacetate included glycolic acid, O-carboxymethyl serine, N-carboxymethyl histidine and O-carboxymethyl tyrosine. Three, as yet unidentified products, were isolated but they only accounted for 8 % of the total radioactivity. The scheme indicated in eq. (6.1) accounts for the various products formed.

The reaction of greatest biochemical significance is represented by process 3 in which the carbene reacts with a tyrosine residue of another chymotrypsin molecule. This finding is consistent with the known ability of chymotrypsin to form dimers at acidic *p*H and indicates that this approach is capable of delineating the nearest

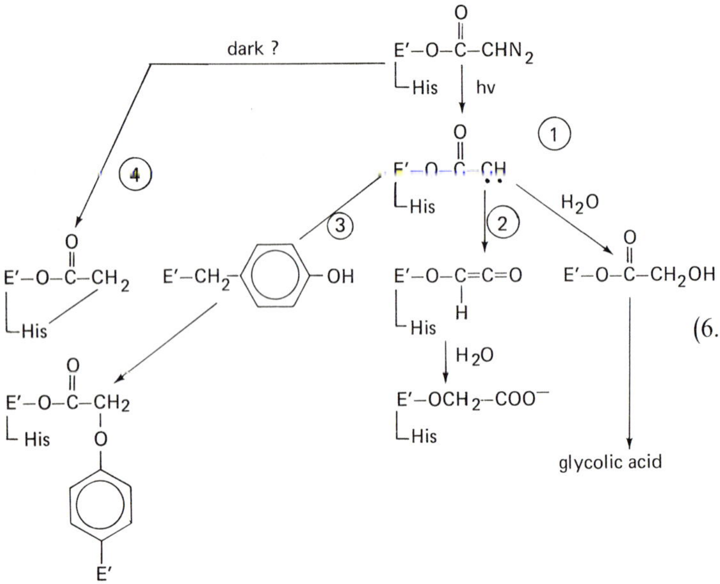

(6.1)

neighbor of a protein in a multicomponent system.

The generation of glycolic acid represents an insertion of the carbene into the O–H bond of water (process 4 eq. 6.1) and indicates a complexity which hopefully can be minimized with other light-activated modification reagents. Furthermore, the formation of O-carboxymethylserine is a rearrangement of the reactive intermediate generated by photolysis which limits the amount of important information which can be extracted from studies of this type. The design of photoactivated groups which are not subject to rearrangement comparable to the Wolff rearrangement (process 2) is most important.

One approach to the rearrangement problem for carbenes has been partially solved with the use of ethyl 2-diazomalonyl esters which are not as susceptible to rearrangements as diazoacetates (Hexter and Westheimer 1971). Vaughan and Westheimer (1969) have prepared the nitrophenyl ester of ethyl 2-diazomalonate and used it to acylate the reactive serine of trypsin. Photolysis at 253 nm has yielded a glutamic acid residue which presumably arises from the insertion of the generated carbene into the methyl group of alanine. The substituted malonyl derivative thus formed was transformed into glutamic acid after acid hydrolysis. Although the glutamic acid formed accounted for only 3% of the total radioactivity, these experiments demonstrate that the insertion of a carbene into a hydrophobic residue can take place. Hexter and Westheimer (1971) have further shown that photolysis of the ethyl diazomalonyl derivative of both trypsin and chymotrypsin at 254 nm at 0°C for 120 sec yields S-carboxymethyl cysteine. Since neither of these proteins contains cysteine residues, this amino acid residue must arise from the insertion of the carbene into a disulfide linkage.

Cooperman and his associates have used the ethyl diazomalonyl group in the synthesis of a series of reversibly bound photoaffinity labels (Brunswick and Cooperman 1971, 1973; Cooperman and Brunswick 1973). The synthesis and use of these compounds will be described below.

6.1.2. Nitrenes

Nitrenes, the nitrogen analogs of carbenes have been introduced as a reactive group in photoaffinity labels for antibodies by Fleet et al. (1969). Nitrenes tend to be more selective in their reactions and possibly will provide fewer products than carbenes (but see also § 6.2.3). The types of reaction that they can undergo (eq. 6.2, Knowles 1972) include insertions into C–H bonds to yield secondary amines, cycloadditions to double bonds to form cyclic 3-member imines and

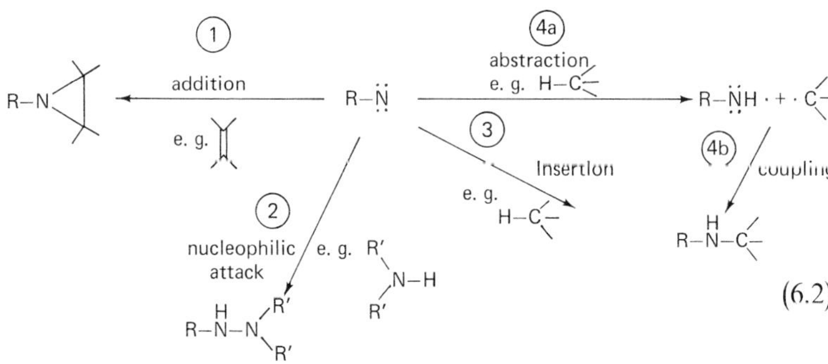

(6.2)

hydrogen atom abstractions followed by coupling of the free radicals, and addition to nucleophiles.

Several types of precursors can yield nitrenes upon photolysis: acyl azides, alkyl azides or aryl azides. Acyl azides cannot be used in affinity labels since they are effective acylating agents and the nitrenes that may be generated from them readily rearrange. Alkyl azides are unstable and require 290 nm light to be activated to the corresponding nitrene and are therefore not ideal. Aryl azides are stable in the absence of light and, depending on their structure, can be photolyzed at long wavelengths. In addition, they are not very susceptible to rearrangements. As a result, aryl azides, if they can be made to bind tightly to a receptor site, are the most promising precursors of nitrenes. They are routinely synthesized by diazotization of the corresponding aniline, followed by treatment with sodium azide at −20°C.

Fleet et al. (1969) have prepared compound XXIV, coupled it to bovine γ-globulin and used the resulting product as their antigen. Following isolation of the antibody fraction, a solution of XXV and the antibody fraction was photolyzed (§6.2.1) at 4°C for 18 hr, with light from two Mazda 125 W MB/V pearl glass lamps. This was filtered by a solution of sodium nitrite to absorb short wavelength light. Most of the label incorporated (1.1 moles per mole of protein) was associated with the heavy chain.

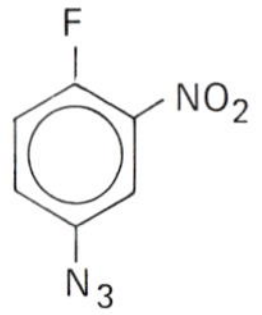

XXIV

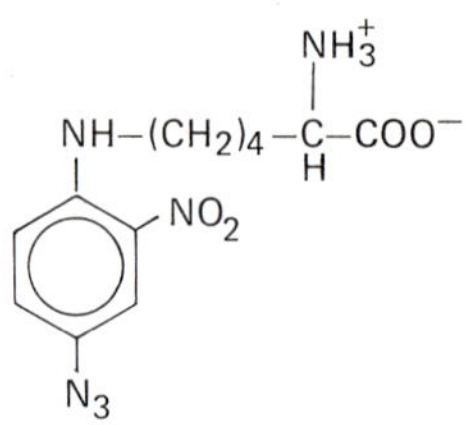

XXV

6.1.3. *Benzophenones and acetophenones*

Recently, Galardy et al. (1973) have suggested the use of benzophenone derivatives as functional groups for photoactivatable affinity labels. Upon irradiation at wavelengths greater than 320 nm, benzophenone in water and benzene adds to acetyl glycine methyl ester to yield compound XXVI. Presumably, the benzophenone triplet produced by irradiation, abstracts a hydrogen from glycine and then combines with the resulting free radical to yield the indicated product. The useful feature of aromatic ketones is that in their triplet state, they do not react with water. The incorporation of acetophenone and benzophenone groups into affinity labels promises to be a fruitful approach in the design of photoactivated affinity labels.

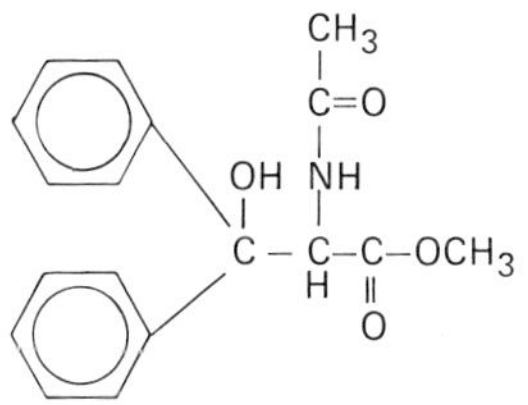

XXVI

6.2. *Conditions of photolysis*

6.2.1. *Excitation wavelength*

The use of reversibly-bound photoaffinity labels presents unique problems that are not presented by ordinary affinity labels or indeed by those reagents in which the photoactivatable groups are attached covalently to the protein prior to photolysis. However, one problem common to both the latter type modification reagents as well as the reversibly-bound photoaffinity labels is the choice of the wavelength for photolysis.

Clearly, the choice is restricted by the absorption spectrum of the label. However, diazoketone and diazoacetyl derivatives, for example, possess two absorption bands – one at 254 nm (ε 7000) and one at 350 nm (ε 10). Since carbenes may be produced by irradiation at either wavelength the question which immediately arises is which absorption should be used. The potential gain from irradiating with the shorter wavelength is that the intermediate formed is more reactive than that generated at the longer wavelength. This would enhance the likelihood of derivatization of the protein (Vaughan 1970). However, the major factor which restricts the use of the lower wavelength is that most proteins are susceptible to photodecomposition. Cooperman and Brunswick (1973) have recently emphasized, however, that proteins with low cystine or tryptophan content should not be extremely sensitive to irradiation at 253.7 nm. In their studies on phosphofructokinase, they found that irradiation at this wavelength did not produce any pronounced destruction in the absence of the photoaffinity label $O^{2'}$-(ethyl-2-diazomalonyl)adenosine 3′:5′-cyclic monophosphate (XXVII) and that the extent of incorporation of the affinity label into phosphofructokinase was four-fold greater upon irradiation at 253.7 nm rather than at 350 nm. Clearly, prior to any study with a photoaffinity label, the sensitivity of the particular protein to photodecomposition should be examined.

Various irradiation procedures have been reported. In their initial studies, Singh et al. (1962) irradiated diazoacetyl-chymotrypsin for 90 min with three G.E. sunlamps and filtered out all radiation below 315 nm using a solution of 420 g of copper sulfate pentahydrate in 2000 ml of water. More recently Hexter and Westheimer (1971) have used a Rayonet photochemical reactor model with an RPR-3500 Å lamp as the light source. Photolyses have been carried out at 253.7 with a RPR 253.7 lamps by Hexter and Westheimer (1971) and Cooperman and Brunswick (1973). Fleet et al. (1969) used light from two Mazda 125 W MB/V pearl glass lamps and Ruoho et al. (1973) used light from a HBO 200 W super pressure mercury lamp (Osram). In the former case, a sodium nitrite solution was used to filter out light below 400 nm, while in the latter case a monochromator was used to select the appropriate wavelength.

6.2.2. *Quantitative labelling*

One limitation in several studies with photoaffinity labels has been incomplete labelling of the target site (Converse and Richards 1969; Browne et al. 1971; Brunswick and Cooperman 1971). Recently Cooperman and Brunswick (1973) have explained these low yields in terms of the following series of reactions (eq. 6.3)

$$E + D \underset{}{\overset{K_D}{\rightleftharpoons}} ED \tag{6.3.1}$$

$$E + A \overset{K_A}{\rightleftharpoons} EA \tag{6.3.2}$$

$$h\nu + D \rightarrow A \tag{6.3.3}$$

$$h\nu + ED \rightarrow EA \tag{6.3.4}$$

$$h\nu + ED \rightarrow EA' \tag{6.3.5}$$

where A is the stable product of D, the photoaffinity label, obtained from photolysis in solution and EA′ represents the derivatized form of the protein. Low yields of the derivatized protein EA′ can be explained in terms of these equilibria in the following manner. Prior to photolysis, the native protein E, and the photoaffinity label are the sole species present. As photolysis proceeds, the concentration of A increases. Since this stable product has affinity for the ligand-binding site of interest, a competitive inhibitor or protecting agent of the modification reaction is generated and the extent of labeling (concentration of EA′) is reduced.

Cooperman and Brunswick (1973) have shown that with phosphofructokinase, the extent of derivatization can be markedly increased if A is continually eliminated from the solution being photolyzed and fresh D is added. They suggested two possible approaches to accomplish this goal. The first is continuous dialysis of the protein with a solution of the photoaffinity label during photolysis. The second procedure, preferred by these authors, involved 3 quartz columns (26 mm × 5 mm) ($V_T = 0.3$ ml) packed with a relatively transparent resin such as DEAE Sephadex and linked in parallel. If a buffer is chosen such that the protein of interest is adsorbed to the resin, the affinity label can then be passed through the assembled columns while the UV lamp is focussed on the gel. The ligand can be easily recirculated if care is taken to prevent the photolysis of the ligand when it is not in the gel. At the conclusion of the desired photolysis period, the protein can then be eluted from the resin and the extent of incorporation determined. Whereas Westheimer and his colleagues and Cooperman and

carbon tetrachloride as eluent, 17 g of ethyl diazoacetate was added and the reaction mixture was allowed to stand for 3 hr. Then benzene and excess phosgene were removed at reduced pressure. Concentrated alkali was used to trap the phosgene. Ethyl diazomalonyl chloride distilled from the reaction mixture at 58–60°C/15 mm and could be redistilled at 50–52°C/0.5 mm. Infrared spectra of liquid films of the compound showed the following characteristics: 4.61 μ(s), 5.62 μ(br) 5.86 μ.

The synthesis of XXVII, which has been used by Brunswick and Cooperman (1971, 1973) as a photoaffinity label for cyclic AMP (cAMP) binding sites, is indicated below.

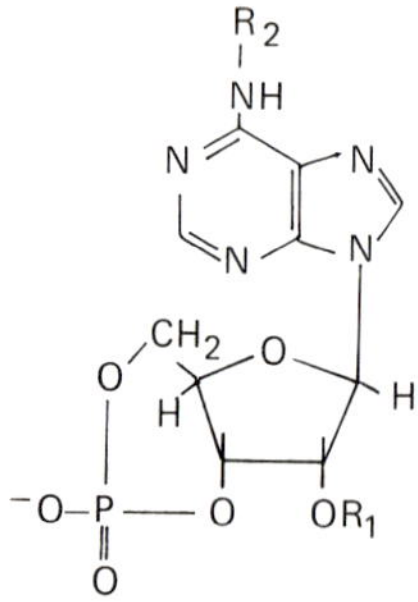

XXVII R_1 = CO–CN_2–CO_2Et
R_2 = H

XXVIII R_2 = R_1 = CO–CN_2–CO_2Et

To prepare XXVII, cAMP (0.1 g, 0.3 mmole) and (^{3}H) cAMP (25 μCi of specific activity 20–30 Ci/mmole) were dissolved in 3.4 ml of 0.38 M aqueous triethylamine. The mixture was evaporated to dryness, dissolved in dry pyridine, again evaporated to dryness and finally redissolved in 2.0 ml of dry pyridine with gentle warming. After cooling the resulting solution to 0°C, ethyl 2-diazomalonyl chloride (0.15 ml, 1.14 mmoles) was added dropwise with stirring. After the 5 min addition was complete, the reaction mixture was allowed to stand at room temperature for 10 min. It was then cooled to 0°C and treated with 2 ml of absolute ethanol in order to quench the reaction. After 30 min the solution was evaporated to dryness, the resulting residue was twice dissolved in absolute ethanol (5 ml) and again evaporated to dryness.

The residue then was dissolved in 30 ml of 0.04 M aqueous triethylammonium bicarbonate buffer (*p*H 7.5), (resulting *p*H 5.6). It was chromatographed on a DEAE cellulose column (HCO_3^- form) (3.4 × 15.0 cm), with elution first with 500 ml of water and then with a linear gradient of trimethylammonium bicarbonate at *p*H 7.2 (0–0.07 M). XXVII was completely resolved from some of XXVIII which was formed under the above reaction conditions. However, it was still contaminated by small amounts of cAMP and ethyl 2-diazomalonic acid. These impurities were apparently generated from the hydrolysis of some XXVII when the triethylammonium bicarbonate was removed. Pure samples of XXVII were obtained by preparative paper chromatography on either Whatman #40 or 3 MM paper with overnight development with ethanol: 0.5 M ammonium acetate, *p*H 7.0 (5:2, v/v).

6.3.2. Synthesis of aryl azides

To synthesize 4-fluoro-3-nitrophenyl azide (XXIV, § 6.1.2) (Fleet et al. 1969), 4-fluoro-3-nitroaniline was diazotized in the usual manner and subsequently treated with sodium azide at −20°C to give a 70% yield of XXIV (m.p. 52°C) as light-sensitive straw colored needles which could be recrystallized from petroleum ether.

Appendix I

High voltage paper electrophoresis

High voltage electrophoresis (2000–4000 V) on Whatman 3 MM paper (57 cm in length) is carried out in an apparatus in which the ends of the paper are immersed in the two buffer chambers and the rest of the paper is supported on a rack that is completely immersed in an inert solvent (e.g. Varsol), cooled by circulating tap water. In our laboratory we use a Savant apparatus, but others are also suitable.

The origin is generally marked on the paper (with pencil) at $3\frac{1}{2}$ inches from one end for electrophoresis at *p*H 1.9 and at 9–10 inches for electrophoresis at *p*H 3.6, 4.7 or 6.5, although certain procedures may require a shift in the position of the origin. Samples are usually applied to the dry paper, and if volumes larger than 10–20 μl are to be applied at the same point, the paper should be dried (with a hair dryer or other type of fan) between applications. In some instances, the samples (in less than 25 μl) may be applied directly to papers saturated with the electrophoresis buffer (after air drying for 5–10 min). If the samples are applied to dry papers, the papers are then placed on the electrophoresis racks and saturated with a stream of buffer (a squeeze bottle is convenient) in such a way that the solvent will approach the sample areas by capillary action at about the same rate from both sides.

Once the sample areas have also become saturated with buffer, the papers (on the racks) are allowed to air dry for 5–10 min and are then placed in the tanks so that the origins are closest to the positive electrodes. If adequate cooling is provided, voltages up to 4000 volts (80 volts/cm) may be used. However, we have usually found that full-width sheets of paper usually require voltage settings in the range of 2000–3000 volts (40–60 volts/cm) to prevent excessive current flow and overheating (this results in faster migrations and instrument shut-down). The runs are usually made at about 100 000 volt-min (e.g. 25 min at 4000 volts, 35 min at 3000 volts). Salts, urea and other substances may cause streaking, slowing or other aberrant migration patterns. In some instances the effects of salts can be minimized by leaving the papers at 100–200 volts for 10–20 min before beginning the high voltage run.

The buffers commonly used for high voltage electrophoresis are: (a) *p*H 1.9; 87 ml of glacial acetic acid and 25 ml of 99% formic acid, diluted to 1 liter with water; (b) *p*H 3.6; 10 ml of pyridine, 100 ml of glacial acetic acid and 890 ml of H_2O; (c) *p*H 4.7; 20 ml of pyridine and 20 ml of glacial acetic acid, diluted to 1 liter with water; (d) *p*H 6.4; 100 ml of pyridine, 4 ml of glacial acetic acid and 1.8 liters of H_2O. Except for the *p*H 4.7 buffer, all buffers used to saturate the paper are the same as those present in the buffer chambers. The *p*H 4.7 buffer is used in the buffer chamber as given above, but a dilution of 1:5 of 1:10 may often be necessary for saturating the papers to prevent excessive current flow. It is preferable to use pyridine that has been redistilled from ninhydrin (1 g/l).

After electrophoresis for the appropriate time, the papers are placed on glass rods in an oven at 60°C (the oven should preferably be equipped with a fan venting to a fume hood or to the outside) and dried (usually requires 20–30 min). They are then dipped in a ninhydrin reagent (see p. 183) and again heated in the oven for 15–60 min for color development.

Paper chromatography

Separations of amino acids and peptides can be carried out by descending paper chromatography on sheets of Whatman 3 MM paper (57 cm in length). Samples are applied as described above at the origin, which is generally $3\frac{1}{2}$ inches from one end of the paper. A fold is made across the full width of the paper at $2\frac{1}{2}$ inches from the same end; this fold is the place where the paper is supported by a glass rod. Another fold (in the opposite direction) is made 1 inch from the same end to allow the paper to dip into the solvent tray. The bottom edge of the paper is cut with 'pinking shears' to allow many drip points and more uniform solvent flow after the solvent reaches the bottom of the paper. Although few substances will migrate at or near the solvent front, the first time an unknown is run in a solvent system, the run should be ended before the solvent reaches the end of the paper (usually 12–15 hr). Later, runs for 24 hr or more may give better separations or prove to be more convenient.

After chromatography for the appropriate time, the papers are dried and stained as described under high voltage electrophoresis. Salts, urea and other substances often interfere with the migrations of amino acids and peptides.

Of the many solvents that can be used for paper chromatography some of those commonly used are: (a) 1-butanol:glacial acetic acid:water (200:30:75 v/v); (b) 1-butanol: pyridine:glacial acetic acid:water (15:10:3:12 v/v); (c) 1-butanol:pyridine:water (1:1:1 v/v). It is preferable to use pyridine which has been redistilled from ninhydrin (1 g/l). Solvent (a) is good for separations of amino acids and hydrophobic peptides, solvent (b) is a good one for separating many types of peptides, and (c) is often used where peptides do not migrate well at more acidic *p*H. An infinite number of variations in these and other solvents are possible, but some changes may result in phase separation. For example, solvent (a) is near the saturation point for 1-butanol and water;

addition of either will result in the formation of 2 phases. Freshly made solvents may give different results than solvents which have been stored for prolonged periods. For example, solvent (a) forms butyl acetate on standing, and this fourth component enhances the separation of leucine and isoleucine. As an example of varying the solvent composition and its effect on migration of peptides, the amount of butanol in the solvent may be varied from 70–130 parts by volume to obtain the optimum chromatographic resolution for the particular peptide mixture under study; thus in one case the solvent mixture was 1-butanol : glacial acetic acid : water (70–130 : 60 : 75) and this allowed large peptides to migrate whereas in the original solvent they remained at the origin (DeLange et al. 1969a).

Paper chromatography or electrophoresis on a preparative scale

Several μmoles (generally 1–3) of peptide mixture can often be fractionated on one paper by any of the electrophoretic and chromatographic systems given above. Preliminary experiments should be made to determine the best systems. The preparative papers are made as described above except that the origin is extended to a total length of 4 to 12 inches (depending on the amount of material to be purified) and the sample is applied uniformly over the entire length. A μl pipette (e.g. 100 μl) is usually convenient for applying the sample in a narrow streak; the paper should be dried between applications of sample. Guide strips of $\frac{1}{8}$ to $\frac{1}{4}$ inch are marked at the ends of the applied material (and also in the center for the longer streaks) and are extended the entire length of the paper. After the electrophoretic or chromatographic step these guide strips are cut out and stained with ninhydrin reagent to locate the peptides. The unstained regions, containing the peptides of interest, are cut out and eluted with 30% acetic acid (or other solvent) for 1–2 days at room temperature. These peptide solutions may be concentrated by rotary evaporation and reapplied to another paper to check the purity or to separate any mixtures in another system.

Peptide mapping ('fingerprints')

Combinations of 2 paper electrophoretic and chromatographic systems are usually superior for the analytical separation of peptides or amino acids in a mixture. Although two electrophoretic systems (e.g. *p*H 6.4 followed by *p*H 1.9 at right angles to each other) or two chromatographic systems can be used, we have generally found that chromatography in solvent (b) is often best for the first direction, followed (after drying the paper at room temperature for 2–4 hr) by electrophoresis at *p*H 3.6 (or *p*H 6.4) in the second direction (right angles to the first). Electrophoresis at *p*H 1.9 is often not satisfactory after chromatography in pyridine solvents, due to the formation of a front that develops during electrophoresis. Thorough drying (e.g. for 24 hr) of the paper after chromatography has lessened this problem. Electrophoresis after chromatography is usually better than chromatography after electrophoresis. Amino acids are best separated by chromatography in solvent (a) followed by electrophoresis at *p*H 1.9. Chromatography should be in the short direction of the paper, so that electrophoresis can be in the long (57 cm) direction. The electrophoresis buffer is applied as described under High Voltage Electrophoresis.

Detection reagents for peptides and amino acids

Ninhydrin reagent. Most peptides and amino acids can be detected on papers by dipping the paper in a solution containing ninhydrin (or spraying the paper with this solution) and heating in an oven at 60°C for 15–60 min. Further color development will sometimes occur overnight. Various colors ranging from yellow to violet are often observed and can be used to help identify certain peptides or amino acids.

Ninhydrin reagents in common use include: (a) 0.1% ninhydrin in 95% ethyl alcohol: collidine (95:5 v/v); (b) 0.1% ninhydrin in 95% ethyl alcohol: glacial acetic acid: collidine (50:15:2 v/v); and (c) 1 g $CdCl_2$ (or cadmium acetate) dissolved in 100 ml H_2O; add 50 ml of glacial acetic acid and 1000 ml of acetone containing 1 g of dissolved ninhydrin. Reagent (a) is one that can be used for most purposes. Reagent (b) may be preferable to Reagent (a) when papers have been run at alkaline *p*H, particularly if the buffer is not volatile. Reagent (c) can be used to estimate quantities of material present, since it gives a more uniform color with most peptides and amino acids. The use of Technical grade collidine in Reagents (a) and (b) will usually give enhanced color differentiation.

Hypochlorite reagent for detection of ninhydrin-negative peptides. Certain peptides (e.g. those containing α-N-acetyl or other groups on the α-amino group and those containing NH_2-terminal glutamine which has cyclized) do not give a colored product with ninhydrin. These may be detected by the use of a reagent which detects peptides and other substances with N-H bonds (see Mazur et al. 1962). After fractionation of peptide mixtures on paper, the paper is dried and sprayed with 1% *tert*-butyl hypochlorite in cyclohexane and then air-dried at room temperature for 1 hr in a hood or other place with rapid air movement. The sheet is then sprayed with an aqueous solution of KI (1%) and soluble starch (1%). Compounds with N–H bonds will give blue-black spots on a white or light blue background. Greater sensitivity can be obtained by placing the paper in a sealed jar with *tert*-butyl hypochlorite in a beaker at the bottom for 1 hr. The paper should then be air dried for 6 hr before spraying with the starch-iodide solution. The background color is usually stronger with this method.

Reagents for detection of specific residues in peptides. Many reagents give specific color reactions with certain types of residues in peptides. Among the more useful of these are:

a) Ehrlich reagent for detection of tryptophan: 1 g of *p*-dimethylaminobenzaldehyde, dissolve in 90 ml of acetone, add 10 ml of concentrated HCl, dip paper immediately; tryptophan gives a violet color.

b) Pauly reagent for histidine and tyrosine: 10 ml of stock solution (4.5 g sulfanilic acid, 5 ml concentrated HCl, diluted to 500 ml with H_2O), cool to 0°C, add 1.0 ml of 4.5% $NaNO_2$ dropwise with stirring, wait 2–3 min and add 11 ml of Na_2CO_3 (10%, w/v); spray paper, histidine gives a bright red-orange color; tyrosine (free) gives a pale, orange color; tyrosine (in peptides) gives a blue-violet color.

c) Sakaguchi reagent for arginine: equal volumes of 1.1% diacetyl (2,3-butanedione), 20% KOH and 2.5% α-naphthol in absolute ethanol; mix in order shown with brief stirring before adding third reagent; dip paper immediately; arginine gives a pink to red color on a brown background.

These reagents can be used after the peptides have been stained with ninhydrin, but all collidine must be removed from the paper (thorough drying for several hours) before the Pauly reagent is used. The Sakaguchi reagent cannot be used after the Pauly reagent, and we have generally found the sensitivity to be less when the Sakaguchi reagent is used after ninhydrin than when it is used directly.

d) Phenanthrenequinone reagent, an alternative test for arginine: equal volumes of 0.02% phenanthrenequinone in absolute ethanol and 10% NaOH in 60% ethanol, freshly prepared; dip the paper in the reagent and after 20 min of air drying at room temperature the peptides containing arginine appear as brilliant green or blue-white fluorescent spots against a dark-blue background under 366 nm ultraviolet light; (Easley et al. 1969). This reaction can be used first, followed by either the ninhydrin stain or the Pauly reagent, but papers should be air dried for 2–3 hr. Peptides containing tryptophan give a darker blue fluorescence with the phenanthrenequinone reagent and they can often be detected by examining the unstained paper under ultraviolet light (366 nm).

Appendix II

LIST OF SUPPLIERS

Source	Specific items mentioned in the text
Ion-exchange resins and gel filtration materials	
Beckman Instruments Inc. Spinco Division 1117 California Ave. Palo Alto, California 94304, USA.	PA-28, PA-35 and AA-15
Beckman-RIIC Ltd. Eastfield Industrial Estate Glenrothes, Fife KY7 4NG Scotland.	
Bio-Rad Laboratories 32nd & Griffin Ave. Richmond, California 94804, USA.	Aminex A-5, Dowex 1-X8 Dowex 2-X8 Dowex 50-X12
Bio-Rad Laboratories Ltd. 27 Homesdale Road, Bromley, Kent, England.	
Durrum Chemical Corporation 3950 Fabian Way Palo Alto, California 94303, USA.	Durrum DC-2, Durrum DC-2A
Kenneth R. Arsenault Durrum International Sales Corp. 30 Rue Racins 78220 Viroflay, France.	

Subject index p. 201

LIST OF SUPPLIERS

Source	Specific items mentioned in the text
Pharmacia Fine Chemicals Inc. 800 Centennial Ave. Piscataway, N. J. 10017, USA.	Sephadex beads for gel filtration; ion-exchange Sephadex resins
Pharmacia Fine Chemicals Box 604 S-75125 Uppsala 1, Sweden.	
Reeve Angel 9 Bridewell Place Clifton, N.J. 07014, USA.	DEAE-cellulose, CM-cellulose
H. Reeve Angel & Co. Ltd. 14 New Bridge Street London EC4V 6AY, England.	
Equipment	
Beckman Instruments Inc. Spinco Division 1117 California Ave. Palo Alto, California 94304, USA.	Amino acid analyzers and associated equipment and supplies
Beckman-RIIC Ltd. Eastfield Industrial Estate Glenrothes, Fife KY7 4NG Scotland.	
Radiometer 72, Emdrupvej Copenhagen NV, Denmark.	pH-Stat and accessories
Savant Instruments Inc. 221 Park Avenue Hicksville, N.Y. 11901, USA.	High voltage electrophoresis equipment
Supports for the preparation of water-insoluble proteins	
Bio-Rad Laboratories 32nd & Griffin Avenue Richmond, California 94804, USA.	Agarose derivatives

Source	Specific items mentioned in the text
Bio-Rad Laboratories Ltd. 27 Homesdale Road Bromley, Kent England.	
Pierce Chemical Co., Inc. P.O. Box 117 Rockford, Illinois 61105, USA.	Corning activated silica glass
Pierce & Warringer (U.K.) Ltd. 44 Upper Northgate Street Chester, Cheshire England.	
Proteolytic enzymes	
Henley & Co., Inc. 202 East 44th Street New York, NY 10017, USA	Citrus leaf carboxypeptidase C (Rohm and Haas) Aminopeptidase M (Rohm and Haas)
Miles Laboratories Inc. 1127 Myrtle Street Elkhart, Indiana 46514, USA.	Prolidase
Miles-Seravac (Pty) Ltd. Moneyrow Green Holyport, Maidenhead Berkshire, England.	
Bureau Lausanne Chemin de Messidor 5 CH-1006 Lausanne, Switzerland.	
Sigma Chemical Co. P.O. Box 14508 St. Louis, Mo. 63178, USA.	Subtilisin
Sigma London Chemical Co. Norbiton Station Yard Kingston-upon-Thames, Surrey, England.	

Source	Specific items mentioned in the text
Worthington Biochemical Corp. Freehold, NJ 07728, USA.	Chymotrypsin, trypsin, elastase, carboxypeptidases A and B, pepsin, papain.
Worthington Biochemical Corp. 6078 Neu-Isenburg 2 Am Forsthaus Gravenbruch 73 Germany.	

Aspergillopeptidase A (E.C. 3.4.4.17) is an acid proteinase from *Aspergillus saitoi*. This enzyme may be prepared and assayed by the procedures described by E. Ichishima, Methods Enzymol. *19*, 397 (1970).

References

ALEXANDER, J., I. B. WILSON and R. KITZ (1963) J. Biol. Chem. *238*, 741.

AMBLER, R. P. (1965) Biochem. *96*, 32P.

ANDRES, S. F. and M. Z. ATASSI (1973) Biochemistry *12*, 942.

ARNDT, F., (1943), Organic Syntheses, Collect., Vol. 2 (Wiley, New York) p. 165.

ASATOOR, A. M. and M. D. ARMSTRONG, (1967), Biochem. Biophys. Res. Commun. *26*, 168.

AVIRAM, I. and A. SCHEJTER (1971) Biochim. Biophys. Acta *229*, 113.

BAKER, B. R. (1969) Accts. Chem. Res. *2*, 129.

BAKER, B. R. and G. J. LOURENS (1967) J. Med. Chem. *10*, 1113.

BAKER, R. B. (1967) Design of Active-Site Directed Irreversible Enzyme Inhibitors (Wiley, New York).

BALDWIN, G. S. and P. R. CARNEGIE (1971) Biochem. J. *123*, 69.

BANASZAK, L. J. and F. R. N. GURD (1964) J. Biol. Chem. *239*, 1836.

BANKS, T. E. and J. A. SHAFER (1970) Biochemistry *9*, 3343.

BANKS, T. E. and J. A. SHAFER (1972) Biochemistry *11*, 110.

BARMAN, T. E. and D. E. KOSHLAND, JR. (1967) J. Biol. Chem. *242*, 5771.

BAYLISS, R. S., J. R. KNOWLES and G. B. WYBRANDT (1969) Biochem. J. *113*, 377.

BEELEY, J. G. and H. NEURATH (1968) Biochemistry 7, 1239.

BELL, E. A. (1962) Biochem. J. *83*, 225.

BELLAMY, L. J. (1956) The Infrared Spectra of Complex Molecules (Methuen, London) p. 273.

BENASSI, C. A., E. SCOFFONE and F. M. VERONESE (1965) Tetrahedron Letters *49*, 4389.

BENESCH, R. and R. E. BENESCH (1962) Methods Biochem. Anal. *10*, 43.

BENESCH, R. E., R. BENESCH, R. D. RENTHAL and N. MAEDA (1972) Biochemistry 11, 3576.

BENISEK, W. F. and F. M. RICHARDS (1968) J. Biol. Chem. *243*, 4267.

BENOITON, N. L., R. E. DEMAYO, G. J. MOORE and J. R. COGGINS (1971) Can. J. Biochem. *49*, 1292.

BENSON, J. V., JR., M. J. GORDON and J. A. PATTERSON (1967) Anal. Biochem. *18*, 228.

BICKLE, T. A., J. W. B. HERSHEY and R. R. TRAUT (1972) Proc. Natl. Acad. Sci. (Wash.) *69*, 1327.

Subject index p. 201

BLUMENFELD, O. O. and P. M. GALLOP (1962) Biochemistry *1*, 947.

BOHAK, Z. (1964) J. Biol. Chem. *239*, 2878.

BOLTON, A. E. and W. M. HUNTER (1973) Biochem. J. *133*, 529.

BOOKCHIN, R. M. and P. M. GALLOP (1968) Biochem. Biophys. Res. Commun. *32*, 86.

BORNSTEIN, P. and G. BOLIAN (1970) J. Biol. Chem. *245*, 4854.

BRADBURY, A. F. and D. G. SMYTH (1973) Biochem. J. *131*, 637.

BRADBURY, S. L. (1969) J. Biol. Chem. *244*, 2002.

BRAUN, V. and V. BOSCH (1972) Eur. J. Biochem. *28*, 51.

BRAUNITZER, G., K. BEYREUTHER, H. FUJIKI and B. SCHRANK (1968) Z. Physiol. Chem. *349*, 265.

BROSTOFF, S. and E. H. EYLAR (1971) Proc. Natl. Acad. Sci. (Wash.) *68*, 765.

BROWN, W. E. and F. WOLD (1973) Biochemistry *12*, 835.

BROWNE, D. T., S. S. HIXSON and F. H. WESTHEIMER (1971) J. Biol. Chem. *246*, 4477.

BRUICE, T. C., J. J. GREGORY and S. L. WALTERS (1968) J. Amer. Chem. Soc. *90*, 1612.

BRUNSWICK, D. J. and B. S. COOPERMAN (1971) Proc. Natl. Acad. Sci (Wash.) *68*, 1801.

BRUNSWICK, D. J. and B. S. COOPERMAN (1973) Biochemistry *12*, 4074.

BUTLER, P. J. G. and B. S. HARTLEY (1972) Methods Enzymol. *25B*, 191.

BUTLER, P. J. G., J. I. HARRIS, B. S. HARTLEY and R. LEBERMAN (1967) Biochem. J. *103*. 78P.

BUTLER, P. J. G., J. I. HARRIS, B. S. HARTLEY and R. LEBERMAN (1969) Biochem. J. *112*, 679.

CANDIDO, E. P. M. and G. H. DIXON (1972) Proc. Natl. Acad. Sci. (Wash.) *69*, 2015.

CARNEGIE, P. R. (1971) Nature (Lond.) *229*, 25.

CARRAWAY, K. L. and D. E. KOSHLAND (1972) Methods Enzymol. *25B*, 616.

CARSTEN, M. E. and J. G. PIERCE (1963) J. Biol. Chem. *238*, 1724.

CAVINS, J. F. and M. FRIEDMAN (1970) Anal. Biochem. *35*, 489.

CERAMI, A. and J. M. MANNING (1971) Proc. Natl. Acad. Sci (Wash.) *68*, 1180.

CHAN, W. W. C., (1968) Biochemistry 7, 4247.

CHANGEUX, J.-P., T. P. PODLESKI and L. WOFSY (1967) Proc. Natl. Acad. Sci. (Wash.) *58*, 2063.

CHASE, J. F. A. and P. K. TUBBS (1969) Biochem. J. *111*, 225.

CHENG, K. W. and J. G. PIERCE (1972) J. Biol. Chem. *247*, 7163.

CHIBNALL, A. C., J. L. MANGAN and M. W. REES (1958) Biochem. J. *68*, 114.

CHRISTENSEN, B. G., W. J. LEANZA, T. R. BEATTIE, A. A. PATCHETT, B. H. ARISON, R. E. ORMOND, F. A. KUEHL, JR., G. ALBERS-SCHONBERG and O. JARDETZKY (1969) Science *166*, 123.

CLAMP, J. R., G. DAWSON and L. HOUGH (1967) Biochim. Biophys. Acta *148*, 342.

COHEN, L. A. (1968) Ann. Rev. Biochem. *37*, 695.

COHEN, L. A. (1970) The Enzymes *1*, 147.

COLETTI-PREVIERO, M. A., A. PREVIERO and E. ZUCKERKANDL (1969) J. Mol. Biol. *39*, 493.

COMB, D. G., N. SARKAR and C. J. PINZINO (1966) J. Biol. Chem. *241*, 1857.

CONVERSE, C. A. and F. F. RICHARDS (1969) Biochemistry *8*, 4431.
COOPERMAN, B. S. and D. J. BRUNSWICK (1973) Biochemistry *12*, 4079.
COVELLI, I. and J. WOLFF (1966) J. Biol. Chem. *241*, 4444.
COVELLI, I., L. FRATI and J. WOLFF (1973) Biochemistry *12*, 1043.
CRESTFIELD, A. M., S. MOORE and W. H. STEIN (1963) J. Biol. Chem. *238*, 622.
CRESTFIELD, A. M., W. H. STEIN and S. MOORE (1963) J. Biol. Chem. *238*, 2413, 2421.
CUATRECASAS, P., S. FUCHS and C. B. ANFINSEN (1969) J. Biol. Chem. *244*, 406.
CUATRECASAS, P., M. WILCHEK and C. B. ANFINSEN (1968) Proc. Natl. Acad. Sci. (Wash.) *61*, 636.
CUATRECASAS, P., M. WILCHEK and C. B. ANFINSEN (1969) J. Biol. Chem. *244*, 4316.
DAVIES, G. E. and G. R. STARK (1970) Proc. Natl. Acad. Sci. (Wash.) *66*, 651.
DAWID, I. B., T. C. FRENCH and J. M. BUCHANAN (1963) J. Biol. Chem. *238*, 2178.
DE CAT, A. H. and R. K. van POUCHE (1963) J. Org. Chem. *28*, 3426.
DEGANI, Y., and A. PATCHORNIK (1971) J. Org. Chem. *36*, 2727.
DEGANI, Y. and A. PATCHORNIK (1974) Biochemistry *13*, 1.
DEGANI, Y., H. NEUMANN and A. PATCHORNIK (1970) J. Am. Chem. Soc. *92*, 6969.
DEIBLER, G. E. and R. E. MARTENSON (1973) J. Biol. Chem. *248*, 2387.
DELANGE, R. J. (1970) J. Biol. Chem. *245*, 907.
DELANGE, R. J. and E. L. SMITH (1971) Ann. Rev. Biochem. *40*, 279.
DELANGE, R. J. and E. L. SMITH (1974) The Proteins *4*, in press.
DELANGE, R. J., D. M. FAMBROUGH, E. L. SMITH and J. BONNER (1969a) J. Biol. Chem. *244*, 319.
DELANGE, R. J., A. N. GLAZER and E. L. SMITH (1969b) J. Biol. Chem. *244*, 1385.
DELANGE, R. J., A. N. GLAZER and E. L. SMITH (1970) J. Biol. Chem. *245*, 3325.
DEMPSEY, W. B. and H. N. CHRISTENSEN (1962) J. Biol. Chem. *237*, 1113.
DEMPSEY, W. B. and E. E. SNELL (1963) Biochemistry *2*, 1414.
DIXON, H. B. F. and R. N. PERHAM (1968) Biochem. J. *109*, 312.
DOOLITTLE, R. F. (1965) Biochem. J. *94*, 742.
DOOLITTLE, R. F. and R. W. ARMENTROUT (1968) Biochemistry *7*, 516.
DORNER, F. (1971) J. Biol. Chem. *246*, 5896.
DUS, K., S. LINDROTH, R. PABST and R. M. SMITH (1966) Anal. Biochem. *14*, 41.
EASLEY, C. W., B. J. M. ZEGERS and M. DE VIJLDER (1969) Biochim. Biophys. Acta *175*, 211.
EDELHOCH, H. (1967) Biochemistry *6*, 1948.
EDMAN, P. (1960) Ann. N.Y. Acad. Sci. *88*, 602.
EDMAN, P. (1970) Sequence determination. *In*: Needleman, S. B., ed., Protein Sequence Determination (Springer-Verlag, Berlin) p. 211.
EDMAN, P. and G. BEGG (1967) Eur. J. Biochem. *1*, 80.
EISELE, B. and K. WALLENFELS (1968) Eur. J. Biochem. *6*, 29.
ELLMAN, G. L. (1959) Arch. Biochem. Biophys. *82*, 70
ELZINGA, M. (1970) Biochemistry *9*, 1365.
ELZINGA, M. (1971) Biochemistry *10*, 224.

ESHDAT, Y., J. F. McKELVY and N. SHARON (1973) J. Biol. Chem. *248*, 5892
FAHRNEY, D. E. and A. M. GOLD (1963) J. Am. Chem. Soc. *85*, 997.
FANGER, M. W. and H. A. HARBURY (1965) Biochemistry *4*, 2541.
FIELDS, R. (1971) Biochem. J. *124*, 581.
FIELDS, R. (1972) Methods Enzymol. *25B*, 464.
FIRNAU, G. and K. FRITZE (1972) Bioinorg. Chem. *2*, 167.
FISCHER, E. H., A. W. FORREY, J. L. HEDRICK, R. G. HUGHES, A. B. KENT and E. G. KREBS (1963) Chemical and Biological Aspects of Pyridoxal Catalysis (Pergamon Press, New York) p. 544.
FLEET, G. W. J., R. R. PORTER and J. R. KNOWLES (1969) Nature (Lond.) *224*, 511.
FONTANA, A. (1972) Methods Enzymol. *25B*, 419.
FONTANA, A. and E. SCOFFONE (1972) Methods Enzymol. *25B*, 482.
FONTANA, A., F. M. VERONESE and E. BOCCU (1973) FEBS Letters *32*, 135.
FONTANA, A., F. M. VERONESE and E. SCOFFONE (1968) Biochemistry 7, 3901.
FORMAN, H. J., H. J. EVANS, R. L. HILL and I. FRIDOVICH (1973) Biochemistry *12*, 823.
FOSTER, J. A., E. BRUENGER, W. R. GRAY and L. B. SANDBERG (1973) J. Biol. Chem. *248*, 2876.
FRAENKEL-CONRAT, H. (1944) J. Biol. Chem. *154*, 227.
FRAENKEL-CONRAT, H. and C. M. TSUNG (1967) Methods Enzymol. *11*, 151.
FRAENKEL-CONRAT, H., J. I. HARRIS and A. L. LEVY (1955) Methods Biochem. Anal. *2*, 359
FRANTZ, W. L. and R. W. TURKINGTON (1972) Endocrinology *91*, 1545.
FREEDMAN, R. B. (1971) Quart. Revs. *25*, 431.
FRENCH, T. C., I. B. DAWID and J. M. BUCHANAN (1963) J. Biol. Chem. *238*, 2186.
FRIEDMAN, M., L. H. KRULL and J. F. CAVINS (1970) J. Biol. Chem. *245*, 3868.
FRIEDMAN, M., K. H. SHULL and E. FARBER (1969) Biochem. Biophys. Res. Commun. *34*, 857.
FROEDE, H. C. and I. B. WILSON (1971) Enzymes *5*, 87.
GALARDY, R. E., L. C. CRAIG and M. P. PRINTZ (1973) Nature New Biol. *242*, 126.
GENNARI, G. and G. JORI (1970) FEBS Letters *10*, 129.
GERSHEY, E. L., G. W. HASLETT, G. VIDALI and V. G. ALLFREY (1969) J. Biol. Chem. *244*, 4871.
GETHING, M. J. and B. E. DAVIDSON (1972) Eur. J. Biochem. *30*, 352.
GIROT, I. L., T. A. SMITH and R. H. ABELES (1969) J. Biol. Chem. *244*, 6341.
GLAZER, A. N. (1970) Ann. Rev. Biochem. *39*, 101.
GLAZER, A. N. (1975) The Proteins *2*, in press.
GLAZER, A. N., R. J. DELANGE and R. J. MARTINEZ (1969) Biochim. Biophys. Acta *188*, 164.
GLIMCHER, M. J., G. L. MECHANIC and U. A. FRIBERG (1964) Biochem. J. *93*, 198.
GOLD, A. H. and H. L. SEGAL (1964) Biochemistry *3*, 778.
GOLD, A. H. and H. L. SEGAL (1965) Biochemistry *4*, 1506.
GOLD, A. M. and D. FAHRNEY (1964) Biochemistry *3*, 783.

GOLDBERGER, R. F. (1967) Methods Enzymol. *11*, 317.
GOLDBERGER, R. F. and C. B. ANFINSEN (1962) Biochemistry *1*, 401.
GOOD, A. H., P. S. TRAYLOR and S. J. SINGER (1967) Biochemistry *6*, 873.
GOODWIN, T. W. and R. A. MORTON (1946) Biochem. J. *40*, 628.
GORBUNOFF, M. J. (1972) Methods Enzymol *25B*, 506.
GOREN, H. J., D. M. GLICK and E. A. BARNARD (1968) Arch. Biochem. Biophys. *126*, 607.
GOUNARIS, A. D. and G. E. PERLMANN (1967) J. Biol. Chem. *242*, 2739.
GREGORY, H., P. M. HARDY, D. S. JONES, G. W. KENNER and R. C. SHEPPARD (1964) Nature (Lond.) *204*, 931.
GROSS, E. and J. L. MORELL (1966) J. Biol. Chem. *241*, 3638.
GUIDOTTI, G. and W. KONIGSBERG (1964) J. Biol. Chem. *239*, 1474.
GUNDLACH, H. G., W. H. STEIN and S. MOORE (1959) J. Biol. Chem. *234*, 1754, 1761.
HABEEB, A. F. S. A. (1960) Can. J. Biochem. Physiol. *38*, 493.
HABEEB, A. F. S. A. (1972) Methods Enzymol. *25B*, 558.
HAMILTON, P. B. (1963) Anal. Chem. *35*, 2055.
HARDING, H. W. J. and G. E. ROGERS (1971) Biochemistry *10*, 624.
HARRINGTON, W. F. and P. H. VON HIPPEL (1961) Adv. Prot. Chem. *16*, 1.
HARRIS, G. M. and R. L. HILL (1969) J. Biol. Chem. *244*, 2195.
HARTMANN, S. C. (1963) J. Biol. Chem. *238*, 3036.
HASS, G. M. and H. NEURATH (1971a) Biochemistry *10*, 3535.
HASS, G. M. and H. NEURATH (1971b) Biochemistry *10*, 3541.
HAYASHI, R., S. MOORE and W. H. STEIN (1973) J. Biol. Chem. *248*, 2296.
HEINRICH, C. P., S. ADAM and W. ARNOLD (1973) FEBS Letters *33*, 181.
HEINRIKSON, R. L. (1971) J. Biol. Chem. *246*, 4090.
HEINRIKSON, R. L., W. H. STEIN, A. M. CRESTFIELD and S. MOORE (1965) J. Biol. Chem. *240*, 2921.
HEXTER, C. S. and F. H. WESTHEIMER (1971) J. Biol. Chem, *246*, 3928, 3934.
HILL, R. L. and W. R. SCHMIDT (1962) J. Biol. Chem. *237*, 389.
HIRS, C. H. W. (1956) J. Biol. Chem. *219*, 611.
HIRS, C. H. W. (1967) Methods Enzymol. *11*, 197.
HIRS, C. H. W. and S. N. TIMASHEFF (1972) Methods Enzymol. *25B*.
HOFMANN, T. (1964) Biochemistry *3*, 356.
HOLBROOK, J. J. and R. JECKEL (1969) Biochem. J. *111*, 689.
HOLBROOK, J. J. and G. PFLEIDERER (1965) Biochem. Z. *342*, 141.
HOLMGREN, A. (1972) Eur. J. Biochem. *26*, 528.
HORTON, H. R. and D. E. KOSHLAND, JR. (1972) Methods Enzymol. *25B*, 468.
HUGLI, T. E. and S. MOORE (1972) J. Biol. Chem. *247*, 2828.
HUGLI, T. E. and W. H. STEIN (1971) J. Biol. Chem. *246*, 7191.
HULTQUIST, D. E., R. W. MOYER and P. D. BOYER (1966) Biochemistry *5*, 322.
HUNT, L. T. and M. O. DAYHOFF (1970) Biochem. Biophys. Res. Commun. *39*, 757.
HUNTER, M. J. and M. L. LUDWIG (1972) Methods Enzymol. *25B*, 585.

Subject index p. 201

HUSZAR, G. and M. ELZINGA (1971) Biochemistry *10*, 229.

INAGAMI, T. and K. MURAKAMI (1972) Anal. Biochem. *47*, 501.

INGLIS, A. S. and T.-Y. LIU (1970) J. Biol. Chem. *245*, 112.

IRREVERRE, F., K. MORITA, A. V. ROBERTSON and B. WITKOP (1962a) Biochem. Biophys. Res. Commun. *8*, 453.

IRREVERRE, F., K. MORITA, S. ISHII and B. WITKOP (1962b) Biochem. Biophys. Res. Commun. *9*, 69

ITANO, H. A. and E. A. ROBINSON (1972) J. Biol. Chem. *247*, 4819.

JACOBSON, G. R., M. H. SCHAFFER, G. R. STARK and T. C. VANAMAN (1973) J. Biol. Chem. *248*, 6583.

JAKOBY, W. B. (1971) Methods Enzymol. *22*.

JAMES, G. T. and E. A. NOLTMANN (1973) J. Biol. Chem. *248*, 730.

JANATOVA, J., J. K. FULLER and M. J. HUNTER (1968) J. Biol. Chem. *243*, 3612.

JANSEN, E. F., M. D. F. NUTTING and A. K. BALLS (1949) J. Biol. Chem. *179*, 189.

JEPPSSON, J.-O. and J. SJÖQUIST (1967) Anal. Biochem. *18*, 264.

JEVONS, F. R. (1963) Biochem. J. *89*, 621.

JOHNSON, P., C. I. HARRIS and S. V. PERRY (1967) Biochem. J. *105*, 361.

JORI, G., G. GALIAZZO, A. MARZOTTO and E. SCOFFONE (1968) J. Biol. Chem. *243*, 4272.

KAPLAN, H., K. J. STEVENSON and B. S. HARTLEY (1971) Biochem. J. *124*, 289.

KENNER, R. A. and H. NEURATH (1971) Biochemistry *10*, 551.

KIEFER, H., J. LINDSTROM, E. S. LENNOX and S. J. SINGER (1970) Proc. Natl. Acad. Sci. (Wash.) *67*, 1688.

KIM, J. H., B. SHOME, T.-H. LIAO and J. G. PIERCE (1967) Anal. Biochem. *20*, 258.

KIMMEL, J. R. (1967) Methods Enzymol. *11*, 584.

KING, L. and R. N. PERHAM (1971) Biochemistry *10*, 981.

KING, T. P. (1966) Biochemistry *5*, 3454.

KIRSCHNER, M. W. and H. K. SCHACHMAN (1973) Biochemistry *12*, 2987.

KLAPPER, M. H. and I. M. KLOTZ (1972) Methods Enzymol. *25B*, 536.

KLEE, C. B. and J. A. GLADNER (1972) J. Biol. Chem. *247*, 8051.

KLOTZ, I. M. (1967) Methods Enzymol. *11*, 576.

KNOWLES, J. R. (1972) Accts. Chem. Res. *5*, 155.

KNOX, R., G. O. KOHLER, R. PALTER and H. G. WALKER (1970) Anal. Biochem. *36*, 136.

KOKESH, F. C. and F. H. WESTHEIMER (1971) J. Amer. Chem. Soc. *93*, 7270.

KONIGSBERG, W. H. (1972) Methods Enzymol. *25B*, 185.

KREIL, G. and P. D. BOYER (1964) Biochem. Biophys. Res. Commun. *16*, 551.

KUROSKY, A. and T. HOFMANN (1972) Can. J. Biochem. *50*, 1282.

LAINE, R. A., W. J. ESSELMAN and C. C. SWEELEY (1972) Methods Enzymol. *28B*, 159.

LEACH, S. J. and E. M. J. PARKHILL (1955) Proceedings of the International Wool Textiles Research Conference, Australia, vol. C, p. 92.

LEE, C. K. and J. M. MANNING (1973) J. Biol. Chem. *248*, 5861.

LEVITZKI, A., W. B. STALLCUP and D. E. KOSHLAND, JR. (1971) Biochemistry *10*, 3371.

LEVY, D. and R. A. PASELK (1973) Biochim. Biophys. Acta *310*, 398.
LI, S.-L. and C. YANOFSKY (1972) J. Biol. Chem. *247*, 1031.
LIGHT, A. and E. L. Smith (1963) The Proteins *1*, 1.
LINDLEY, H. (1956) Nature (Lond.) *178*, 647.
LIU, T.-Y. (1967) J. Biol. Chem. *242*, 4029.
LIU, T.-Y. (1972) Methods Enzymol. *28B*, 48
LIU, T.-Y. and Y. H. CHANG (1971) J. Biol. Chem. *246*, 2842.
LUDWIG, M. L. and M. J. HUNTER (1967) Methods Enzymol. *11*, 595.
LUNDBLAD, R. L. and W. H. STEIN (1969) J. Biol. Chem. *244*, 154.
MAGNUSSON, S., L. SOTTRUP-JENSEN, T. E. PETERSEN, H. R. MORRIS and A. DELL (1974) FEBS Letters *44*, 189.
MAIN, A. R. (1964) Science *144*, 992.
MARCUS, F. and E. HUBERT (1968) J. Biol. Chem. *243*, 4922.
MARON, E., Y. ESHDAT and N. SHARON (1972) Biochim. Biophys. Acta *278*, 243.
MATSUBARA, H. and R. M. SASAKI (1969) Biochem. Biophys. Res. Commun. *35*, 175.
MATTHEWS, B. W., P. B. SIGLER, R. HENDERSON and D. M. BLOW (1967) Nature (Lond.) *214*, 652.
MAURER, H. R. (1971) Disc Electrophoresis and Related Techniques of Polyacrylamide Gel Electrophoresis (Walter de Gruyter, New York).
MAZUR, R. H., B. W. ELLIS and P. S. CAMMARATA (1962) J. Biol. Chem. *237*, 1619.
MCELVAIN, S. M. and J. P. SCHROEDER (1949) J. Am. Chem. Soc. *71*, 40.
MCMURRAY, C. H. and D. R. TRENTHAM (1969) Biochem. J. *115*, 913.
MEANS, G. E. and R. E. FEENEY (1968) Biochemistry *7*, 2192.
MEANS, G. E. and R. E. FEENEY (1971) Chemical Modification of Proteins (Holden-Day, San Francisco).
MEANS, G. E., W. I. CONGDON and M. L. BENDER (1972) Biochemistry *11*, 3564.
MEIGHEN, E. A. and H. K. SCHACHMAN (1970) Biochemistry *9*, 1163.
MELCHIOR, W. B. and D. FAHRNEY (1970) Biochemistry *9*, 251.
MILLER, E. J. and K. A. PIEZ (1966) Anal. Biochem. *16*, 320.
MILLER, E. J., G. R. MARTIN, C. E. MECCA and K. A. PIEZ (1965) J. Biol. Chem. *240*, 3623.
MILSTEIN, C. (1964) Biochem. J. *92*, 410.
MOON, A. Y., J. MERCOUROFF and G. P. HESS (1965) J. Biol. Chem. *240*, 717.
MOORE, S. (1963) J. Biol. Chem. *238*, 235.
MOORE, S. (1972) The prescision and sensitivity of amino acid analysis. *In:* Meienhofer, J., ed., Chemistry and Biology of Peptides (Ann Arbor Science Publishers Inc., Ann Arbor) p. 629.
MOORE, S., D. H. SPACKMAN and W. H. STEIN (1958) Anal. Chem. *30*, 1185, 1190.
MORRISON, M. and G. S. BAYSE (1970) Biochemistry *9*, 2995.
MOULT, J., Y. ESHDAT and N. SHARON (1973) J. Mol. Biol. *75*, 1.
MURACHI, T. and K. KATO (1967) J. Biochem. *62*, 627.
MURRAY, K. and C. MILSTEIN (1967) Biochem. J. *105*, 491.

Subject index p. 201

NAIDER, F. and Z. BOHAK (1972) Biochemistry *11*, 3208.
NAKAJIMA, T. and B. E. VOLCANI (1969) Science *164*, 1400.
NAKAJIMA, T. and B. E. VOLCANI (1970) Biochem. Biophys. Res. Commun. *39*, 28.
NAKAJIMA, T., Y. MATSUOKA and Y. KAKIMOTO (1971) Biochim. Biophys. Acta *230*, 212.
NEUMANN, N. P., S. MOORE and W. H. STEIN (1962) Biochemistry *1*, 68.
NOLAN, C., W. B. NOVOA, E. G. KREBS and E. H. FISCHER (1964) Biochemistry *3*, 542.
NORMAN, A. W., R. T. WEDDING and M. K. BLACK (1965) Biochem. Biophys. Res. Commun. *20*, 703
OGLE, J. D., R. B. ARLINGHAUS and M. A. LOGAN (1962) J. Biol. Chem. *237*, 3667.
OKUYAMA, T. and K. SATAKE (1960) J. Biochem. (Tokyo) *47*, 454.
O'LEARY, M. H. and F. H. WESTHEIMER (1968) Biochemistry 7, 913.
PAIK, W. K. and S. Kim (1967) Biochem. Biophys. Res. Commun. *27*, 479.
PAIK, W. K. and S. KIM (1970) Biochem. Biophys. Res. Commun. *40*, 224.
PAIK, W. K. and S. KIM (1971) Science *174*, 114.
PERHAM, R. N. and J. O. THOMAS (1971) J. Mol. Biol. *62*, 415.
PETERSON, J. D., S. NEHRLICH, P. E. OYER and D. F. STEINER (1972) J. Biol. Chem. *247*, 4866.
PHILLIPS, D. R. and M. MORRISON (1970) Biochem. Biophys. Res. Commun. *40*, 284.
PIEZ, K. A. (1968) Ann. Rev. Biochem. *37*, 547.
PIEZ, K. A. and L. MORRIS (1960) Anal. Biochem. *1*, 187.
PIHL, A. and R. LANGE (1962) J. Biol. Chem. *237*, 1356.
PISANO, J. J. (1972) Methods Enzymol. *25*, 27.
PISANO, J. J. and T. J. BRONZERT (1969) J. Biol. Chem. *244*, 5597.
PISANO, J. J., J. S. FINLAYSON and M. P. PEYTON (1969) Biochemistry *8*, 871.
PISZKIEWICZ, D. and E. L. SMITH (1971) Biochemistry *10*, 4538.
PISZKIEWICZ, D., M. LANDON and E. L. SMITH (1970) J. Biol. Chem. *245*, 2622.
PISZKIEWICZ, D., M. LANDON and E. L. SMITH (1971) J. Biol. Chem. *246*, 1324.
PLAPP, B. V., S. MOORE and W. H. STEIN (1971) J. Biol. Chem. *246*, 939.
PLUMMER, T. H., JR. and C. H. W. HIRS (1964) J. Biol. Chem. *239*, 2530.
POPENOE, E. A. and V. DU VIGNAUD (1954) J. Amer. Chem. Soc. *76*. 6202.
PORTER, W. H., L. W. CUNNINGHAM and W. M. MITCHELL (1971) J. Biol. Chem. *246*, 7675.
PREVIERO, A., M. A. COLETTI-PREVIERO and J. C. CAVADORE (1967a) Biochim. Biophys. Acta *147*, 453.
PREVIERO, A., M. A. COLETTI-PREVIERO and P. JOLLÈS (1967b) J. Mol. Biol. *24*, 261.
RAFTERY, M. A. and R. D. COLE (1963) Biochem. Biophys. Res. Commun. *10*, 467.
RAFTERY, M. A. and R. D. COLE (1966) J. Biol. Chem. *241*, 3457.
RAJAGOPALAN, T. G., W. H. STEIN and S. MOORE (1966) J. Biol. Chem. *241*, 4295.
RAY, W. J., JR. (1967) Methods Enzymol. *11*, 490.
RAY, W. J., JR. and D. E. KOSHLAND, JR. (1960) Brookhaven Symp. Biol. *13*, 135.
REES, M. W. (1946) Biochem. J. *40*, 632.
REPORTER, M. and J. L. CORBIN (1971) Biochem. Biophys. Res. Commun. *43*, 644.

RICE, R. H. and G. E. MEANS (1971) J. Biol. Chem. *246*, 831.
RILEY, M. and R. N. PERHAM (1970) Biochem. J. *118*, 733.
RIMON, S. and G. E. PERLMANN (1968) J. Biol. Chem. *243*, 3566.
RIORDAN, J. F. (1973) Biochemistry *12*, 3915.
RIORDAN, J. F. and M. SOKOLOVSKY (1971) Accts. Chem. Res. *4*, 353.
RIORDAN, J. F. and B. L. VALLEE (1972a) Methods Enzymol. *25B*, 500.
RIORDAN, J. F. and B. L. VALLEE (1972b) Methods Enzymol. *25B*, 521.
RIORDAN, J. F. and B. L. VALLEE (1972c) Methods Enzymol. *25B*, 515.
RIPPA, M., L. SPANIO and S. PONTREMOLI (1967) Arch. Biochem. Biophys. *118*, 48.
ROBERTUS, J. D., R. A. ALDEN, J. J. BIRKTOFT, J. KRAUT, J. C. POWERS and P. E. WILCOX (1972) Biochemistry *11*, 2439.
ROCHAT, C., H. ROCHAT and P. EDMAN (1970) Anal. Biochem. *37*, 259.
ROHOLT, O. A. and D. PRESSMAN (1972) Methods Enzymol. *25B*, 438.
RONCHI, S., M. C. ZAPPONI and G. FERRI (1969) Eur. J. Biochem. *8*, 325.
ROSE, I. A. and E. L. O'CONNELL (1969) J. Biol. Chem. *244*, 6548.
ROSS, W. C. J. (1950) J. Chem. Soc. 2257.
RUOHO, A. E., H. KIEFER, P. E. ROEDER and S. J. SINGER (1973) Proc. Natl. Acad. Sci. (Wash.) *70*, 2567.
SALVATORE, G. and H. EDELHOCH (1973) Hormonal Proteins and Peptides *1*, 201.
SANGER, F., (1949) Biochem. J. *44*, 126.
SANGER, F., (1963), Proc. Chem. Soc., *76*.
SANGER, F. and E. O. P. THOMPSON (1963) Biochim. Biophys. Acta *71*, 468.
SCHELLENBERG, K. (1963) J. Org. Chem. *28*, 3259.
SCHOELLMANN, G. and E. SHAW (1963) Biochemistry *2*, 252.
SCHNACKERZ, K. D. and E. A. NOLTMANN (1971) Biochemistry *10*, 4837.
SCHROEDER. D. D. and E. SHAW (1971) Arch. Biochem. Biophys. *142*, 340.
SCHROEDER, W. A. (1972a) Methods Enzymol. *25B*, 298.
SCHROEDER, W. A. (1972b) Methods Enzymol.*25B*, 138
SCHROEDER, W. A., J. R. SHELTON and B. ROBBERSON (1967) Biochim. Biophys. Acta *147*, 590.
SCHROEDER, W. A., J. B. SHELTON and J. R. SHELTON (1969) Arch. Biochem. Biophys. *130*, 551.
SCOFFONE, E., A. FONTANA and R. ROCCHI (1968) Biochemistry *7*, 971.
SCOFFONE, E., G. JORI and G. GALIAZZO (1970) Biochem. Soc. Symp. *31*, 163.
SEELY, J. H., R. EDATTEL and N. L. BENOITON (1969) J. Chromatog. *44*, 618.
SHAFER, J., P. BARNOWSKY, R. LAURSEN, F. FINN and F. H. WESTHEIMER (1966) J. Biol. Chem. *241*, 421.
SHAW, E. (1970a) The Enzymes *1*, 91.
SHAW, E. (1970b) Physiol. Rev. *50*, 244.
SHECHTER, Y., Y. BURNSTEIN and A. PATCHORNIK (1972) Biochemistry *11*, 653.
SHOTTON, D. and B. S. HARTLEY (1973) Biochem. J. *131*, 643.
SIGLER, P. B., B. A. JEFFREY, B. W. MATTHEWS and D. M. BLOW (1966) J. Mol. Biol. *15*, 175.

Subject index p. 201

SIGMAN, D. S. and E. R. BLOUT (1967) J. Amer. Chem. Soc. *89*, 1747.

SIGMAN, D. S., D. A. TORCHIA and E. R. BLOUT (1969) Biochemistry *8*, 4560.

SIGNOR, A. G., M. BONORA, L. BIONDI, D. NISATO, A. MARZOTTO and E. SCOFFONE (1971) Biochemistry *10*, 2748.

SINGER, S. J. (1967) Adv. Protein Chem. *22*, 1.

SINGH, A., E. R. THORNTON and F. H. WESTHEIMER (1962) J. Biol. Chem. *237*, PC3006.

SLOBIN, L. I. and S. J. SINGER (1968) J. Biol. Chem. *243*, 1777.

SMITH, D. L., B. B. BRUEGGER, R. M. HALPERN and R. A. SMITH (1973) Nature *246*, 103.

SMYTH, D. G. (1967) J. Biol. Chem. *242*, 1579.

SMYTH, D. G., F. C. BATTAGLIA and G. MESCHIA (1971) J. Gen. Physiol. *44*, 889.

SMYTH, D. G., O. O. BLUMENFELD and W. KONIGSBERG (1964) Biochem. J. *91*, 589.

SPACKMAN, D. H., W. H. STEIN and S. MOORE (1958) Anal. Chem. *30*, 1190, 1185.

SPANDE, T. F. and B. WITKOP (1967) Methods Enzymol. *11*, 498.

SPANDE, T. F., B. WITKOP, Y. DEGANI and A. PATCHORNIK (1970) Adv. Protein Chem. *24*, 97.

SPIES, J. R. (1967) Anal. Chem. *39*, 1412.

SPIES, J. R. and D. C. CHAMBERS (1948) Anal. Chem. *20*, 30.

SPIRO, R. G. (1965) Methods Enzymol. *8*, 3.

SPIRO, R. G. (1970) Ann. Rev. Biochem. *39*, 599.

SPIRO, R. G. (1972) Methods Enzymol. *28B*, 3.

STARK, G. R. (1967a) Methods Enzymol. *11*, 125.

STARK, G. R. (1967b) Methods Enzymol. *11*, 590, 594.

STARK, G. R. (1970) Adv. Protein Chem. *24*, 261.

STARK, G. R. (1972a) Methods Enzymol. *25B*, 103.

STARK, G. R. (1972b) Methods Enzymol. *25B*, 369.

STARK, G. R. and D. G. SMYTH (1963) J. Biol. Chem. *238*, 214.

STEFANINI, S., E. CHIANCONE, C. H. MCMURRAY and E. ANTONINI (1972) Arch. Biochem. Biophys. *151*, 28.

STEIN, M. J. and I. E. LIENER (1967) Biochem. Biophys. Res. Commun. *26*, 376.

STEINERT, P. M., H. W. J. HARDING and G. E. ROGERS (1969) Biochim. Biophys. Acta *175*, 1.

STENFLO, J., P. FERNLUND, W. EGAN and P. ROEPSTORFF (1974) Proc. Natl. Acad. Sci. (Wash.) *71*, 2730.

STEVENSON, K. J. and L. B. SMILLIE (1965) J. Mol. Biol. *12*, 937.

STEWART, I. (1963) J. Chromatog. *10*, 404.

STRUMEYER, D. H., W. N. WHITE and D. E. KOSHLAND, JR. (1963) Proc. Natl. Acad. Sci. (Wash.) *50*, 931.

TAKAHASHI, K. (1968) J. Biol. Chem. *243*, 6171.

TAKAHASHI, K., W. STEIN and S. MOORE (1967) J. Biol. Chem. *242*, 4682.

TANG, J. and B. S. HARTLEY (1967) Biochem. J. *102*, 593.

TANG, J. and B. S. HARTLEY (1970) Biochem. J. *118*, 611.

THOMAS, E. W. (1970) Carbohydrate Res. *13*, 225.

THOMPSON, E. O. P. (1954) Biochim. Biophys. Acta *15*, 440.
THORELL, J. I. and B. G. JOHANSSON (1971) Biochim. Biophys. Acta *251*, 363.
TOENNIES, G. and R. P. HOMILLER (1942) J. Amer. Chem. Soc. *64*, 3054.
TOWER, D. B. (1967) Methods Enzymol. *11*, 76.
TRAUB, W. and K. A. PIEZ (1971) Adv. Protein Chem. *25*, 243.
TRAUT, R. R., A. BOLLEN, T.-T. SUN, J. W. B. HERSHEY, J. SUNDBERG and R. L. PIERCE (1973) Biochemistry *12*, 3266.
TRAYLOR, P. S. and S. J. SINGER (1967) Biochemistry *6*, 881.
UDENFRIEND, S., S. STEIN, P. BOHLEN and W. DAIRMAN A., (1972) In: Meienhofer, J., ed., Chemistry and Biology of Peptides (Ann Arbor Science Publishers Inc., Ann Arbor) p. 655.
UYEDA, K. (1969) Biochemistry *8*, 2366.
VALLÈE, B. L. and J. F. RIORDAN (1969) Ann. Rev. Biochem. *38*, 733.
VANAMAN, T. C., S. J. WAKIL and R. L. HILL (1968) J. Biol. Chem. *243*, 6420.
VAUGHAN, R. J. (1970) Ph.D. Dissertation, Harvard University.
VAUGHAN, R. J. and F. H. WESTHEIMER (1969) J. Amer. Chem. Soc. *91*, 217.
VERONESE, F. M., E. BOCCU and A. FONTANA (1972) FEBS Letters *21*, 277.
VICKERY, H. B. (1972) Adv. Protein Chem. *26*, 81.
VISSER, L., D. S. SIGMAN and E. R. BLOUT (1971) Biochemistry *10*, 735.
WALEY, S. G., J. C. MILLER, I. A. ROSE and E. L. O'CONNELL (1970) Nature (Lond.) *227*, 181.
WÅLINDER, O. (1968) J. Biol. Chem. *243*, 3947.
WĂLINDER, O. (1969) J. Biol. Chem. *244*, 1065.
WALKER, W. H. and T. P. SINGER (1970) J. Biol. Chem. *245*, 4224.
WAXDAL, M. J., W. H. KONIGSBERG, W. L. HENLEY and G. M. EDELMAN (1968) Biochemistry 7, 1959.
WESTHEAD, E. W. (1972) Methods Enzymol. *25B*, 401.
WHITAKER, J. R. and J. PEREZ-VILLASENOR (1968) Arch. Biochem. Biophys. *124*, 70.
WICKNER, R. B., C. W. TABOR and H. TABOR (1970) J. Biol. Chem. *245*, 2132.
WILCOX, P. E. (1967) Methods Enzymol *11*, 605.
WINZLER, R. J. (1955) Methods Biochem. Anal. *2*, 279.
WITTER, A. and H. TUPPY (1960) Biochim. Biophys. Acta *45*, 429.
WOFSY, L. and D. MICHAELI (1967) Proc. Natl. Acad. Sci. (Wash.) *58*, 2296.
WOLFF, J. and I. COVELLI (1969) Eur. J. Biochem. *9*, 371.
YANKEELOV, J. A., JR (1970) Biochemistry *9*, 2433.
YANKEELOV, J. A., JR., C. D. MITCHELL and T. H. CRAWFORD (1968) J. Amer. Chem. Soc. *90*, 1664.

Subject index p. 201

Subject index

SEPARATION METHODS FOR NUCLEIC ACIDS AND OLIGONUCLEOTIDES

HANNAH GOULD

Department of Biophysics,
King's College, London, U.K.

and

H. R. Matthews

Department of Biophysics,
Portsmouth Polytechnic, Portsmouth, U.K.

Chapter 9. Practice of preparative gel electrophoresis of nucleic acids 408

Chapter 10. Applications of gel electrophoresis 419

List of abbreviations

BD-	benzoylated DEAE-
Bis	N,N′-methylene *bis* acrylamide
C_0t	initial concentration × time
CPM	counts per minute
DEAE-	diethylaminoethyl-
DEAEC	diethylaminoethyl cyanide
CMAEC	dimethylaminoethyl cyanide
DMPN	dimethylproprionitrile
DNA	deoxyribonucleic acid
DNase	deoxyribonuclease
dV/dx	voltage gradient
EDTA	ethylenediamine tetra acetic acid (versine)
HAP	hydroxyapatite
mA	milliamperes
MAK	methylated albumin on Kieselguhr
mequiv.	milliequivalents
n	number of nucleotides per molecule
PEI	polyethylenimine
PTFE	polytetrafluoroethylene (Teflon)
PVC	polyvinylchloride
R_f	relative mobility
R_{fBPB} / R_B	mobility relative to bromophenol blue

Subject index p. 487

RNA	ribonucleic acid
RNase	ribonuclease
RPC	reversed phase chromatography
rRNA	ribosomal RNA
S	sedimentation coefficient
SDS	sodium dodecyl sulphate
sRNA	soluble RNA
TEMED	tetramethyl ethylenediamine
tRNA	transfer RNA
Tris	Tris-(hydroxymethyl)-amino methane

Oligonucleotide nomenclature

NXYZ	any nucleoside
Pu	any purine nucleoside
Py	any pyrimidine nucleoside
A	adenosine
dA	deoxyadenosine
C	cytidine
dC	deoxycytidine
G	guanosine
dG	deoxyguanosine
rT	ribothymidine
T	thymidine
U	uridine
diHU	dihyrouridine
5MeC	5-methyl cytidine
Ψ	pseudouridine

I	inosine
dI	deoxyinosine

A 'p' added to the left of any of the above indicates the corresponding 5′ nucleotide and a 'p' added to the right corresponds to the 3′ nucleotide; e.g.

pA	adenosine 5′ phosphate (sometimes abbreviated 'AMP')
Ap	adenosine 3′ phosphate (or sometimes adenosine 2′ or 3′ monophosphate)

An oligonucleotide is abbreviated by the correct sequence of nucleotides although the intermediate 'p's may be omitted in long sequences. The presence or absence of terminal phosphate group is indicated by the presence or absence of terminal 'p's; e.g. ApUp dinucleotide written in the 5′ to 3′ direction having 3′ terminal phosphate but no 5′ terminal phosphate.

Extra 'p's can be added to indicate pyrophosphate bonds, e.g. pppGp guanosine tetraphosphate.

An olignucleotide of known composition but unknown sequence can be written with brackets e.g. (Ap_2GpUp) oligonucleotide, 4 nucleotides long with molar composition adenosine (50%), guanosine (25%) uridine (25%), cytidine (0%).

If part of the sequence is known it can be removed from the brackets, e.g. (Ap_2Gp)Up an oligonucleotide with 3′ terminal Up and the indicated length and composition of the remainder.

$(dAT)_n$	alternating copolymer of adenylic and thymidylic acid
poly (A)	polyriboadenylic acid
poly (U)	polyribouridylic acid

Choice of method

1.1. General

Although practically every known molecular separation technique has at some time been applied to nucleic acids and oligonucleotides there are quite specific guide-lines to the best method in particular circumstances. To use these guide-lines in a specific instance it must be known: a) whether a preparative or purely analytical result is required; b) how much material is available or the amount of material required to be separated; c) the order of magnitude of the chain lengths in the initial sample and in the fractions required; and d) whether the sample is ribonucleic acid (RNA), double stranded deoxyribonucleic acid (DNA) or single stranded DNA. (c) is most easily determined by analytical ultracentrifugation (§ 11.2) or acrylamide gel electrophoresis (ch. 7). RNA and DNA can be distinguished chemically or enzymatically (Chargaff and Davidson 1955), and single and double stranded DNA can be assayed by hydroxyapatite chromatography (§ 11.4) or by their density in CsCl gradients, single stranded DNA being denser (§ 11.3). When these parameters are known it may still be necessary to decide between methods based on chain-length differences, composition differences or other characteristics.

The methods covered in detail in this manual are mainly those of chromatography and electrophoresis. Although isopycnic centrifugation is covered (§ 11.3), sedimentation velocity methods are only touched on (§ 11.2). It is intended to cover these in a future manual. The other major omission is the use of cellulose acetate and DEAE-paper electrophoresis in the analysis of high specific activity radioactively labelled oligonucleotides. This powerful analytical method is excellently described by Brownlee (1972) in this series. Gel filtration is mentioned (§ 2.3.3; § 4.1; § 6.7; § 11.1) but the technical details are fully described by Fischer (1969) also in this series. These methods are included in the discussion in this chapter. Other parallel laboratory manuals are by Peterson (1971) and Gordon (1969).

1.2. Oligonucleotides (degree of polymerisation, $n \leqslant 100$)

A variety of powerful methods is available for fractionating short oligonucleotides. Work on nucleotide sequence analysis of small RNA molecules ($n=80$ or 120) and more recently viral RNA molecules ($n \simeq 3000$) and even ribosomal precursor RNAs (up to 45 s) (Holley et al. 1965a; Brownlee 1972; Maden et al. 1972) has stimulated the development of these procedures. They can also be used for synthetic oligonucleotides (e.g. Hachman and Khorana, 1969). The methods depend largely on chromatography and electrophoresis on filter papers, diethylaminoethyl(DEAE)paper, cellulose acetate, thin layers of cellulose or polyethyleneimine (PEI)-cellulose, or columns.

The general criterion, that paper and thin layer methods are useful in the analysis of small (up to a few mg) chemical quantities in concentrated solutions (<1 ml total volume), is applicable here. These methods possess other limitations in that larger oligonucleotides ($n > 10$) often move slowly, if at all, and that guanine-rich oligonucleotides often move slowly and trail over paper at the usual concentrations. This makes traditional paper chromatography and paper electrophoresis useful for mixtures of the smaller oligonucleotides such as those obtained from specific enzyme digests of larger oligonucleotides ($n < 1000$), those obtained as single fractions in another fractionation procedure, and those obtained in *in vitro* synthesis of oligonucleotides.

Many of the fractionation problems can be overcome by the careful use of cellulose acetate and DEAE-paper electrophoresis (Brownlee 1972) but the methods are limited to radio-chemical quantities.

Other mixtures of oligonucleotides must be fractionated in larger quantities or are too complex to be separated by traditional paper chromatography and electrophoresis. Large quantities (>1 mg) of material arise in preparative procedures, in nucleotide sequence analysis of nucleic acids which are not radioactively labelled, and in mixtures where the components of interest are present in very small proportions. Column chromatography is widely used in these cases.

Gel filtration columns can be used to give a coarse separation on the basis of size or for fractionation of mono-nucleotides. Generally, ion-exchange columns provide much greater resolution and have the further advantage that the volume of the original oligonucleotide solution need not necessarily be small, indeed the volumes of the fractions may be relatively large and contain high concentrations of inorganic salts and, maybe, urea. Dowex (polystyrene based) resins are used for mononucleotides but only occasionally for oligonucleotides. DEAE-cellulose and DEAE-Sephadex (dextran based) are widely used for oligonucleotides.

1.3. Nucleic acids (degree of polymerisation, $n > 10$)

Three general properties of long polynucleotide chains are used for their fractionation: size, composition, and reassociation or hybridisation. The main size dependent methods are gel electrophoresis, gel filtration and sedimentation; the main composition dependent methods are isopycnic centrifugation and hydroxyapatite (HAP) although counter current distribution and methylated albumin kieselguhr (MAK) columns have been important during the development of the subject. Transfer RNA (tRNA) fractionation is usually carried out by ion-exchange chromatography on DEAE-Sephadex, benzoylated DEAE-cellulose (BD-cellulose) or a quaternary ammonium chloride. Hydroxyapatite, isopycnic centrifugation and affinity chromatography can be used in conjunction with reassociation and hybridisation.

Gel electrophoresis is of very wide application and is described in detail in chs. 7–10.

TABLE 1.1

Recommended methods for separation of nucleic acids and nucleotides.

Molecular weight	Degree of poly-merisation (nucleotides)	Quantity*	Fractionation principle	Method
300	1	<10 mg	composition	paper chromatography or electrophoresis thin layer chromatography
		>0.1 mg	composition	column chromatography (multi-component methods)
<30000	<100	radio-chemical amounts	size composition sequence	cellulose acetate and DEAE-paper electrophoresis
		<10 mg	size composition	paper chromatography or electrophoresis thin layer chromatography
		<10 mg	sequence	paper chromatography thin layer chromatography
		>1 mg	size composition sequence	column chromatography on DEAE-cellulose at *p*H 8.6 or in 7 M urea at *p*H 7.5 for tRNA use BD-cellulose or RPC5 or RPC6

		> 1 mg	size	DEAE-columns 7 M urea *p*H 7.5
		> 1 mg	composition	DEAE-Sephadex *p*H 2.7 7 M urea DEAE columns *p*H 4,4 to 4,0. 7 M urea
		> 1 mg	sequence	DEAE columns without urea
> 3000	> 10	< 10 mg	size	gel electrophoresis
		> 1 mg	size	gel filtration, sedimentation
		< 100 mg	composition	hydroxyapatite columns
> 30000	> 100	< 10 mg	sequence	DNA reassociation RNE-DNA hybridisation affinity chromatography
> 300000	> 1000	> 1 μg < 100 mg	composition	isopycnic centrifugation

* The limits are by no means absolute but usually extra precautions are needed to exceed them. Where the ranges overlap both methods are applicable. Where no lower limit is given it will be set by the ability to detect the compounds. Where no upper limit is given the methods are applicable at the level of 1 g or more.

Its main limitations are that it is not usually the best method for small oligonucleotides ($n < 10$), it does not distinguish nucleotide composition differences clearly, and it is difficult to scale up for preparative use. It is widely used for analytical and small scale preparative separations because it is quick, sensitive and has high resolving power. Very little specialised apparatus is required and routine fractionation can be carried out by a technician.

Gel filtration and sedimentation generally have less resolving power and sensitivity than gel electrophoresis but they can be more easily scaled up for moderate and large scale preparative use. Thin layer gel filtration can be moderately sensitive for analytical applications and analytical ultracentrifugation can provide the fastest analysis as well as being reasonably sensitive.

Isopycnic centrifugation is limited to high molecular weight polynucleotides ($n > 10^5$) and its resolving power is limited. It is, however, the best method available for fractionating large polynucleotides on the basis of nucleotide composition and can be used on small and intermediate scales. Ion exchange chromatography, particularly on BD-cellulose or RPC5 or RPC6, affords very high resolution of tRNA species and can be applied simply and both on a small and large scale. Hydroxyapatite is an unusual material with an application in DNA fractionation. It can be used to separate DNA fractions differing in thermal stability or rate of reassociation because it separates single and double stranded DNA. It is used preparatively on a small scale but is difficult to scale up. The resolving power is limited by the statistical nature of the reassociation reaction.

1.4. Summary

Table 1.1 summarises the most likely methods to try for a given fractionation problem. The divisions are fairly sharp but by no means absolute and in some cases methods not mentioned here will be applicable.

Nucleotide composition of nucleic acids

2.1. Methods of hydrolysis

The nucleotide composition of oligonucleotides is usually measured by digesting the oligonucleotide to its constituents, in the form of nucleotides, nucleosides or bases and then estimating the proportion of each substance in the mixture either directly or by separating and estimating the components. Alkali, acid and enzyme digestion are commonly used.

2.1.1. Alkali hydrolysis (RNA and oligoribonucleotides only)

The oligonucleotide is incubated in 0.3 N KOH for 18 hr at 37°C (Markam and Smith 1952). Variations of these conditions are possible, e.g. Zamir et al. (1965) used 1.0 N KOH at 80°C for 1 hr. The main products of digestion are nucleoside (mixed 2′, 3′) mono-phosphates (e.g. Michelson 1963). A phosphorylated 5′ end of an oligonucleotide will yield a nucleoside 3′, 5′ diphosphate; and a free 3′-OH of an oligonucleotide will yield a nucleoside. A 2′-0-methyl ribose (which is found, for example, in tRNA, Smith and Dunn 1959; Hall 1963; Sanger et al. 1965) in the oligonucleotide gives rise to an alkali-resistant dinucleotide. A slight deamination of cytidylic acid to uridylic acid occurs. Some minor bases are degraded, for example, dihyrouridylic acid decomposes to β-ureidopropionic acid N-ribosyl phosphate (Cohn and Doherty 1956). In general the reactions are as follows:

$$\mathrm{ApBp} \ldots \mathrm{YpZp} \xrightarrow{\mathrm{KOH}} \mathrm{Ap}+\mathrm{Bp} \ldots +\mathrm{Yp}+\mathrm{Zp}$$

$$\mathrm{pAp} \ldots \mathrm{Z} \xrightarrow{\mathrm{KOH}} \mathrm{pAp}+\mathrm{Bp}+ \ldots +\mathrm{Yp}+\mathrm{Z}$$

An alkaline digest must normally be desalted before the nucleotides can be successfully fractionated. This may conveniently be carried out by neutralising the digest with 6 N perchloric acid (10 min at 0°C) or Dowex 50 H^+ and spinning the solution clear in a bench centrifuge.

An alternative is to use a volatile alkali such as piperidine. Bishop and Bradly (1965) digested ^{32}P labelled RNA with 1 M piperidine in sealed tubes at 60°C for 30 hr. They added some unlabelled ribosomes as carrier and found that the presence of an Oxoid membrane filter during digestion did not affect the subsequent separation and estimation, by ^{32}P radioactivity, of the nucleotides. The piperidine was removed by drying in a current of warm air.

2.1.2. Acid hydrolysis

Digestion of RNA and oligoribonucleotides under acid conditions (e.g. 1–10 mg RNA, 0.25 ml 1.0 N HCl at 100°C for 60 min Leech et al. 1968) produced purine bases and pyrimidine mononucleotides. Variation of the conditions is possible (Michelson 1963). For example, in a study of the methylated constituents of RNA Bjork and Svensson (1967) used a 30 min digestion time. The solution may be desalted by drying.

Hydrolysis of DNA yields free purine bases and, under mild conditions, apurinic acid which can be further degraded by more severe conditions to pyrimidine sequences: pPyp…Pyp (Michelson 1963, p. 368). Kirk (1963, 1967) used mild hydrolysis to liberate the purines which were then estimated after separation by column chromatography:

0.7 mg calf thymus DNA 1 ml 15 mM KCl 0.1 ml 0.33 N HCl	} in Pyrex test-tube (10 × 75 mm)

The mixture was placed in a boiling water bath for 1 min then sealed tightly and kept at 100°C for 40 min. All four bases can be liberated by extensive acid hydrolysis (Chargaff 1955), e.g. 70% perchloric acid for 60 min at 100°C (Marshak and Vogel 1951) or anhydrous formic acid at 175°C for 0.5 to 2 hr (Vischer and Chargaff 1948), but this is likely to degrade the bases and/or give erroneous base compositions through interactions with other decomposition products (Kirk 1967; Abrams 1951; Wyatt 1955).

2.1.3. Enzymic hydrolysis

This has the distinct advantage that the hydrolysis is very specific and takes place under mild conditions so that side reactions are minimised. Usually small volumes of dilute buffer solutions are used so that desalting may be unnecessary. Nucleoside 5′ monophosphates may be obtained.

Miyazawa and Thomas (1965) used the following conditions in a study of the nucleotide composition of oligonucleotides from phage DNA. Pancreatic DNase digestion: the DNA was dialysed into 0.01 M NaCl, 5 mM Tris *p*H 7.3 and made 2 mM $MgCl_2$. 0.10 μg pancreatic DNase per ml DNA solution was added from a stock solution of enzyme (Worthington Biochemical Corp.) (1.5 mg/ml in 0.10 M NaCl containing 0.1% bovine serum albumin) and the digestion proceeded for 2 hr at 37°C. This yielded a mixture of small oligonucleotides (Laskowski 1966a) which were finally degraded to 5′-mononucleotides by snake venom diesterase: 0.05 vol 1.0 M Tris *p*H 9.0 was added, the digest made 5 mM Ca^{2+}, and 6 units/ml snake venom phosphodiesterase added before incubation at 45°C for 2 hr (Laskowski 1966b). Nucleosides may then be prepared by digestion with phosphomonoesterase (Bernardi 1966; Chersi et al. 1966; Carraro and Bernardi 1968a, b).

Exhaustive digestion with T 2 ribonuclease (Uchida and Egami 1966) has been used to prepare 3′-ribonucleotides (e.g. Pratt et al. 1964; Leder and Nirenberg 1964; Rushizky and Miller 1967). Trinucleotides may be digested by incubating 50 μg oligonucleotide with 3.5×10^{-3} units T_2 RNase in 0.02 ml of 0.5 M ammonium acetate, *p*H 4.5, for 2.5 hr at 45°C (Rushizky and Sober 1963).

Hall (1964) used whole snake venom and bacterial alkaline phosphatase to prepare nucleosides from mixed sRNA in a search for minor bases (Hall 1965).

2.2. 'Paper' methods

The experimental techniques relevant to this section are described later (§ 3.1.3; § 3.2.2; § 3.4).

2.2.1 Paper electrophoresis (Smith 1955)

This is a very popular method particularly for ribonucleotides.

The paper and the electrode chambers contain 0.05 M or 0.1 M ammonium formate made *p*H 3.5 with 88% formic acid. With a voltage gradient of 100 volt cm^{-1} the nucleotides are separated in 1 to 3 hr, Up having run a distance of approximately 30 to 90 cm respectively. The order of migration towards the anode is Up (fastest), Gp, Ap and Cp. Except for Gp the 2′ and 3′ isomers migrate together.

The spots can be seen in near ultraviolet light in a dark room because they quench the fluorescence of the paper. (*Wear protective goggles when using ultraviolet light*). For quantitative analysis the spots are cut out, the nucleotides eluted with water or dilute buffer or 0.05 N HCl and their optical densities measured. The extinction coefficients at *p*H 7 are given in Table 2.1.

TABLE 2.1

Photometric determination of nucleotides (Sober 1968).

Nucleotide	Extinction coefficient $\varepsilon_{max}(\times 10^{-3})$ 1 M^{-1} cm^{-1}	Wavelength nm (λ_{max})
Ap	15.4	259
Cp	9.2	270
Gp	13.4	252
Up	10.0	262

Radioactivity can be determined by counting either the paper directly or the eluted nucleotides. Carrier nucleotides are used, if necessary, to make the spots visible.

2.2.2. Paper chromatography

This method is cheaper than paper electrophoresis in terms of capital equipment but slower (one or two days, but many samples can be run simultaneously).

The two-dimensional system (§ 3.3) uses descending chromatography in isobutyric acid : 0.5 M NH_3 : 0.1 M EDTA, 100 : 1 : 6 for 19 hr on Whatman No. 1 chromatography paper at least 45 cm square. The order of migration is $U \simeq G < C < A$. The solvent for the second dimension, which requires 13 hr, is prepared by adding 600 g $(NH_4)_2SO_4$ and 20 ml *n*-propanol to 1 l of 0.05 M KH_2PO_4 + 0.05 M K_2HPO_4. The order of migration is $A < G < U \simeq C$. The paper is dried between the two stages.

The spots are visualised as for paper electrophoresis and eluted with 0.05 N HCl (§ 2.2.1).

The mixed 2′ and 3′ ribonucleotides, Cp, Gp, Ap and Up, can be separated in one dimension (Lane 1963). Sheets of Whatman No. 1 filter paper are impregnated by dipping them through a solution made by diluting 1 vol saturated ammoniumsulphate with 9 vol of water. The sheets are air dried in a fume cupboard and stored. The chromatographic tank, but not the paper, is equilibrated for 24 hr with the developing solvent, 80 vol of 95% ethanol, 20 vol of water. The samples are loaded on the impregnated paper and chromatographed immediately for 15–24 hr at 22°C. The spots can be quantitatively eluted with water.

2.2.3. *Thin layer chromatography*

In general, thin layer methods are quicker and more sensitive than paper methods and in principle paper methods can be directly transferred to cellulose thin layers. In practice these methods have not been widely used for nucleotide fractionation (but see § 1.2 and § 3.4). The following manufacturers for example provide general information on the use of the products for thin layer chromatography: H. Reeve Angel (Whatman); Camlab (Glass) Ltd; Shandon Southern Ltd; Eastman-Kodak. It is not proposed to go into more detail here.

Randerath and Randerath (1967a) have developed a thin layer method specific for nucleotides using PEI-cellulose (polyethyleneimine-cellulose). Commercial thin layers are manufactured by J. T. Baker Chemical Co. and the conditions required with these are slightly different from those used by Randerath and Randerath (1967a) who made their own thin layers. Jacobson (1971) recommends that the sample be thoroughly desalted and the unloaded sheets irrigated with 1 M acetic acid to remove visible impurities. The nucleotides are then spotted on the chromatogram 20 mm from the bottom and ascending chromatography carried out in 1 M acetic acid until the front almost reaches the top of the sheet (200 mm). After evaporating the acetic acid, the ascending chromatography is continued in the same direction using 0.33 M LiCl until the LiCl front has risen 60 to 80 mm above the origin. Cp moves fastest followed by Ap, Up and Gp in that order.

2.3. Column chromatography

Many schemes for fractionating nucleotides, nucleosides and bases on sulphonated polystyrene resins have been published. The main difficulty with these methods is variation between resin batches (e.g. Anderson et al. 1963). Nucleotide separations can be achieved on DEAE-cellulose (Whatman Data Sheet 13, 1967) and DEAE-Sephadex (Fiers et al. 1965b) but these media do not seem to be widely used. Gel filtration columns will separate some nucleotide components. Ligand exchange chromatography and partition chromatography of nucleosides are useful for minor components.

2.3.1. Dowex

The principles of ion-exchange chromatography are discussed in ch. 3. Here, some useful elution systems for nucleotides are described. The descriptions are based on published work and the author's experience but it must be emphasised that variations between batches of Dowex resins may make the methods difficult to repeat and any method should be rigorously tested before use (e.g. Matthews 1968a).

2.3.1.1. Anion exchange at low pH

Ribonucleotides are separated in the order, Cp, Ap, Up, Gp, by elution from a Dowex-2 Cl^- column (2.5 × 0.94 cm) with 5 l 0.003 N HCl at 0.8 ml/min. Deoxyribonucleotides are separated in a similar order, dCp, dAp, Tp, dGp, by elution from Dowex-1 Cl^- (200–400 mesh, 8 × 0.72 cm) with 3 l of 0.002 N HCl (*p*H 7) at 1 ml/min (Cohn 1955).

Ribonucleotides are separated on a column (11 × 0.6 cm) of Dowex-1 formate (× 10, 200–400). The column was washed successively with: 250 ml 3 M sodium formate; 100 ml 1 M sodium formate, 6 N formic acid; 100 ml 88% formic acid; distilled water to effluent pH 4. Nucleotides were loaded in distilled water (20 ml) and then eluted by a gradient from distilled water to 1 N formic acid (30 ml) increasing to 4 N formic acid (150 ml) or sometimes to 0.2 M ammonium formate in 4 N formic acid increasing to 0.4 M ammonium formate in 4 N formic acid. The column may be regenerated with 88% formic acid (200 ml) followed by distilled water (Hurlbert et al. 1954; Bishop and Bradley 1965).

Anderson et al. (1963) have described a more comprehensive system for nucleotide analysis. Their system has been recommended for adaptations of some amino acid analysers. A single column 0.9 × 160 cm of Dowex-1 (× 8, 200–400 hydraulically fractionated to about 60 *μ* particle diameter) washed in acid and alkali was packed in sections in 0.15 M sodium acetate *p*H 4.4. The sample, vol 0.5–1.5 ml in buffer, was eluted by a 1.4-l linear gradient from 0.15–3 M sodium acetate at a constant *p*H (4.4), flow-rate (1 ml/min) and temperature (40°C). The first few peaks were extremely sharp and a lower flow rate could be used here. Good separations of quite complex mixtures were obtained in 28 hr. The triphosphates, UTP, ATP, GTP could be separated more quickly (in 6 hr) on a 0.9 × 50 cm column of the same resin eluted with a 1 l linear gradient from 0.5 M sodium acetate, 0.25 M NaCl to 1.0 M sodium acetate, 0.5 M NaCl *p*H 3.6 at 1.7 ml/min at room temperature. A freshly packed column was used for each determination in both cases.

2.3.1.2. Cation exchange at low pH

Blattner and Erickson (1967) have described two simple systems, one for 2′, 3′ ribonucleotides, and one for 5′ deoxyribonucleotides.

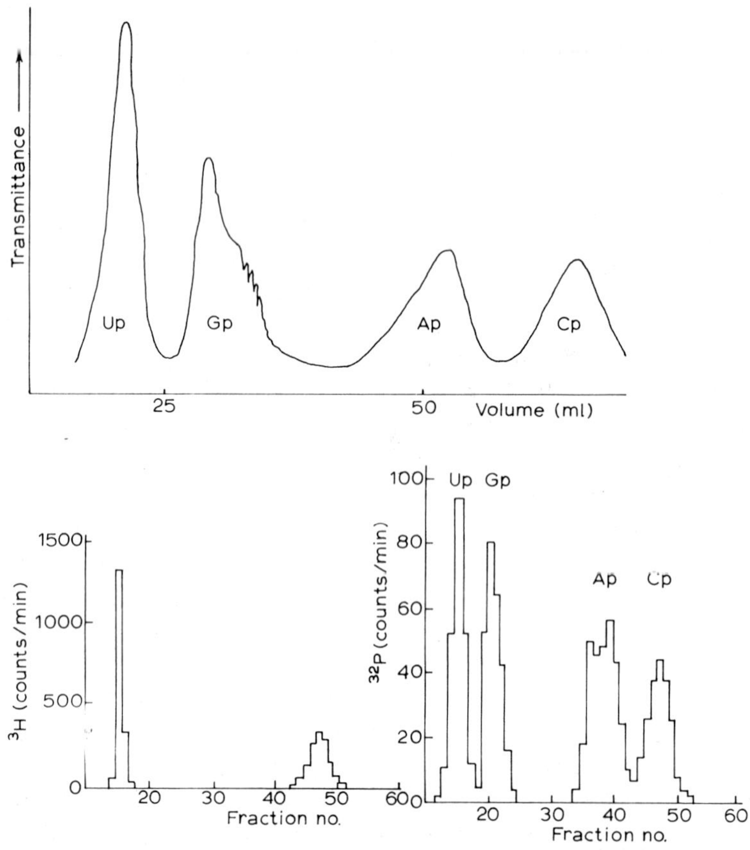

Fig. 2.1. Nucleotide fractionation. A sample of μ2 phage RNA uniformly labelled with ^{32}P and the pyrimidines labelled with ^{3}H was digested with alkali (§ 2.1.1) and separated by column chromatography on Dowex 50 formate eluted with 0.25 M ammonium formate *p*H 4.1. The ultraviolet transmission graph is traced from the record of a Uvicord I ultraviolet monitor output. Radioactivities were measured by dissolving the samples in a scintillation 'cocktail' and counting in a liquid scintillation counter. The peaks were identified from their ultraviolet spectra.

For 2′, 3′ ribonucleotides, they use Dowex 50 (×4, minus 400 mesh washed in acid and alkali) in a 0.8×85 cm column eluted with 0.25 M ammonium formate adjusted to *p*H 4.1 with formic acid at 1 ml/min. This separates the four main ribonucleotides (but not the 2′, 3′ isomers) in about 1 hr (Fig. 2.1). The column can be reused without regeneration since only one buffer is used throughout. It is essential that the loaded sample be in the elution buffer and not more than 1.5 ml in volume (Matthews 1968d). Each nucleotide is eluted in a volume small enough for direct radioactivity measurement by Cerenkov counting (Matthews 1968b). The order of elution given in this reference (Blattner and Erickson 1967) is wrong, it should be Up, Gp, Ap, Cp (Matthews 1968d). This method is slightly quicker, more sensitive and more convenient than that of Katz and Comb (1963). Its principal advantage is that the column can be reused immediately but moderate pressures are required for its operation.

For 5′ deoxyribonucleotides Blattner and Erickson (1967) use the same resin in a 0.8×40 cm column eluted with 0.1 M ammonium formate adjusted to *p*H 3.2 and obtain a performance similar to that obtained for the 2′, 3′ ribonucleotides.

An earlier procedure described by Katz and Comb (1963) separates Up, Gp and (Ap+Cp) in the first stage and then Ap and Cp in the second stage. Because of the different absorption spectra of Ap and Cp only the first stage may be necessary for nucleotide composition determination. Moderate volumes of eluant are used so sensitivity is reasonable (50 to 100 nmoles of each nucleotide, or about 0.1 mg RNA) (Katz and Comb 1963; Nishimura et al. 1967). The first column is 0.9×5.0 cm of Dowex 50 H^+ (×4, 200–400) washed with 3 N HCl, water until neutral, and finally with 20 ml 0.05 N HCl. The sample of nucleotides, in 0.05 N HCl, is loaded onto the column and washed in with 1 ml 0.05 N HCl. Up is eluted with 5 ml 0.05 N HCl. The column is then eluted with water at 1 ml/min or less. Gp is eluted in the first 7.5 ml of water effluent and Ap and Cp in the next 25 ml. The nucleotide composition of the sample may be determined from the extinction co-efficients of the fractions (at 2 wavelengths for the Ap and Cp fraction).

Ap and Cp may be separated if required by loading directly onto a 0.9 × 1.0 cm column of Dowex-1 formate (× 8, 200–400) and eluting with 20 ml 0.05 N HCOOH (Cp) and then 30 ml 0.4 N HCOOH (Ap) at 1 ml/min.

A disadvantage of these methods (Katz and Comb 1963; Blattner and Erickson 1967) is that Up passes straight through the column and is liable to be contaminated with, for example, oligonucleotides, inorganic phosphate or polyphosphate. This is particularly serious with ^{32}P labelled Up but the effect can be reduced by adsorbing the Up on activated charcoal and counting this with a Geiger–Muller counter.

2.3.1.3. *High pH*

Mundry (1965) has described a small column (2 ml packed volume) for separation of ribonucleotides at alkaline *p*H. The column is packed with Dowex-1 Cl^- (× 8, –400) in 0.01 N HCl. After packing it is washed with 0.04 M Tris–HCl *p*H 8.8, 0.06% Brij. The sample is loaded in this buffer and eluted with a 600 ml linear gradient from this buffer to 0.4 M glycine buffer *p*H 9.5, 0.06% Brij. The method suffers from the disadvantage that the *p*H varies during elution (cf. Anderson et al. 1963).

2.3.2. *Other ion-exchangers*

2.3.2.1. *Conventional chromatography*

Mundry (1965) has also described the use of DEAE-Sephadex for the separation of ribonucleotides and nucleosides. Using a 1.1 × 85 cm column and a 1.1-l linear gradient from 0.04 M Tris–HCl *p*H 8.8 to 0.20 M Tris–HCl, 0.25 M NaCl *p*H 9.5 or a linear gradient from 0.04 M triethylamine carbonate *p*H 8.8 to 0.35 M triethylamine carbonate, 0.15 M NaCl *p*H 9.5 he has separated the 8 main ribonucleosides and nucleotides. The nucleoside separation is very sensitive to traces of salt and some difficulty with reproducibility was experienced.

Fiers et al. (1965b) separated Up and Cp on DEAE-Sephadex (1.1 × 53 cm) with a 2-l gradient from 0.03 M to 0.3 M ammonium bicarbonate *p*H 8.6. In this method a large volume of sample may be applied.

Some ribonucleoside and nucleotide separations on 1.5 × 34 cm columns of DEAE-cellulose eluted with 0.09 M sodium acetate, 0.2 M acetic acid *p*H 4.4 have been described (Whatman Data Sheet DS/13).

A column (17 cm × 1 cm) of Zeo-Karb 225 was washed with 0.03 N HCl (at least 20 ml) and an acid hydrolysate of DNA was loaded. Apurinic acids were eluted with 0.03 N HCl (50 ml) and then guanine and adenine were eluted separately with 2 N HCl. This is part of an accurate chemical method for measurement of DNA composition (Kirk, 1967).

2.3.2.2. High performance liquid chromatography

High performance liquid chromatographs can be used for nucleotide separations (Hadden et al. 1971) usually by ion-exchange chromatography on special commercially available resins using gradient elution with phosphate buffers. More recently, Holton et al. (1974) have used a special reversed phase ion-exchange material (RPC-TMSN) and ammonium acetate buffers to obtain good nucleotide separations and some oligonucleotide separations. High performance liquid chromatographs work on the same principles as conventional liquid chromatography, as described in this manual, but analysis times are greatly reduced by using very high resolution columns and column packings with very high flow rates. This requires the use of high pressures, 1000–3000 psi. The equipment is relatively expensive but is becoming more generally available. It is particularly suited to nucleotide separations because of their high extinction coefficients at 254 nm which allows the simplest type of ultraviolet detector to be used. These systems are very good where a large number of samples needs to be analysed and the initial cost and setting up time can be justified. Separation times are reduced by approximately one order of magnitude over conventional liquid chromatography. The equipment and resins are available from suppliers such as Pye Unicam, Dupont, Waters Ass. and Varian.

The special resin (RPC-TMSN) used by Holton et al. (1974) was made by suspending 500 g silica gel (E. Merck 5–25 μm) in 1.5 l toluene with 50 g trimethyl silylchloride (TMS-Cl) and 50 g hexamethyldisilazane (HMDS). The solution was refluxed for 2 days with intermittent addition of an equivalent amount of TMS-Cl and HMDS. The silylated silica was filtered washed with chloroform and methanol with subsequent drying for 10 hr at 100°C under a vacuum of 1 Torr. To 500 g of the product was added a solution of 25 ml of trimethyl c_8–c_{10} alkyl ammonium chloride (Adogen 464, Ashland Chemicals) in 300 ml chloroform, giving a ratio Adogen 464:silica, of 5:100 v/w. The chloroform was removed by stirring vigorously in a fume cupboard for 2 days and by drying under vacuum (0.01 Torr, 25°C). The resin was dry packed into a column 2 foot long by $\frac{3}{8}$ inch internal diameter (approximately 610 × 10 mm) and eluted at 4 ml min^{-1} with 0.1 M ammonium acetate adjusted to *p*H 4.0 with trifluoracetic acid. Good separations of nucleotides were achieved in runs of a few minutes. Oligonucleotides could also be eluted, especially with a more concentrated eluent. The authors state that the method can be used preparatively (Holton et al. 1974).

For the use of commercially available reversed phase ion exchange materials see § 5.2.3.

2.3.3. Gel filtration

Secondary effects in gel filtration columns (cf. Schwartz and Zabin 1966) allow some fractionation of nucleic acid components, particularly nucleosides, on these columns (Hohn and Pollman 1963; Schwartz et al. 1965; Uziel and Cohn 1965; Mezzasoma and Farina 1966a, b; Braun 1967a, b; Dirheimer and Ebel 1967; Hohn and Schaller 1967; Carrara and Bernardi 1968a).

A clean separation of the 4 main nucleosides (either ribo- or deoxyribo-) on cross-linked Dextran (Sephadex G-10) has been described by Braun (1967b). He used a 1.5 × 90 cm column eluted with 0.01 M citric acid Na_2HPO_4, *p*H 3.5 at 25 ml/hr. The sample was loaded in 0.5 ml water and contained 0.1 mg of each nucleoside. The elution took 10 hr and each nucleoside was eluted in a volume of 10–20 ml in the order, C, U, A, G or C, T, A, G for the ribo- and deoxyribo-series respectively. The column can be reused immediately without regeneration.

Carrara and Bernardi (1968a) have described a different system using polyacrylamide gel beads (Biogel P 2). The nucleosides are eluted in smaller volumes but are not all separated in one run. They used a 0.9×80 cm column (which may well account for the smaller volumes) packed with Biogel P 2 which had been washed in 0.1 M EDTA and had the fines decanted. Elution with 2 mM ammonium carbonate, *p*H 10.2 separates dI, dG+T, dC, dA in that order; elution with 0.2 mM sodium phosphate *p*H 7.2 separates dI+dC+T, dA, dG. The unresolved group may be separated by evaporating to dryness, redissolving and running with the other elution system. A useful feature of the neutral pH system is that nucleotides are eluted before dI+dC+T so that nucleosides in the presence of nucleotides may be analysed. This may be particularly useful for identifying nucleoside end groups of oligonucleotides (Carrara and Bernardi 1968b).

2.3.4. Partition chromatography

This is the method used by Hall (1965) in conjunction with paper chromatography for the fractionation of mixtures of minor ribonucleosides. 690 g of Whatman Celite 545-Microcel E (9:1) was soaked in 308 ml of the lower phase of ethyl acetate:2 ethoxyethanol:water (4:1:2) and dry packed in 25 g aliquots in a 5.08×105 cm column. The sample, in the same solvent, mixed with 80 g of support (Celite–Microcel) was placed on top of the column. The column was eluted with the upper phase of the above solvent until uridine (the 3rd peak) was eluted and then the eluent was changed to the upper phase of ethyl acetate:1-butanol:ligroin:water (1:2:1:1). Each of the 6 peaks eluted was desalted and concentrated by repeated evaporation and redissolution in water. Fraction 1 was rechromatographed on a smaller column using 1-butanol:water: concentrated ammonium hydroxide (3:1:0.05), the lower phase being used for the column (150 g Celite–Microcel) and sample and the upper phase for elution.

Fraction 2 was analysed by paper chromatography in 2-propanol: concentrated HCl:water (680:170:155). Fraction 3 was uridine. Fraction 4 was rechromatographed in the same way as Fraction 1 but using ethyl acetate:1-propanol:water (4:1:2). Fraction 5 was dissolved in hot water and then cooled and kept at 4°C for several days to precipitate most of the guanosine and then rechromatographed in the same way as Fraction 1. Finally, Fraction 6 was rechromatographed using ethyl acetate:1-butanol:water (1:1:1).

2.3.5. Ligand exchange chromatography on a copper-loaded chelating resin (Goldstein 1967)

Chelex-100 (Whatman) resin was suspended in 1 M $CuCl_2$ overnight, washed repeatedly in water and suspended in 1 N ammonia overnight. A column (0.9 × 45 cm) was packed with a small volume of non-$CuCl_2$ treated resin at the bottom followed by the copper complexed resin above. After washing the column, the nucleic acid components were loaded in a small volume of water and eluted with water (nucleotides followed by weakly basic nucleosides), 1 N ammonia (other nucleosides) and/or 2.5 N ammonia (bases). The nucleotides are not bound by the column and so are not fractionated. The nucleosides and bases are, however, well fractionated. Several minor components are well separated. The method is relatively quick and the eluants are volatile.

2.4. Multicomponent analyses

Methods of determining nucleotide composition without separating the components are summarised here.

2.4.1. Multi-component spectrophotometric analysis

The composition of mixtures of ribonucleotides, which may be obtained from RNA by alkaline hydrolysis or enzyme digestion, may be determined from the absorption spectrum of the solution in the range 220–300 nm. The calculation may be based on a large number (say 50) of absorptions throughout the spectrum and the spectrum analysed by a least squares, or better, by a linear programming procedure in terms of the standard spectra of the four main nucleotides. The spectra of minor components may also be included but this tends to reduce the accuracy of a determination in some cases. The method is very susceptible to the presence of impurities. This can be partly obviated by analysing spectra taken at several pH values and/or by destroying one component by UV irradiation. The analysis may also be carried out by analysing only the absorptions at a few critical wavelengths.

The spectra of native and denatured DNA as well as the difference spectrum (hyperchromic spectrum) between these two have been studied in some detail. These spectra can be used to determine the DNA base-pair composition (Fresco et al. 1963; Hirschman and Felsenfeld 1966).

These methods undoubtedly work but they must be applied with great care especially as they are extremely sensitive to the presence of impurities. The following two methods are much more widely used.

2.4.2. Thermal denaturation temperature of DNA

The denaturation temperature, T_m, of double helical DNA is a linear function of its base pair composition

$$T_m = 69.3 + 0.41\ (\mathrm{GC}) \qquad (2.1)$$

where T_m°C is the mid-point of the thermal denaturation profile (in a solvent containing 0.2 M Na^+) and GC is the mole per cent guanine + cytosine (Marmur and Doty 1959, 1962) (see § 11.4.4.1).

The solvent used by Marmur and Doty (1962) was 0.15 M NaCl + 0.015 M sodium citrate adjusted to *p*H 7.0 ± 0.3 containing about 20 μg/ml DNA. The optical density with a 1 cm light path at 260 mμ of the solution was measured as a function of temperature using a spectrophotometer equipped with a variable temperature cell. Evaporation must be prevented and a correction for thermal expansion is required. T_m is the temperature at which the absorbance increase is 50% of the final, maximum, absorbance increase. The use of other sodium ion concentrations drastically affects the results. The necessary corrections are described by Owen et al. (1969).

2.4.3. Density of DNA in concentrated CsCl solutions

This is an accurate, simple method for determining the base-pair composition of double-stranded DNA. It is not sensitive to impurities in the sample (although the CsCl must be free from rubidium, at least) and requires only 1 μg of DNA (Sueoka 1959; Marmur and Doty 1959; Rolfe and Meselson 1959; Schildkraut et al. 1962).

The density is found with reference to a DNA of known density using a CsCl density gradient set up in an ultracentrifuge. 0.84 ml of a stock solution of CsCl (130 g CsCl + 70 ml 0.02 M Tris *p*H 8.5) is mixed with 0.23 ml of sample solution (1–2 μg reference DNA). The density is adjusted to 1.710 g/ml by the addition of water as necessary and measurement of the refractive index, *n*, of the solution, which is related to density (eqn. 11.2). This solution (0.75 ml) is spun in an analytical ultracentrifuge at 44,770 rev/min at 25°C. Equilibrium is attained by 20 hr and ultraviolet absorption photographs are taken. The density, ρ, of the sample DNA is found in terms of the density, ρ_0, of the reference DNA (eq. 11.3) (Sueoka 1961; Ift et al. 1961; Schildkraut et al. 1962). The average mole fraction of G + C of the sample DNA is then calculated from:

$$\rho = 1.660 + 0.098\,(\mathrm{GC}) \tag{2.2}$$

These figures are based on *Escherichia coli* DNA as reference which is taken to have a density of 1.710 g/ml. Further details in § 11.3.

The relation has recently been justified for fractions of mammalian DNA (Schildkraut and Maio 1969), but does not hold for DNAs with a highly repeated very simple nucleotide sequence (Filipski et al. 1973).

Paper chromatography, paper electrophoresis and thin layer chromatography

3.1. Paper electrophoresis

3.1.1. Principles of paper electrophoresis

A solute will move through paper under the action of a voltage gradient $\mathrm{d}V/\mathrm{d}x$ with a speed (mobility) proportional to $q(\mathrm{d}V/\mathrm{d}x)/k$ where q is the net charge on the molecule and k represents the retarding effect ('frictional force') of the paper on the motion of the molecule. The charge, q, on an oligonucleotide whose p*K*s are known may be calculated as a function of *p*H (Budovskii and Demushkin 1964) or read from dissociation curves (Smith 1955). For oligonucleotides that have not been characterised in this way, an approximate value for the net charge may be calculated by summing the charges on the individual nucleotides which make up the oligonucleotides. The frictional co-efficient, k, is more difficult to predict, but in general it increases with the size of the molecule. Smith (1955) gives relative values of k for mono-, di- and trinucleotides (1.00; 1.43; 2.00) calculated from diffusion data. Mobilities calculated on these bases agree well with experiment at least for short oligonucleotides.

Relative mobilities are defined with reference to a standard material, which may be the solvent front in chromatography (R_f), as

$$\frac{\text{distance from origin of unknown}}{\text{distance from origin of standard}}$$

Electrophoretic mobility may also be defined as

$$\frac{\text{distance from origin}}{\text{voltage gradient} \times \text{time}}$$

The frictional constant, k, for a given oligonucleotide is not a rapidly varying function of the pH of the electrophoresis buffer. In the region of a pK, however, the charge, q, on the oligonucleotide is a rapidly varying function of pH. The separation of oligonucleotides by paper electrophoresis depends on the exploitation of their different pKs. This is achieved by choosing the pH of the electrophoresis buffer so that differences in pK values of the compounds to be separated are expressed as different charges, q, at this pH.

As an example of the use of paper electrophoresis for the fractionation of oligonucleotides consider the fractionation of some decanucleotides obtained from MS2 viral RNA by T1 ribonuclease digestion. The specificity of the enzyme ensured that each oligonucleotide contained only one Gp residue and the decanucleotides were isolated by column chromatography (§5.2.1.2). The oligonucleotide mixture was electrophoresed for 17 hr at 6 volt/cm in 0.02 M ammonia formate pH 2.7. At this pH the nucleotides, Ap, Cp, Gp, Up have net charges, q, of -0.08, -0.02, -0.66, 0.98 respectively. Thus the mobility of these decanucleotides should depend mostly on the ratio of Ap+Cp to Up in their composition. Good separation in the predicted order has been obtained (Rushizky et al. 1965).

Other useful pH values are: pH 1.9 where fractionation depends mostly on the number of Up residues; pH 3.5 where the four main ribonucleotides may be separated; and higher pH values where differences between Ap and Cp can be exploited, although Rushizky et al. (1965) did not have much success at pH 4.0–4.4 with penta- to heptanucleotides. Degradation of purine nucleotides may occur at pH 1.9, although this is not observed on DEAE-paper electrophoresis and deamination of cytosine to uridine may occur at very high pH values.

In general, large oligonucleotides run faster than small ones of similar composition because the charge differences are greater than the frictional coefficient differences. This can be used to separate the components of a homologous series.

3.1.2. Electrophoresis apparatus and practical considerations

The mobility of uridylic acid in 0.05 M ammonium formate buffer *p*H 3.5 is approximately 0.4 cm hr^{-1} volt cm^{-1}. It is commonly necessary for this nucleotide to run about 40 cm along the paper. So, a potential gradient of 10 volt cm^{-1} would be needed to complete the run in 10 hr, i.e. a potential difference of 400 volts. In practice very much larger voltages, up to about 5 kV may be used and separations are then achieved in an hour or so. Currents up to about 10 mA per cm width of paper are used.

This makes electrophoresis apparatus extremely dangerous and at least one fatal accident has been reported (Spencer et al. 1966a, b). It is essential that the apparatus be built to a high standard of safety and all safety precautions observed. This can be achieved with negligible inconvenience to the operator. In particular it must be impossible to switch on the high voltage before the apparatus is completely enclosed and adequately insulated and earthed. Such large currents also cause considerable heating of the paper. Breakdown of the solutes and charring of the paper are avoided by cooling. This may be done by immersing the paper in a coolant such as white spirit or by placing the paper between two smooth flat metal surfaces held together by air pressure and cooled by tap water. Both methods are in use. Suitable apparatus is available commercially (Michl 1958; Gross 1961; Naughton and Hagopian 1962; for review see Wunderly 1961; Brownlee 1972).

The ionic strength of the buffer needs to be high enough to maintain the *p*H at the chosen value and to make the effect of the sample conductivity on the voltage gradient negligible. However, the heat generated by a given voltage across the paper is proportional to the conductivity of the buffer, so the ionic strength should be low enough to allow reasonable voltages to be used without overheating. As a compromise, 0.05 M buffers are often used, although higher and lower molarities are not infrequent.

The oligonucleotide solution is loaded onto the paper along a line for a 1-dimensional fractionation or in a spot for a 2-dimensional fractionation. The loading volume should be about 10 μl per cm or per spot, containing little or no inorganic salts. The mass of oligonucleotide that may be loaded depends on its solubility in the electrophoresis buffer and the nature of the paper.

In general, the solubility of an oligonucleotide decreases with increasing chain length and those containing guanine residues are particularly insoluble. Too high concentrations lead to 'trailing' of the material over a large area of the paper. This is a common phenomenon with guanine-rich oligonucleotides. The capacity of a paper increases with the amount of water it can absorb so that, for example, Whatman 3MM paper has a higher capacity than the thinner Whatman no. 1 paper. Less flow of buffer is obtained with thin papers and these are preferred where high capacity is not essential.

The trailing of large and guanine-rich oligonucleotides can be reduced by washing the paper with EDTA (Armstrong et al. 1964) and by using cellulose acetate instead of paper. Cellulose acetate has a very low capacity and is difficult to work with because it is brittle when dry, but it has been very successfully used in the fractionation of oligonucleotides labelled at high specific activity with ^{32}P (Sanger et al. 1965).

3.1.3. Experimental procedure for paper electrophoresis

The use of a flat-plate water cooled apparatus is described. Brownlee (1972) describes the 'hanging' or 'up and over' types of tank which use an organic coolant.

The electrophoresis apparatus is prepared by cutting 4 sheets of thick polythene to cover the cooling plates, two sheets below the electrophoresis paper and two above. The electrode vessels are filled with buffer and the wicks prepared. The wicks are 4 small sheets of 3MM filter cut to bridge the gaps between the electrophoresis paper and the electrode vessels. The papers are soaked in buffer and washed dialysis membrane is placed over the edges due to contact the electrophoresis paper (Fig. 3.1).

The electrophoresis paper is cut to the correct size for the apparatus and the position(s) of the starting spot(s) or line measured up and marked in pencil. The loading solution is then applied by supporting the paper so that it has air underneath the loading spot and applying small ($\sim 1\ \mu l$) aliquots which are allowed to dry between applications. A cold air blower (hair dryer) is used to speed drying. When all the sample has been loaded and the spot has dried, the paper is sprayed with buffer in a fume cupboard (Shandon Southern Ltd. market a suitable laboratory spray gun) until it is thoroughly and evenly soaked but not dripping. It is then transferred to the prepared electrophoresis apparatus and the run commenced.

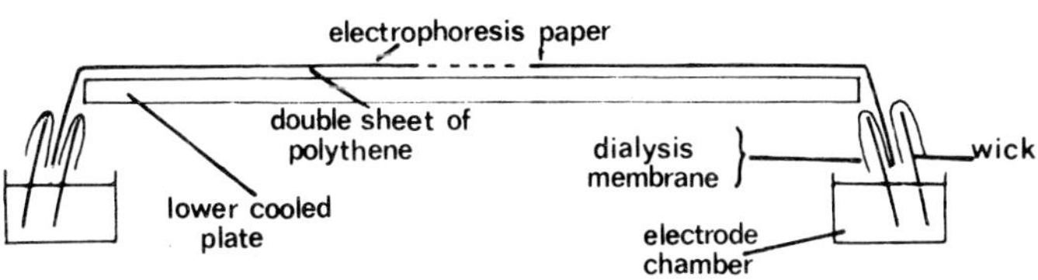

Fig. 3.1. Flat plate high voltage electrophoresis.

After the run the paper is dried in a warm air oven fitted with an extractor fan and racks for hanging the papers. The wicks and polythene sheets can be reused several times.

Detection and elution of the spots have already been described (§ 2.2.1).

3.2. Paper chromatography

3.2.1. Principles of paper chromatography

Paper chromatography can be used instead of, or in 2-dimensional systems as well as, paper electrophoresis. Its principal advantage is that less expensive equipment is required and that some separations, particularly sequence-dependent ones, are difficult to obtain by paper electrophoresis. Its disadvantage is that relatively long development times are required, although simple separations can be accomplished overnight.

The fractionation depends on many factors. The basic process, however, is partition of the solute (oligonucleotides) between a stationary phase (water absorbed by the cellulose fibres of the paper) and a moving phase (the chromatographic solvent). The behaviour of the solute thus depends on its partition coefficient between the water-cellulose complex and the chromatographic solvent. Solutes with relatively high solubilities in the chromatographic solvent will move rapidly and those with relatively low solubilities will move slowly. Thus, in a mixture of solutes separation will occur due to differences in partition coefficient between the components of the solute.

Partition coefficients will, in general, be affected by the water content, the ionic strength, the *p*H and the organic part of the chromatographic solvent. The ionic strength and *p*H will also affect solubility in the stationary phase. In general, increasing ionic strength produces decreasing solubility of oligonucleotides in both the stationary phase and the moving phase. The net result is to reduce the mobility in a selective way, so much so that a solvent containing 80% saturated ammonium sulphate *p*H 6 with only 2% isopropanol will separate nucleotides with the pyrimidine nucleotides moving rapidly and Gp and then Ap more slowly (Markam and Smith 1952).

*p*H affects the degree of ionisation of the solute. Increasing degree of ionisation will usually produce lower mobility because the partition coefficient, 'solubility in stationary phase/solubility in moving phase', will increase. The effect will depend on the p*K*s of the solute. At acid *p*H values, differences in the p*K*s of the $-NH_2$ groups in Ap, Gp and Cp provide variations in the effect of *p*H on mobility; and at alkaline *p*H values the enol –OH of Up and Gp begins to ionise above a *p*H of about 8. These differences are particularly useful in 2-dimensional paper chromatography and might suggest ways of modifying a solvent which does not separate the components of interest.

The solubility of an oligonucleotide in the chromatographic solvent depends on ionic strength and *p*H as above and also on the water content and nature of the organic part of the chromatographic solvent. Increasing the water content of the chromatographic solvent increases the solubility of the oligonucleotide and so increases its mobility. This usually sets a lower limit to the water content below which the mobility of the oligonucleotide is negligible. Slightly higher water contents will give low mobilities but a large effect due to the organic component and hence good separation. In many systems, further increase in water content produces higher mobilities but relatively poorer separation. Higher mobility has the advantage of decreasing the development time of the chromatogram so a compromise is usually struck to give the maximum mobility consistent with sufficient resolution. However, the effect is not the same for all oligonucleotides as more polar molecules will be affected more than less polar ones. So, increasing the water content will increase the mobility of the more polar molecules more than the mobility of the less polar molecules. This will often reduce the resolution, but means that complicated effects can occur.

The effect of the organic component of the chromatographic solvent is important but complicated. Hydrophobic, Van der Waal's and hydrogen bonding forces combine to provide interactions between oligonucleotides, organic molecules and water. In general, oligonucleotides are capable of forming all these types of bonds. Solvents whose properties encourage these bonds will give rise to high mobility; solvents which cannot combine in these ways will give lower mobility. Hydrogen bonds are important in interactions with butyric acid but not with aliphatic alcohols and, indeed, these solvents produce different mobilities for different nucleotides.

In summary, differences in composition, length and nucleotide sequence between oligonucleotides can provide the basis for fractionation by paper chromatography. Increasing length of an oligonucleotide tends to produce a decreasing mobility and decreasing resolution of a given difference in nucleotide composition or sequence. This can sometimes be overcome by very long development times,

Subject index p. 487

but paper electrophoresis is often preferred to paper chromatography for longer oligonucleotides. Paper chromatography has a particular advantage in the separation of sequence isomers where the complicated nature of the interactions of the oligonucleotide with the organic solvent, among other effects, allows sequence effects to be exploited.

The many systems described in the literature usually contain an organic solvent such as *iso*butyric acid or an aliphatic alcohol with an aqueous solution of ammonia, and acid or an inorganic buffer.

3.2.2. *Experimental procedure for paper chromatography*

A chromatography tank capable of taking paper of the order of 50 cm square is used. This is an enclosed tank with troughs at the top and bottom between which the paper hangs. Tanks are widely available commercially (e.g. Shandon Southern Ltd.).

The sample is loaded on the paper as described for paper electrophoresis but the paper is not sprayed before the run (§ 3.1.3). The bottom edge of the paper is serrated to allow buffer to drip off evenly and the paper is loaded, dry, into the chromatography tank. The atmosphere in the tank and the paper are allowed to equilibrate with a beaker of the chromatography buffer placed in the tank for at least 0.5 hr. Then the upper trough (for descending chromatography) is filled with the buffer and chromatography commences.

For the second dimension (§ 3.3.3), if required, the paper is dried as for paper electrophoresis, the original serrated edge is cut off and a serrated edge is cut on the new bottom of the sheet. Then the procedure above is repeated.

Detection and elution of the spots have already been described (§ 2.2.1).

3.3. *Two-dimensional paper chromatography and/or electrophoresis*

A particularly powerful procedure using paper methods is two-dimensional paper electrophoresis and/or chromatography. This is most conveniently applied by loading the oligonucleotide solution in a small spot near one corner and running, by electrophoresis or chromatography, the mixture along one edge of the paper. The paper is then turned through 90° and re-run in the second dimension using a different fractionation procedure. In this way the components of a complex mixture may be spread over the whole area of the paper and the advantages of two separate fractionation systems can be combined.

The paragraphs below mention some of the most useful methods in paper chromatography and electrophoresis. The pattern of spots obtained by fractionation of an enzyme digest of a nucleic acid is often called a 'fingerprint'.

A widely applicable two-dimensional method was introduced by Rushizky and Knight (1960). For the first dimension they used paper electrophoresis at *p*H 2.7 in ammonium formate prepared by adding 7.5 ml formic acid (98%) to 2.5 ml of water and adjusting to *p*H 2.7 with concentrated ammonium hydroxide. This separates oligonucleotides largely according to their Gp and Up content. The second dimension was paper chromatography in a slightly acidic solvent prepared by adjusting the electrophoresis buffer (above) to *p*H 3.8 with concentrated ammonium hydroxide and then adding one volume *tert*-butanol. The final measured *p*H was 4.8. This separates the oligonucleotides largely according to chain length. The method provides good resolution but does not distinguish between Ap and Cp residues nor between sequence isomers. It is particularly useful for the products of pancreatic ribonuclease digestion of RNA or oligonucleotides. Loads of 2–7 mg of the oligonucleotide mixture may be run on Whatman 3MM paper. This system also illustrates the effect of reducing the concentration of the aqueous component: an 87:63 (v/v) ammonium hydroxide:*tert*-butanol mixture gives lower mobility but higher resolution. Partition coefficients are very temperature dependent, and in this system temperatures above the normal 22°C produce higher mobilities but lower resolution.

A similar system has been used by Rushizky and Sober (1962a) to fractionate the products of T1 ribonuclease digestion of RNA. The electrophoresis buffer was dilute formic acid *p*H 2.35; and the chromatography solvent was *tert*-butanol:0.02 M ammonium formate *p*H 2.7 (55:45, v/v). Bayev et al. (1965) have used a *tert*-butanol:formic acid *p*H 3.8 (1:1, v/v) paper chromatography solvent in the second dimension with paper chromatography in *iso*butyric acid:0.5 N ammonia (5:3, v/v) *p*H 3.7 in the first dimension. This *iso*butyric acid system had been previously used by Shapiro and Chargaff (1963) and Spencer and Chargaff (1963a, b) in combination with paper chromatography in *iso*propanol:water (7:3, v/v) in an ammoniacal atmosphere. They fractionated pyrimidine nucleotide sequences from DNA very successfully up to a chain length of about 6 nucleotides. Sequence isomers were not fractionated. Spencer and Chargaff (1963a, b) used *n*-butanol:0.05 N ammonia (6:1, v/v) to resolve pyrimidine deoxyribonucleotide sequences containing 5-methylcytosine.

Lagokvist and Berg (1962) also use the *iso*butyric acid:0.5 M ammonia (5:3, v/v) paper chromatography solvent. They describe a number of other solvents: *iso*propanol:water:ammonia (85:15:1.3, v/v/v); *iso*propanol:acetic acid:water (6:3:1, v/v/v); and *iso*propanol: *n*-butanol:12 N HCl:water (114:56:49:39) which they used in purification of oligoribonucleotides.

Armstrong et al. (1964) used 1-propanol:water:ammonia (55:35:10, v/v/v) in combination with paper electrophoresis to fractionate the products of pancreatic ribonuclease digestion of some specific transfer RNAs.

Felix et al. (1960) and Sulkowski and Laskowski (1962) used the solvents: ethanol:1 M ammonium acetate (75:30, v/v); and saturated ammonium sulphate:*iso*propanol:water (80:2:18, v/v/v) in two dimensions. This provides high resolution of small ribo- and deoxyribo-oligonucleotides. The method distinguishes between Ap and Cp residues.

Bollum (1962) used a substituted cellulose membrane, DEAE-paper, to fractionate oligonucleotides which were eluted with an aqueous solvent, 0.5 to 1.0 M ammonium bicarbonate. Tyndall et al. (1964) used DEAE-paper with aqueous solvents, 0.3 M ammonium bicarbonate in one dimension and 3 M formic acid in the other to fractionate oligoribonucleotides. Ohsaka et al. (1964) used DEAE-paper and 7 M urea solutions and obtained a fractionation comparable with that obtained on DEAE-cellulose columns by Tomlinson and Tener (1962, 1963).

Thach (1967) describes the fractionation of oligoribonucleotides by paper chromatography in a mixture of 1 M ammonium acetate *p*H 7.0–7.3 and 95% ethanol. The composition of this chromatographic solvent is varied according to the homologous series to be fractionated and the method provides high resolution up to chain lengths of 20 nucleotides, Sanger et al. (1965) describe the use of paper electrophoresis at *p*H 3.5 for the fractionation of the oligonucleotides $(Ap)_n Xp$ obtained by combined digestion of larger oligonucleotides with T1 and pancreatic ribonuclease.

3.4. *Thin layer chromatography (TLC)*

Thin layers of silica or other materials on 20 cm square glass or other plates can be used as an alternative to paper chromatography. Although the principles are the same, spots on thin layers are generally smaller so the method can be quicker and more sensitive. Paper chromatography is, however, still widely used for nucleic acid components. Ready spread thin layers can be obtained commercially (e.g. Merck, Serva) except for thin layer gel filtration (special apparatus available from Pharmacia) or the silica paste can be spread by hand using a commercial spreader (e.g. Shandon Southern). The plates are dried and the sample is loaded carefully onto the layer near the bottom. A closed tank is allowed to equilibrate with the developing solvent which is in the bottom and then the thin layer plate is placed vertically in the tank so that the bottom of the plate rests in the solvent. The solvent is allowed to migrate up the plate by capillary action taking the sample with it. Most commercial tanks will accept several plates at once (e.g. Shandon Southern).

The fractionation of simple oligonucleotide mixtures on thin layers of PE1-cellulose (polyethyleneimine – cellulose) has been described by Randerath and Randerath (1967a, b) (see also § 2.2.3). For one-dimensional fractionation up to 10 mg of oligonucleotides may be handled, but only about 0.5 mg may be loaded for 2-dimensional fractionations. The two-dimensional system used 0.09 M $MgCl_2$, 0.18 M Tris, *p*H 8.45 at 24°C for 7 hr 20 min. The sheet was then washed in methanol and 0.5% acetic acid in methanol (to adjust the *p*H) and subjected to chromatography in the second dimension using 0.5 M magnesium acetate *p*H 5.7 at 37°C for a further 7 hr 20 min. This system just separates the four dinucleotides and eight trinucleotides in a pancreatic ribonuclease digest of RNA. The isomers (Ap, Gp) Cp are the most difficult to separate. The separation depends largely on net charge at the two different *p*H values. It is interesting that 5′ terminal Ap reduces the mobility in both dimensions and in both cases: (Ap,Gp)Cp and (Ap,Gp)Up. The oligonucleotides may be located by their ultraviolet absorbance.

Randerath and Randerath (1967b) give an interesting discussion of the problem of aggregation of Gp-rich oligonucleotides. They find that aggregation depends on the buffer anion, being low with Tris and Mg^{2+} for example.

Urea reduces aggregation, even if it is washed out after loading (with magnesium as anion). Aggregation is a function of temperature, being worst at 4°C and lowest at 37°C.

Their system has higher resolution than paper chromatography and electrophoresis and a higher capacity than cellulose acetate. Its value for more complex mixtures remains to be demonstrated but may well be considerable, particularly for mixtures which cannot easily be radioactively labelled, and contain few Gp residues.

Thin layer methods have also been described by Gassen (1969).

Column chromatography

4.1. *Gel filtration*

Oligonucleotides, unlike nucleosides, are separated on gel filtration columns on the basis of size, particularly in high ionic strength buffers containing 8 M urea or if the experiment is confined to the members of a homologous series. Even in these cases the resolution is generally inferior to ion exchange columns. However, a gel filtration column can be calibrated for molecular weight determination of the members of a homologous series in a buffer of fixed ionic strength (Hohn and Schaller 1967). The calibration is of the form

$$\log K_d = k_1 - kn$$

where K_d is the distribution coefficient, n is the degree of polymerisation and k and k_1 are constants. Other authors have found the usual relationship (elution volume is proportional to the logarithm of the molecular weight) satisfactory for oligonucleotides from tRNA (Millar and Byrne 1967) and for synthetic polydeoxyribonucleotides (Hayes et al. 1964).

4.2. *Principles of ion-exchange column chromatography*

Oligonucleotides are examples of polyelectrolytes that bind firmly to ion-exchangers, in aqueous solutions of low ionic strength. Above about *p*H 2 oligonucleotides in aqueous solution are negatively charged. Since some nucleotides are liable to de-purination below *p*H 2, anion exchange is usually used, the most popular ion-exchange group being a dimethylaminoethyl group bound to an insoluble matrix of either cellulose (DEAE-cellulose) or cross-linked dextran (e.g. DEAE-Sephadex)*. These ion-exchange resins have largely replaced the polystyrene based resins such as Dowex except for mononucleotides. Resins of high quality are available commercially.

Successful fractionation of oligonucleotides requires, in general, that the elution positions of different oligonucleotides are significantly different (zone separation) and that each oligonucleotide is eluted in a sharp band (zone spreading). These factors are affected by the characteristics of the ion-exchange resin, by the design and packing of the column, and by the operation of the column.

4.2.1. Zone separation

Zone separation depends on the selectivity of the ion-exchange resin. The strength of binding of an oligonucleotide to the ion-exchanger depends on the net charge on the oligonucleotide, on the relation between the charge distribution of the oligonucleotide and the charge distribution of the ion-exchanger, on the accessibility of the ion-exchange groups, and on non-ion-exchange processes.

The net charge on an oligonucleotide depends on its nucleotide composition and to a lesser extent, probably, on its nucleotide sequence and secondary structure. The net charge can be varied in a selective manner by adjusting the *p*H and other factors of the environment. The charges on some mononucleotides are shown as functions of *p*H in Chargaff and Davidson (1955). The charge distribution of the oligonucleotide depends on the nucleotide sequence and on the secondary structure of the oligonucleotide. The secondary structure effect can be varied by using different solvents and/or temperatures (e.g. Tomlinson and Tener 1963; Mirzabekov et al. 1966).

In general, it is desirable that the ion-exchange groups be readily accessible to the oligonucleotide. The groups are located in the interior of the resin beads or fibres and so the degree of cross-linking must be low enough to allow the oligonucleotides to diffuse freely in and

* Registered trade mark of Pharmacia Fine Chemicals AB.

out. In particular, the resin beads must be stable so that they do not contract and trap the oligonucleotides when higher ionic strength eluting buffers are employed.

Non-ion exchange processes seem to be unimportant in ion-exchange chromatography of relatively small oligonucleotides on DEAE-Sephadex (Rushizky et al. 1964; Matthews 1968d). The non-ion-exchange effects on Dowex resins are illustrated by the fractionation of mononucleotides (Katz and Comb 1963; Blattner and Erickson 1967) by cation exchange chromatography. Non-ion-exchange effects are important in chromatography on DEAE-cellulose (§ 4.2.3.1; Rushizky et al. 1964).

The detailed exploitation of the above properties of oligonucleotides is described in later sections (ch. 5) dealing with specific fractionation problems.

4.2.2. Zone spreading

A simplified general analysis of zone spreading in chromatography leads to the following expression (Giddings 1961).

$$H = \frac{2D}{V} + d + \frac{2R(1-R)V}{k_2}$$

H represents the height equivalent to a theoretical plate (HETP) (Martin and Synge 1941) which is a common measure of the zone spreading produced by a given column; D is the diffusion coefficient of the oligonucleotide in the mobile phase; V is the velocity of the solvent passing through the column; d represents the mean length of the channels between individual fibres of the resin and is thus comparable with the mean diameter of these fibres; R is the mobility of the solute in question relative to the solvent mobility; and $1/k_2$ is the average time required for desorption of an adsorbed oligonucleotide from the resin. The first term represents the effect of ordinary diffusion, in the mobile phase only. The second term represents so called eddy diffusion and the third term expresses the contribution to zone broadening arising from the fact that equilibrium does not exist in the column during chromatography.

The effect of ordinary diffusion would be reduced by having large solvent flow velocity, V and small diffusion constant, D. Large V is restricted by non-equilibrium considerations (see below) and D cannot be reduced as this would reduce the rate with which the solute migrated in and out of the particle beads, thus increasing the time needed for equilibrium to be approached, i.e. increasing $1/k_2$.

To reduce eddy diffusion, the size of the resin particles, d can be varied. In high resolution work small resin particles are used. This has the disadvantage of restricting the solvent velocity, V, which can be obtained with pressures that do not distort the particles. So, when high resolution is not needed larger particles may be used. With all columns, better results are obtained if a uniform particle size is used, and it is necessary to remove the very fine particles sometimes produced during the washing procedures so that a reasonable flow rate may be obtained and a narrow particle size distribution used.

The non-equilibrium effect is decreased by decreasing the solvent flow velocity V. So low solvent flow rates are used in high resolution work, but not so low that the diffusion term becomes large. The best compromise is $V^2 = k_2 D/[R(1-R)]$. In practice the values of the variables are such that flow rates of a few ml/hr cm^2 (sometimes written cm hr^{-1}) cross sectional area of the resin bed will give low zone spreading with excellent resolution. In many applications where speed is more important than resolution, higher flow rates are used.

The transition rate for desorption, k_2, also affects the non-equilibrium term. Large values of k_2 are required which can only be obtained if diffusion in and out of the resin beads is reasonably rapid. This cannot occur if the cross-linking in the resin is too dense, and the acid and alkali washing procedures recommended by the manufacturers are often needed to attain the correct amount of cross-linking as well as for purification of the resin. When using DEAE-Sephadex very large oligonucleotides may experience considerably restricted diffusion into the beads. This can be overcome to some extent by using the A50 type instead of the A25 type for large oligonucleotides.

Another factor affecting the resolution in the column effluent is the column shape and packing. One consequence of a non-uniformly packed column is that the zone of a solute becomes uneven and skew as it progresses down the column. This effect can be seen by running a coloured substance through the column. In short wide columns the height of a zone is small and the probability of remixing on elution is high. In long, narrow columns the height of a zone is large and the probability of remixing on elution is smaller. In a long, narrow column, too, the size of the resin particles is small compared with the length of the column. These considerations suggest a high column length-diameter ratio, which must, however, be consistent with the flow rate desired. Good resolution may often be obtained with ratios of the order 50:1, but very high resolution requires ratios of the order 1000:1.

4.2.3. Choice of resin

4.2.3.1. General considerations

The choice between substituted cellulose, substituted dextran, substituted polystyrene or other resins depends on the fractionation problem. In particular, ion-exchange chromatography of oligonucleotides on DEAE-cellulose and DEAE-Sephadex depends on interactions between the DEAE-groups and the oligonucleotides and between the cellulose or Sephadex matrix and the oligonucleotides. In general, interactions with the Sephadex matrix are small, provided the degree of cross-linking does not exclude the oligonucleotides from the interior of the Sephadex beads. Normal gel filtration (§ 4.1) does not occur. Interactions with the cellulose matrix are not small. Purine nucleotides, particularly Gp, show a tendency to bind more strongly to the matrix than do pyrimidine nucleotides (Bartos et al. 1963; Staehlin 1963). The effects are, however, very complicated and depend on nucleotide sequence as well as composition and also on the secondary structure of the oligonucleotide.

Whatever the resin, it should have a uniform particle size distribution and a size as small as is consistent with the required flow rate. It should have a high 'chromatographically available' capacity.

This is a complicated function of the small ion capacity (usually 1 to 10 mequiv/g) and the physical properties of the resin (because the ion-exchange groups must be readily accessible to the polyelectrolytes under the conditions of the chromatography). Also important is the rate at which equilibration occurs.

DEAE-Sephadex is available in bead form in two porosity types, A25 and A50. Although molecular sieve effects do not occur in ion-exchange chromatography on DEAE-Sephadex the capacity and flow properties are affected by the porosity type. A25 has better flow properties and is recommended by Pharmacia for solutes up to 10,000 molecular weight (approximately 33 nucleotides). It works well for oligonucleotides at least up to 26 nucleotides long (e.g. Lloyd and Mandeles 1970). A50 is used for larger oligonucleotides.

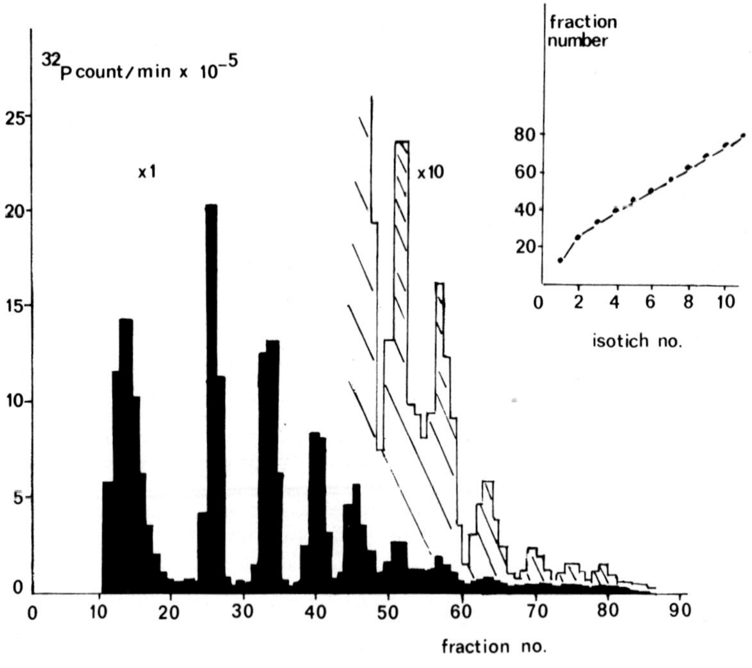

Fig. 4.1.a

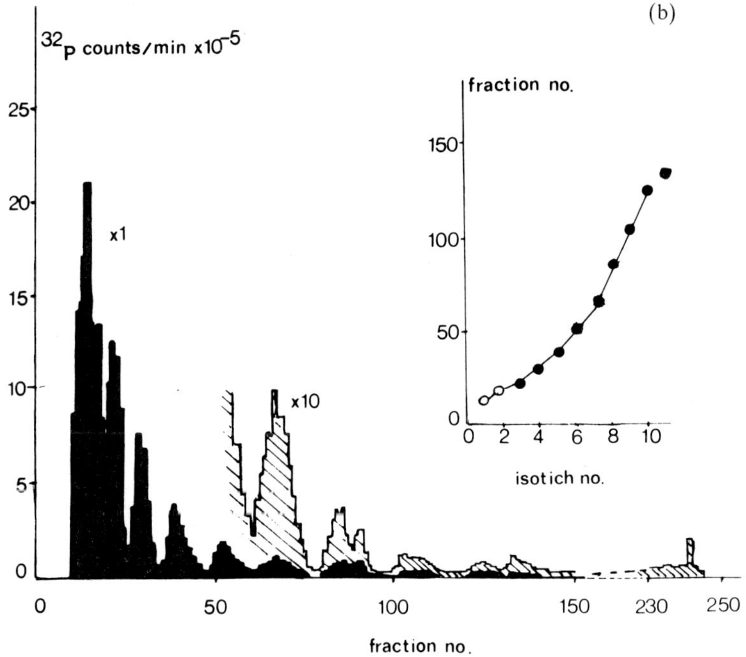

Fig. 4.1. Column chromatography of oligonucleotides on DEAE-cellulose. A complete pancreatic ribonucleose digest of μ2 phage RNA labelled with ^{32}P was fractionated on a 9×500 mm column of DEAE-cellulose in 10 mM Tris, 1 mM EDTA, 7 M urea *p*H 7.9 with a linear gradient from 0.1 M to 1.0 M sodium acetate. The effluent was collected into polyethylene vials and the Cerenkov radiation of each fraction was measured in the liquid scintillation counter. The main figures show the radioactivities of the fractions as functions of elution times. The insets show the position of elution of each isoplith as a function of degree of polymerisation. a) 20 mg RNA was fractionated; b) 40 mg of RNA. Note effect on resolution at beginning due to overloading the column.

Large RNA and DNA molecules would enter neither A25 nor A50 and so A25 would be chosen for its better flow properties but the available capacity is very low.

Even with one type of resin, performance may vary greatly from sample to sample of the resin. This has been clearly shown for DEAE-cellulose by Himmelhoch and Petersen (1966). The characteristics of ion-exchange resins are drastically altered by the washing procedures carried out in the laboratory. Different resins require different treatment and the best course is usually to follow the manufacturers' instruction concerning washing of an ion-exchange resin.

4.2.3.2. *Capacity of resin*

In general, in high resolution applications, the load of oligonucleotides applied to the column is a small fraction of the capacity of the column to bind oligonucleotides. As an example of the amounts which can be used Fig. 4.1. shows two isoplith separations (§ 5.2.1) performed under identical conditions on 0.9×50 cm DEAE-cellulose columns. Increasing the load from 20–40 mg seriously affects the resolution of the main components.

If a column shows satisfactory resolution with a small load then its capacity can be increased by increasing the diameter rather than the length. The capacity is approximately proportional to the $(\text{diameter})^2$. Conversely, if the small load resolution is inadequate then the length of the column should be increased rather than the diameter.

4.3. *Equipment for column chromatography*

Although an ion-exchange experiment is basically very simple to perform it may last several days and nights and so some automatic equipment is generally used. Fig. 4.2 shows a block diagram of a common laboratory arrangement; the items involved are discussed below.

4.3.1. *Gradient formers*

A gradient former is not required for step-wise elution procedures, but most oligonucleotide fractions need gradient elution to achieve the required resolution. That is, the ionic strength, or other property, of the eluting buffer is varied continuously as the elution proceeds.

The simplest type of gradient former is made from two open tall

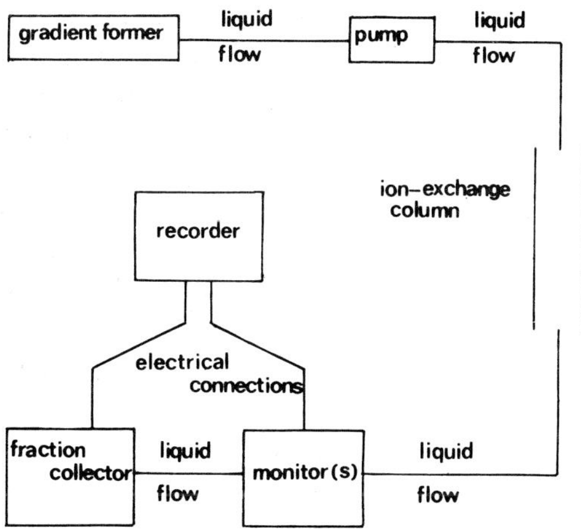

Fig. 4.2. Block diagram showing buffer flow from gradient former through pump, column, and monitor(s) to fraction collector and electrical connections from monitor(s) and fraction collector to recorder. The mains power supply to the pump and other accessories may be obtained from the fraction collector mains output which is automatically cut off when a pre-set number of fractions has been collected if the fraction collector has these facilities.

cylindrical vessels, A and B, connected at the bottom by a narrow tube (Fig. 4.3). The connecting tube should be short and horizontal. If it is made by placing tubing in the tops of the vessels then an air-lock is very likely to form but once a short horizontal tube is free of air a new air-lock is most unlikely. This tube must also be

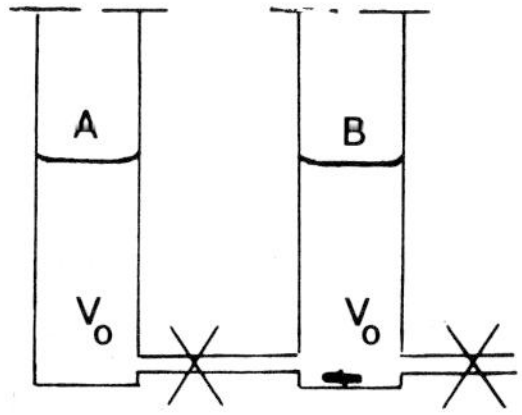

Fig. 4.3. Linear gradient maker.

equipped with an on–off valve or gate clip so that the vessels can be filled. One of the vessels, B, has another tube running out of it, also equipped with a valve or clip, to the pump or column and a magnetic stirring bar or overhead stirrer. The vessels are filled with the valve or clip-closed.

Vessel A contains buffer of the final composition required and vessel B contains buffer of the initial composition. The hydrostatic pressures at the bottoms of the vessels must be equal. For liquids of equal density this means the heights of liquid must be the same. If the densities are not equal then the masses of liquid in each vessel must be the same assuming the cross-sectional areas of each vessel are equal. The valves are then opened and the stirrer switched on. The gradient is withdrawn through the tube leading from vessel B. If air is present in the tube connecting A and B it must be removed, for example with a bent Pasteur pipette.

As gradient is withdrawn from B the hydrostatic pressure in B falls and so liquid from A is forced through into B where it is mixed in. The composition of the buffer in B thus gradually changes towards the final composition in A. If the cross-sectional area of vessel A at any given height is the same as the cross-sectional area of vessel B at the same height and the two liquids have the same density then the gradient will be linear beginning with the composition in B, finishing with the composition in A. If, however, one vessel has a different shape or different cross-sectional area from the other, convex or concave gradients can be generated. The linear gradient is given by:

$$I_{\mathrm{v}} = \frac{I_{\mathrm{A}} - I_{\mathrm{B}}}{2V_0} V + I_{\mathrm{B}}$$

where I_{v} is the composition of the gradient after a volume V has been delivered, V_0 is the initial volume in A or in B, and I_{A} and I_{B} are the compositions of the buffers in A and B respectively.

Although such a device is easily made it can also be purchased in several sizes, for example from MSE Ltd.

A linear gradient generated like this is suitable for many applications. However, for separating complex mixtures of oligonucleotides a very complicated gradient may be required. It may also be necessary to make empirical refinements of the gradient after the initial run of a complicated mixture of oligonucleotides.

Sophisticated gradient makers capable of generating complex gradients are now on the market (e.g. LKB). The simplest ones to operate generate the gradient using two variable speed pumps and two buffer reservoirs. The pump speeds are automatically controlled by the device so that the gradient follows any pre-determined curve. One other type, which has been used in this field and can be fairly simply constructed is shown in Fig. 4.4. A number, maybe 9, of

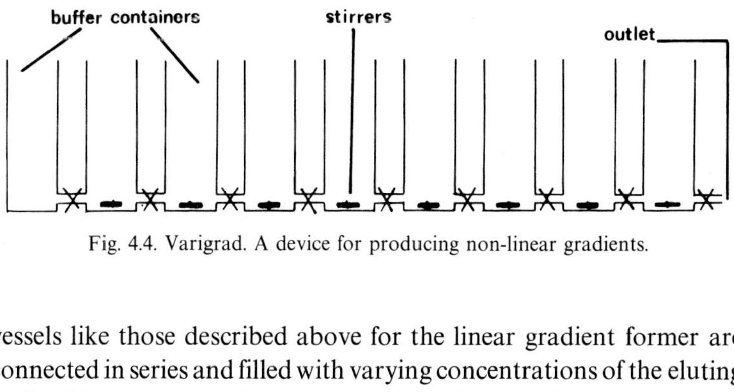

Fig. 4.4. Varigrad. A device for producing non-linear gradients.

vessels like those described above for the linear gradient former are connected in series and filled with varying concentrations of the eluting buffer. The gradient is drawn off at one end and buffer runs from one vessel to another under the influence of hydrostatic pressure. The apparatus is called a varigrad (Peterson and Sober 1959; Peterson and Rowland 1961; Peterson 1970, this series, vol. 2). The gradient produced may be measured empirically or calculated.

In the calculation, the contribution of each chamber to the gradient is determined and the sum of the contributions gives the actual gradient. The contribution due to the buffer L in the nth chamber (the numbers start from the chamber where the gradient leaves the varigrad) is given by:

$$\frac{C}{L} = \frac{(N-n)!}{(N-n)!(n-1)!}\left(1 - \frac{v}{V}\right)^{N-n}\left(\frac{v}{V}\right)^{n-1}$$

where C = concentration of solution L emerging from the varigrad at any point; N = total number of chambers in the system; v = volume of gradient that has emerged from the varigrad up to this point; V = total volume of gradient.

In practice, the best shape of gradient is usually determined empirically. A trial separation may be run with a linear gradient, using a linearly increasing concentration of elution buffer in each chamber. If the results of this trial run suggest that the gradient should be refined to increase or decrease the resolution at particular points then the buffer concentration in the appropriate chambers may be altered (Peterson and Sober 1959).

4.3.2. Pumps or gravity feed

In many cases flow under gravity is satisfactory and in this case a pump is not needed. A constant head may be obtained using a Mariotte flask (e.g. Fischer, this series, 1969) such as that obtainable from Pharmacia Fine Chemicals AB. The principle is shown in Fig. 4.5.

However, in ion exchange chromatography there are two main reasons for using pumps. Firstly, the columns are often operated under larger pressures than are feasible with gravity feed. Secondly, the resistance of the column to flow may vary with the ionic strength and *p*H of the eluting buffer and from one column to another so a pump may be used to maintain a constant flow rate.

For very high pressures specially designed piston pumps such as those in amino acid analysers must be used. For moderate and low pressures a peristaltic pump is satisfactory. Care must be taken to use the correct tubing, silicone rubber or Tygon, with the recommended dimensions for the pump in use and the tubing should be changed regularly to avoid holes developing. The flow rate obtained from these pumps may vary slightly, particularly on changing the tubing, but is accurate enough for most laboratory chromatography.

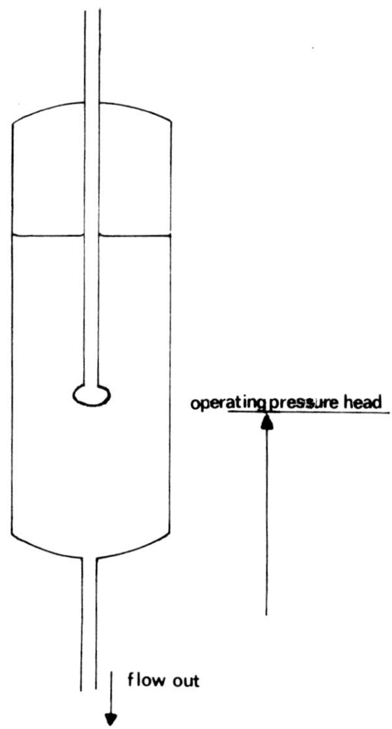

Fig. 4.5. Mariotte flask. A constant pressure head device.

The pulsation introduced by the pump probably does not adversely affect the resolution obtained. When the operating pressure is low the pump may also be placed immediately before the fraction collector instead of before the column, but this can easily cause the column to run dry if there is even a small air leak in the connections above the column.

The column must not be allowed to run dry. This can be prevented by close attention to the column but it may also be sensible to provide a system to prevent this happening. This can be arranged with gravity feed by placing the outlet of the system above the top of the column or by looping the tube connecting the buffer reservoir to the column below the outlet of the system (Fig. 4.6).

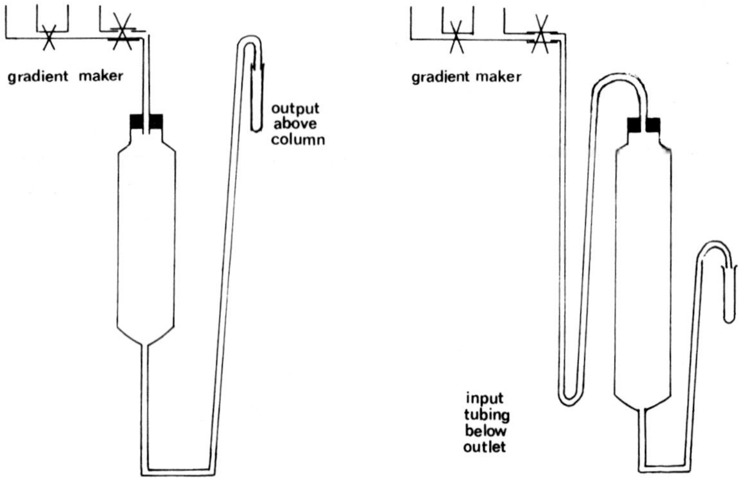

Fig. 4.6. Column chromatography. Two arrangements which help prevent the column running dry.

When a pump is used these methods are not applicable. The pump can be timed to shut down automatically after a given time, or given volume delivered, for example by using the facilities of a fraction collector like the LKB Ultrorac or a level detector like the Fimonitor (Fisons). Alternatively, the gradient may be designed to extend well beyond the point required for the chromatography and the column can then be shut down manually at a convenient time.

4.3.3. Column design and connecting tubing

The liquid circuit in a column chromatography experiment should be as short as reasonably practical and contain a minimum of sharp corners or other regions where mixing can occur. Connecting tubing usually has an internal diameter of 1 mm and may be made of polyethylene, PVC, PTFE or other materials. For low pressure operation satisfactory joints can be made with silicone rubber tubing of intermediate wall thickness and an internal diameter smaller than the outer diameter of the tubes to be joined. Connectors for higher pressures are available from manufacturers such as LKB, Pharmacia and Chromatronix.

The main feature of good column design is the absence of large 'dead spaces' at the top and bottom of the column, particularly the bottom. Suitable columns are available commercially, for example from Pharmacia, and these are recommended for the most versatile systems. However, satisfactory results may be obtained using a simple laboratory column which merely has capillary inlet and outlet and a scintered glass (porosity 2) support for the resin (Matthews 1968d).

Blattner and Erikson (1967) have described a good column which is very easily constructed. The column is made of glass tubing. A porous polyethylene disc at the bottom fits precisely inside the column (a suitable disc may be cut from a sheet of porous polyethylene with a hand cork borer). The disc is supported on a cylindrical rubber stopper. The stopper is pierced with a needle which is then withdrawn and a sharpened piece of teflon (polytetrafluoroethylene, PTFE) tubing is pushed through the hole in the stopper. The sharpened end is cut off flush with the top surface of the stopper. This arrangement almost eliminates dead space at the bottom of the column and provides a convenient form of outlet that may be led through monitors and/or to a fraction collector. Buffer is fed into the top through a similar rubber stopper and teflon tube.

Versatile columns should be made from precision bore tubing, preferably glass coated with silicone or methyl cellulose (see below). The positions of the ends should be adjustable and it should be possible to reverse the flow of buffer through the column. The dead space at both ends should be very small and a simple system for connecting plastic inlet and outlet tubing should be supplied. A jacket for circulating water at a constant temperature should be fitted or, at least, available.

It is convenient to have some means, e.g. a gate clip on a section of Tygon or silicone rubber capillary tubing, to stop the flow of buffer at the bottom of the column. These ideas are shown diagrammatically in Fig. 4.7.

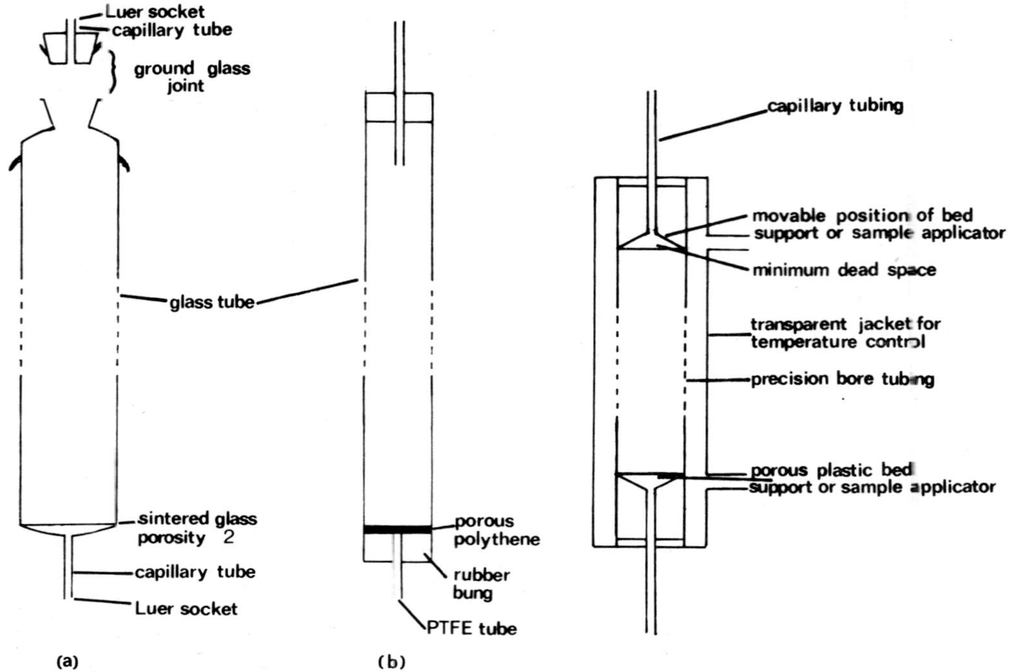

Fig. 4.7. Chromatography columns: a) simple laboratory column; b) easily constructed column; c) diagrammatic representation of a versatile commercial column.

For the best results it is recommended that all the glass parts of the system be siliconised or coated with methyl cellulose. These treatments considerably reduce the surface charge of the glass and improve reproducibility and recoveries. Both coatings need occasional renewing, perhaps once a month for a heavily used system but less often in many cases. The quality of the silicone coating can easily be checked by observing that water will not wet the surface and collects in quite large droplets. The methyl cellulose treatment is recommended by Hjertén (e.g. 1970) but siliconising is probably more widely used in chromatography.

The following method has been found satisfactory (Schwartz and Zabin 1966): prepare a 1% solution of dimethyldichlorosilane [$(CH_3)_2SiCl_2$] in benzene in a fume cupboard. Make sure the glass to be treated is clean and completely dry. Rinse it with the solution several times and then dry it at 250°C. Chlorine is given off during these processes. Protect the hands from the solution. The treatment is now complete and the siliconising can be checked as above. If it is not satisfactory the treatment is repeated, possibly with a higher concentration of dimethyldichlorosilane in benzene.

4.3.4. Monitors

A monitor is not an essential part of a chromatography system. Monitors are, however, widely used and certainly offer a number of advantages although the monitor and its recorder may be the most expensive items in a chromatographic system.

Three types of monitor are important in chromatography of oligonucleotides: ultraviolet absorption or transmission monitors; electrical conductivity monitors; radio-activity monitors.

All three types of monitor may be used in the given system, connected in series. In a system used by the author the output of each of the three monitors was adjusted to range from 0 to 10 mV and all three were fed to a three-channel dot printing potentiometric chart recorder. Three different coloured traces were obtained corresponding to ultraviolet transmission, an approximately linear function of conductivity, and the count rate measured by the radio-activity flow monitor (Matthews 1968a).

A monitor consists of a flow cell, a measuring unit, power supplies and output circuit. Usually the flow cell and measuring unit are in a compact container which can easily be connected in the buffer tubing from the column outlet and are connected electrically to the 'control unit' which contains power supplies and output circuit. The flow cell must be small and designed to avoid mixing and the trapping of air bubbles. If the unit is in a cold room air bubbles are very likely to form as the flow cell is probably slightly warmed by the consumption of electricity in the measuring unit. A rise in temperature reduces the solubility of air in water and so bubbles may form. The problem can be reduced by de-gassing the buffers before use and by arranging for the buffer to flow upwards through the flow cell.

The output circuit may contain a meter to provide immediate visual indication of the measured quantity. This can be useful but is not essential. The main output is intended for current or voltage measuring chart recorders which are briefly discussed below. Some radio-activity monitors provide a print out after preset time intervals; this digital signal cannot easily be presented on a chart recorder.

4.3.4.1. Ultraviolet transmission monitors

Oligonucleotides have a broad absorption band around 260 nm where the extinction coefficient is such that a solution of 30 μg/ml in a 10 mm cell gives an absorbance of the order of 1 (10% transmission). Wavelengths of 254 and 265 nm are not much worse but at 280 nm the extinction coefficient is about half that at 260 nm. This makes ultraviolet monitors working near 260 nm rather sensitive detectors of oligonucleotides and they are widely used in this field.

A more versatile alternative to a flow monitor is a measurement of the absorbance of each of the collected fractions on a spectrophotometer. This can be done automatically at reasonable cost with digital or strip chart recording. The results, of course, are not available as the experiment is in progress and the fractions may be exposed to room temperature for the measurement but this system can be more accurate, versatile and economical on equipment than a conventional monitor and is well worth considering.

The cheapest, and most commonly used, monitors operate at a fixed wavelength and provide an output proportional to the transmission of the sample in the flow cell. This can be recorded directly and gives a good format for locating peaks because the sensitivity for small peaks is high but large peaks will not go off-scale. However, the area under the peak is not directly proportional to the amount of ultraviolet absorbing material in the peak. An absorbance reading can be obtained using a logarithmic recorder or a monitor with a linear absorbance output. These records have the disadvantage that large peaks go off scale or, conversely, the sensitivity to small peaks is low. However, in favourable circumstances, the area of a peak on an absorbance-time record is proportional to the amount of material in a peak.

Records from an ultraviolet monitor can be made quantitative and reasonably accurate, for example in adaptations of amino acid analysers, but in many chromatography experiments their purpose is to locate peaks and provide a qualitative picture of the fractionation as it occurs.

4.3.4.2. Other monitors

These monitors are much less widely used than ultraviolet transmission monitors. However, a flow radio-activity monitor can achieve useful efficiencies for ^{32}P and ^{14}C and even ^{3}H in some cases and then serves much the same purposes as an ultraviolet transmission monitor.

A conductivity monitor is not useful for detecting oligonucleotides because their electrical conductivity is low compared to the solutions used to elute them. Conductivity measurements are used to characterise the elution position of a peak since both conductivity and elution depend on the ionic strength of the solution.

The resistance output of an instrument like the LKB conductolyser can be made more appropriate for conductivity measurements by connecting a resistance in parallel with the conductivity cell. This gives a reasonably linear response, extends the available range and protects the equipment against very low conductivities (Matthews 1968a).

4.3.5. Fraction collectors

In some experiments the column effluent is run to waste after passing through the appropriate monitors. In all other cases some kind of automatic fraction collector is used.

In the simplest system the effluent is stored in a long coil, perhaps with air bubbles to restrict mixing. This neat and compact solution presents difficulties with large volumes and very high resolution, for example the pressure required to move the solution through the coil becomes very large.

There is a large number of mechanical fraction collectors on the market. Reliability is the most important criterion in selecting one since the experiments described in this manual do not require fraction collectors with many facilities although these may sometimes be useful. In practice a timer has been found to be the most reliable fraction cutting method. With a constant flow rate this gives equal volume fractions. Drop counters are not always satisfactory when used over long periods (more than a few hours) with concentrated urea solutions because the urea crystallises out and changes the geometry of the dropper or blocks it up altogether. Two other points to be borne in mind are: firstly, with many circular or spiral moving rack collectors the cutter may be set or the rack modified so that more than one column may be used simultaneously with the same fraction collector; secondly, if an automatic sample changer, for radio-activity or absorbance measurements, is to use the fractions then the containers should be interchangeable (Vestergaard et al. 1967; Matthews 1968b).

4.3.6. Electrical connections and recorders

Connections for buffer tubing have been discussed above (§ 4.3.3). Electrical connections, other than mains power supplies, are required when a monitor is used and/or when automatic shut down is required.

For automatic shut-down the pump power supply is taken from the appropriate socket on the fraction collector and a valve or some other device is used to prevent the column syphoning dry.

Two types of recorder are in common use potentiometric and galvanometric. Potentiometric recorders are more expensive and more versatile but galvanometric recorders are usually adequate for the experiments described in this manual. The writing system may use ink, capillary flow or pad, or temperature or pressure sensitive paper. Capillary flow pens are particularly unreliable.

Fig. 4.8 shows how to connect a current (milliamp) output from a monitor to a millivolt input on a recorder. The positive side of the monitor output is usually connected to the positive side of the recorder input but in some cases better results are obtained with the polarity reversed.

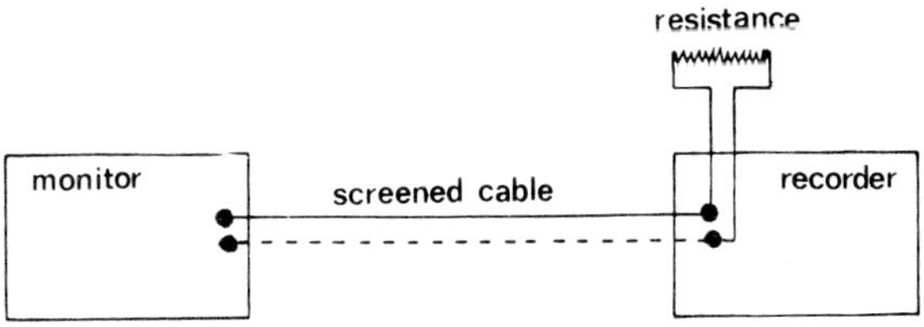

Fig. 4.8. Connecting a current output monitor to a voltage input recorder. Monitor output: 0 to i mA e.g. 0 to 1 mA. Recorder input: 0 to v mV e.g. 0 to 10 mV. Resistance required: v/i ohm e.g. 10/1 = 10 ohm.

In order to identify the fractions in the fraction collector with the peaks on the recorded chart an event marker is required. Continuous trace recorders can use a main trace event marker. Dot printing recorders must have a separate event marker. When event marking facilities are provided on the recorder it is usually necessary to connect the event marker to an external switch which is located in the fraction collector. When event marking facilities are not provided on the recorder the switch in the fraction collector can still be used in most circumstances to provide a blip on the recorder main trace as the fractions change. Fig. 4.9 shows some possible arrangements.

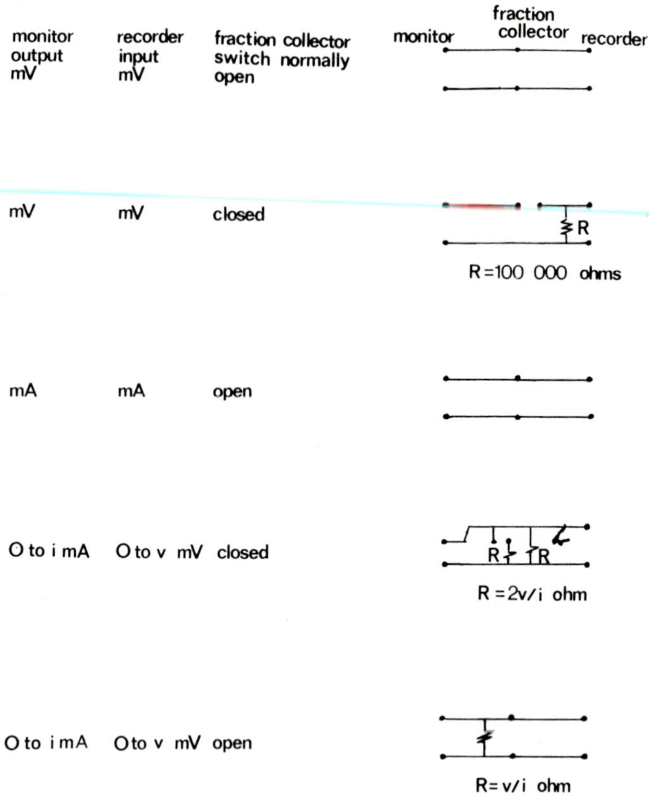

Fig. 4.9. Event marker circuits.

Of course, if the fractions are collected on a time basis an event marker may not be strictly necessary. It is, however, a very useful check on the whole system and provides good identification of the fractions.

The volume of eluent between the monitor and the fraction collector should be small otherwise a correction will be necessary to position the event marker blip. This correction is determined by timing a marker, such as a small air bubble, as it moves from the monitor to the fraction collector.

4.4. Experimental procedures

4.4.1. Preparation of resin

Resins should be washed as directed by the manufacturers. The washing, or 'pre-cycling' is usually necessary to remove impurities and to convert the resin to the appropriate physical and chemical form for chromatography. The washed resin must then be equilibrated with the initial buffer to be used in the chromatography. Pre-cycling is unnecessary with pre-swollen resins, supplied wet.

As an example, the following procedure is recommended for Whatman* DEAE-cellulose DE22 and has been used successfully in oligonucleotide fractionation. The dry resin is suspended in about 15 vol 0.5 N NaOH and washed either by allowing the suspension to settle for 15 to 20 min in a measuring cylinder and then decanting or sucking off the supernatant, or by collecting the resin on a sintered glass filter. This may elute some ultraviolet absorbing yellow material and the washing should be repeated until no more is eluted. The resin is then rinsed several times with distilled water (strictly, until the *p*H falls to 8); washed once quickly with 0.5 N HCl (DEAE-cellulose is unstable in strong acid) and rinsed again with distilled water. The resin is finally washed in 0.5 N NaOH before equilibration.

If the fines have not already been removed by decantation during the later stages of the washing they should be removed by decantation as described above, before equilibration.

The resin may be equilibrated by washing with the initial buffer, titrating to the correct *p*H in the initial buffer (this may take some time as the exchanger does not equilibrate instantaneously) and then washing with the initial buffer until the *p*H and conductivity of the suspended resin is the same as that of the pure buffer. Equilibration can be achieved simply by washing the resin with the initial buffer but this requires a very large volume of buffer.

4.4.2. Packing the column

There are several methods of packing the resin into the column. Here

* Registered Trade mark of W. and R. Balston Ltd.

again the manufacturers' instructions should be heeded (cf. Himmelhoch and Peterson 1966). One method, which may be used for columns up to 90 cm long requires an extension tube to be fitted to the top of the column to increase its length by about 50%. A plumb line is used to set up the column vertically and some 10 cm of buffer are placed in the bottom. The equilibrated resin is in a total volume of about 150 times the wet settled volume of the resin. This gives a reasonably thick slurry. All the slurry is stirred gently and poured gently into the column. The first few cm of bed are allowed to settle by gravity (this gives a layer of coarse particles at the bottom which will not block the filter). Then buffer is allowed to flow from the bottom of the column, and replaced by adding buffer at the top. The flow rate should be maintained at or above that to be used in the chromatography. If necessary pressure may be applied with a liquid pump in the buffer line, or with a small air pump. With a little practice this method gives reproducibly well packed columns in an hour or two. Before use, at least one column volume of initial buffer should be passed through the column. This 'settling' of the column can often be carried out overnight.

Another method, applicable to all lengths of columns, requires slightly more practice than the above but is essential for long columns. A slightly more concentrated slurry (total volume about 125% of the wet settled volume of the exchanger) is used and no column extension is needed. As before, packing is begun with some 10 cm of buffer in the column. An aliquot of the slurry (enough for several cm of bed) is added carefully and allowed to settle under gravity. Then further aliquots are added at intervals, with buffer flowing from the bottom of the column. As each aliquot is added the top few cm of the packed bed are stirred with a glass rod. This process is continued until the bed reaches the required height. The bed is then 'settled' by passing at least one column volume of buffer through it, as before. (For further details see Peterson 1970, this series.)

4.4.3. Loading the column

The oligonucleotide solution is pumped into the column. Usually the *p*H and ionic strength of the solution are comparable with the *p*H and ionic strength of the initial buffer, and the loaded material is washed in with the initial buffer.

Normally the loading conditions are chosen so that the oligonucleotides initially bind firmly to the resin. In this case the volume in which these oligonucleotides are loaded is not critical. In general the loaded volume should be as small as convenient. In the case where the oligonucleotides are not strongly bound, in particular where they are eluted with the initial buffer, then the initial loaded volume is critical and must be small.

The amount of oligonucleotide that may be loaded cannot be calculated directly from the quoted capacity of the resin. For high resolution it is necessary to work at a few per cent of the nominal capacity of the resin so that the absorption isotherms are relatively linear and so that equilibrium is established rapidly.

It is usual to quote both shape and size of a chromatographic column and the quantity of material loaded. The capacity for a given fractionation can be increased by increasing the column diameter and *vice versa*. It is advantageous to work with as small a column as reasonably possible as this usually gives smaller elution volumes.

Applications of column chromatography

5.1. *One-step columns*

5.1.1. *DEAE-cellulose at pH 8.6*

Moderately complex mixtures of oligonucleotides such as those obtained by specific enzymic digestion of nucleic acids about 100 nucleotides long can be extensively fractionated by DEAE-cellulose column chromatography at *p*H 8.6 using gradients of ammonium bicarbonate. This method gives resolution worse than some paper methods (Brownlee 1972) and takes longer, but will accept much larger quantities of material. It has been successfully used in nucleotide sequence studies of specific amino acid transfer RNAs.

A long column is needed for high resolution. Zachau et al. (1966a) used a 1 × 50 cm column at 4°C and RajBhandary et al. (1966) used a 1 × 104 cm column at room temperature. The oligonucleotides are eluted with a gradient from 0.01 M ammonium bicarbonate to about 0.5 M ammonium bicarbonate *p*H 8.6. The shape of the gradient depends on the composition of the oligonucleotide mixture. A 9 chambered varigrad (§ 4.3.1) can be used to obtain a gradient which will provide optimum fractionation.

The ion-exchange process depends largely on the charge on the oligonucleotide. At *p*H 8.6, Cp and Ap have a charge −2 while Up and Gp have charges approximately −2.2 due to the dissociation of their enol –OH groups. So, Cp and Ap containing oligonucleotides would be eluted before the corresponding Up and Gp containing oligonucleotides. This process is affected by the preferential binding of purine nucleotides to the cellulose matrix which would cause oligonucleotides containing Up and Cp to be eluted before the corresponding oligonucleotides containing Gp and Ap.

In Zachau's system at 4°C (1966a) the charge effect is demonstrated by the elution of GpCp (charge $\simeq$ 4.2) before GpUp (charge $\simeq$ 4.4) and the purine binding effect by the elution of CpCpG (charge $\simeq$ 6.2) before CpApG (charge $\simeq$ 4.2). The behaviour of the column is, however, more complicated than this since, for example, GpGpCp (charge $\simeq$ 6.4) is eluted together with ApApApUp (charge $\simeq$ 8.2) although this may be 'explained' as a stronger binding of Gp to the cellulose matrix than of Ap. Nucleotide sequence effects are also present since UpCpCpUpG is well separated from CpUpCpUpG.

5.1.2. Use of 7 M urea for DEAE-cellulose columns

T1 ribonuclease digests of RNA may be fractionated on DEAE-cellulose columns at neutral *p*H in 7 M urea. The purine/pyrimidine ratio is not fixed for a given chain length so the peaks of equal chain length (§ 5.2.1) are very broad and overlap considerably because of the different binding of purine and pyrimidine nucleotides to the cellulose matrix (Bartos et al. 1963). So these columns are not used for fractionation of complex T1 ribonuclease digests according to chain length. They are used for fractionation of T1 ribonuclease digests of transfer RNAs which contain a relatively small number of components. RajBhandary et al. (1966) used a 1 × 110 cm column and eluted with a gradient from 0.2–0.3 M NaCl in 7 M urea and Tris to *p*H 7.5 and they separated most of the oligonucleotides in the complete T 1 RNase digest of specific transfer RNA. Similarly Madison et al. (1966a) used a 250 × 0.3 cm column eluted with a sodium acetate gradient in 7 M urea at *p*H 6.

5.2. Multi-stage column chromatography

The above powerful procedure becomes less useful as the mixture becomes more complex. Peaks are no longer clearly resolved and the interpretation of the elution profile becomes increasingly difficult.

Such complex mixtures are dealt with in a different way, which aims at suppressing most of the differences between oligonucleotides and exploiting only one factor at a time.

Currently, this approach involves the following stages: 1) fractionation according to chain length; 2) fractionation according to nucleotide composition; 3) fractionation according to nucleotide sequence.

These procedures owe much to the work of Tomlinson and Tener and to Rushizky and Sober and their collaborators. They have been largely worked out using specific enzyme digests of ribosomal and viral RNAs. Shapiro and Chargaff and their collaborators have worked with mixtures of oligodeoxyribonucleotides.

5.2.1. Isopliths

An isoplith (or isotich) is a mixture of oligonucleotides each of which has the same length in nucleotides (Hall and Sinsheimer 1963).

Although gel filtration and ion-exchange chromatography on Dowex resins have been used for the first stage the preferred procedure is ion exchange chromatography on DEAE-cellulose or DEAE-Sephadex. The four mononucleotides have similar charges at *p*H values between about 5.5 and 8 so that ion-exchange chromatography at these *p*H values should be independent of the nucleotide composition of the oligonucleotide. This is complicated by the effect of secondary structure of the oligonucleotide. The secondary structure effect can, however, be eliminated by the use of a non-polar solvent such as 7 M urea, 8 M formamide, 8 M ethylene glycol or 8 M propylene glycol (Tomlinson and Tener 1963). These solvents destroy hydrogen bonds and hydrophobic forces which are probably the main forces involved in stabilising the secondary structures of oligonucleotides. 7 M urea is widely used for this purpose.

The oligonucleotides in a pancreatic ribonuclease digest of RNA have the general formula (purine nucleotide)$_{n-1}$ pyrimidine nucleotide, $n=1, 2, 3,\ldots$ Thus for each value of the chain length, n nucleotides, the charge at neutral *p*H and the purine:pyrimidine ratio are functions of n only and both increase monotonically with n. This means that at neutral pH in a pure ion-exchange experiment, all oligonucleotides with a given chain length, $n=r$ nucleotides, are eluted together and before all oligonucleotides with a chain length $n=r+1$ nucleotides.

5.2.1.1. Terminal dephosphorylation

The oligonucleotides from the ends of the original RNA molecule may not fit the general formula. Tobacco mosaic virus and MS2 phage both have adenosine as 3′-OH terminal (Sugiyama 1965; Sugiyama and Fraenkel-Conrat 1971). RNA molecules are synthesised from nucleoside 5′ triphosphates so that di- or triphosphates may be present at 5′ phosphate ends of RNA molecules. In the above chromatography the position of the oligonucleotide depends on the number of phosphate groups and not on the number of nucleosides since the nucleosides are uncharged at this pH (Bell, Tomlinson and Tener 1964).

For the oligonucleotides which do obey the general formula: (purine nucleotide)$_{n-1}$ pyrimidine nucleotide, $n=1, 2, 3\ldots$ the total charge on the oligonucleotide can be reduced by dephosphorylating the 3′-terminal pyrimidine nucleotide. This reduces the molarity of the buffer required to elute a given oligonucleotide and it has been suggested that the more even charge distribution gives sharper peaks. Dephosphorylating does improve resolution, particularly of the longer oligonucleotides. The procedure has been particularly used in the analysis of T1 ribonuclease digests (e.g. Zachau et al. 1966a; Brownlee and Sanger 1967). However, many authors have not found it necessary, as sufficient resolution could be obtained without dephosphorylation and any extra incubation with enzyme exposes the oligonucleotides to possible degradation by contaminating enzymes in the oligonucleotide preparation or in the dephosphorylating enzyme preparation (e.g. Peterson and Reeves 1966).

One useful application of terminal dephosphorylation is in the isolation of terminal nucleotide sequences (Bell, Tomlinson and Tener 1964). For example, a pancreatic ribonuclease fragment containing a 3′-terminal nucleoside will be eluted from a neutral DEAE-cellulose

Unless large quantities of material are required two-dimensional paper chromatography and electrophoresis is a good method for fractionating these shorter oligonucleotides (Rushizky and Sober 1962a, b). This does, however, require extensive desalting and concentration of the fractions before loading.

The longer oligonucleotides in the mixture can also be further fractionated either by paper methods or by column chromatography. For example, Rushizky et al. (1965) separated five decanucleotides (or groups of decanucleotides) each containing only one Gp residue by paper electrophoresis at *p*H 2.7 in 0.02 M ammonium formate using 6 volt/cm for 17 hr. (They also ran a second dimension of paper chromatography using *t*-butyl-alcohol:0.02 M ammonium formate, 17:23, but this did not much improve the separation. This electrophoresis produced a fractionation comparable with column chromatography at *p*H 2.7 to be described below.

5.2.2.1. DEAE-Sephadex at pH 2.7

Pancreatic ribonuclease digests of RNA yield the oligonucleotides (Gp_r, Ap_{n-1-r})Up and (Gp_r, Ap_{n-1-r})Cp, $r=0, 1, 2, \ldots n-1$. Fractionation of these compounds by ion-exchange chromatography should thus seek to exploit the differences in Ap/Gp ratio between oligonucleotides of a given chain length, n nucleotides, as well as whether they contain Up or Cp as the 3′-terminal pyrimidine nucleotide. The ionisation curves suggest a *p*H of 2.7, and this is successful (Rushizky et al. 1964, 1965; Madison et al. 1966b; Vandenbussche and Fiers 1966; Matthews 1968d).

DEAE-Sephadex is used as the interactions with the cellulose matrix of DEAE-cellulose are not needed. 7 M urea is used to obtain good yields and because it is desired to obtain sharp peaks each containing all the isomers with a given chain length, independent of nucleotide sequence. Good fractionation in the chain length region $n=7, 8, 9, 10$ nucleotides is obtained using 0.9×50 cm columns eluted at room temperature with a NaCl linear gradient from 0.0–0.2 M NaCl, both in 7 M urea, 1 mM EDTA adjusted to *p*H 2.7 with HCl. 1 l of each buffer with a flow rate of 15 ml/hr gives a good gradient.

The residue, if any, may be eluted from the column with 2 M NaCl.

The heptanucleotide isoplith from a pancreatic ribonuclease digest of μ2 viral RNA contains the oligonucleotides (Gp_r, Ap_{6-r})Cp, $r=1$, 2, 3, 4, 5 and (Gp_r, Ap_{6-r})Up, $r=1$, 2, 3, 4. These 9 groups of oligonucleotides are all clearly separated by the above column (Fig. 5.1). The column will also clearly separate the 5 octanucleotides

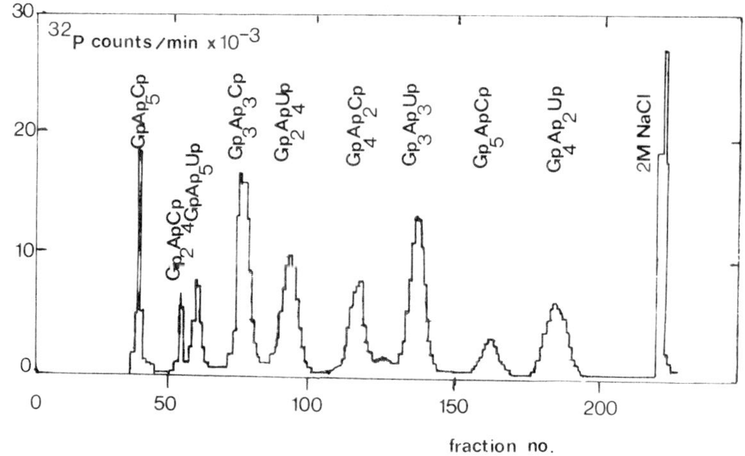

Fig. 5.1. Fractionation of heptanucleotides. Heptanucleotides were isolated from a pancreatic ribonuclease digest of μ2 phage RNA by chromatography on DEAE-cellulose, Fig. 4.1. They were dialysed against distilled water, loaded onto a 9×500 mm column of DEAE-Sephadex previously equilibrated with 7 M urea + 1 mM EDTA + HCl to *p*H 2.7 and eluted with a linear gradient from 0 to 0.2 M NaCl in 7 M urea + 1 mM EDTA + HCl to *p*H 2.7. The eluent was collected directly into polyethylene vials and the Cerenkov radiation from the ^{32}P label in each fraction was measured in the liquid scintillation counter.

found in μ2 viral RNA; (Gp_r, Ap_{7-r})Cp, $r=2$, 3, 4, 5 and (Gp_2Ap_5)Up (Matthews 1968d) (Fig. 5.2).

Vandenbussche and Fiers (1966) have used this method for the fractionation of tetranucleotides from a pancreatic ribonuclease digest of MS2 RNA. Very surprisingly, they found Ap_3Cp and (Ap_2Gp)Cp chromatographed together as did Ap_3Up and ($ApGp_2$)Cp. However, a similar experiment with tetranucleotides from a pancreatic ribonuclease digest of μ2 viral RNA gave the expected chromatogram with all the possible base compositions in well separated peaks (Lee and Deniset 1967).

These two columns, DEAE-cellulose at neutral *p*H followed by DEAE-Sephadex at *p*H 2.7, suffice to separate all the components with different nucleotide compositions present in complete pancreatic ribonuclease digests of RNA molecules with at least about 10^4 nucleotides before digestion. Sometimes, these fractions contain only

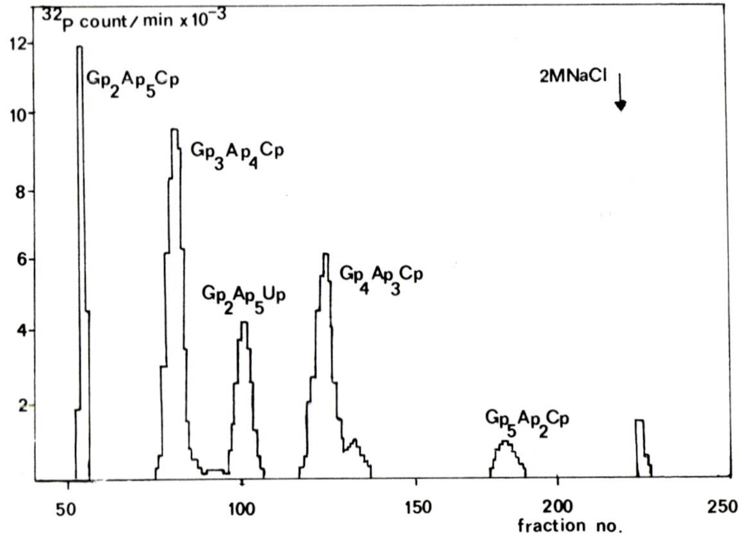

Fig. 5.2. Fractionation of octanucleotides. The conditions are the same as for Fig. 5.1.

one nucleotide sequence. In general, they contain a mixture of nucleotide sequence isomers. Suggestions for fractionating these are given in § 5.2.4.

The DEAE-Sephadex *p*H 2.7 fractionation gives reproducible elution positions for oligonucleotides, and the nucleotide compositions of an oligonucleotide from a pancreatic ribonuclease digest can sometimes be deduced from its relative position on the chromatogram.

The use of DEAE-Sephadex and 7 M urea is designed to eliminate sequence-dependent effects in the chromatography and so, if this has been successful, the elution position of an oligonucleotide will depend only on its net charge at the *p*H of the chromatography. An approximate value for the net charge may be obtained from the algebraic sum of the charges due to the ionisations of each constituent mononucleotide. In general, the net charge will also be affected by interactions between adjacent residues along the phosphate chain but in 7 M urea these interactions may be small. To a first approximation,

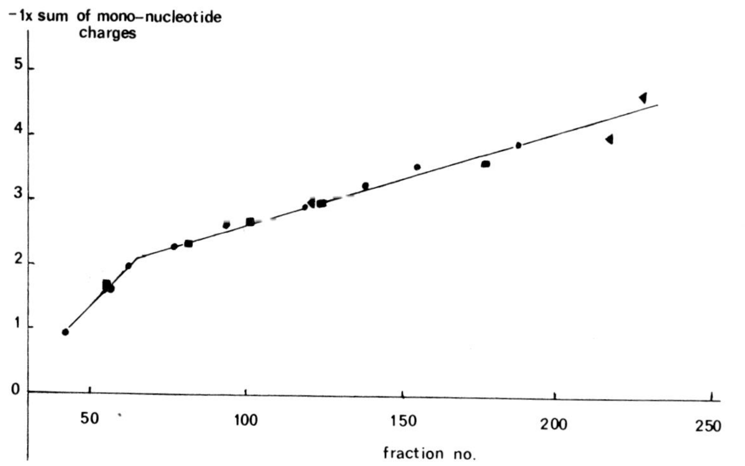

Fig. 5.3. Dependence of elution position on charge. Oligonucleotides in 7 M urea on DEAE-Sephadex columns at *p*H 2.7.

then, the total charge on an oligonucleotide may be calculated by summing the contributions from each mononucleotide. At *p*H 2.7 these contributions are: −0.08 (Ap); −0.02 (Cp); −0.66 (Gp); and −0.98 (Up). The total charge, calculated in this way, is plotted as a function of elution position from DEAE-Sephadex in 7 M urea at *p*H 2.7 in Fig. 5.3, for 17 oligonucleotides isolated from a pancreatic ribonuclease digest of $\mu 2$ viral RNA. These results taken from 3 different columns show that there is a quantitative relationship between elution position and sum of mononucleotide charges and that this is independent both of chain length for $n=7$, 8, 9 nucleotides and of purine/pyrimidine ratio in the same range. In one case, however (5Gp, 3Ap)Up, an anomalous elution position is recorded which presumably represents a particularly strong nucleotide sequence effect which is not completely destroyed in 7 M urea. The deviation from a straight line relationship for the first few oligonucleotides probably represents incomplete ionisation due to the low (< 0.1 M) ionic strength of the elution buffer in this region.

It is interesting, and instructive, to note that Stockx and Vandendriessche (1963) report that the p*K* values of mononucleotides in 7 M urea are approximately 0.5 *p*H unit above their values in aqueous buffers. If, however, the oligonucleotide charges are calculated on this basis, no satisfactory relationship between elution position and charge appears, even the order of elution is incorrect. This is the justification for ignoring the effect of 7 M urea on p*K* values throughout this chapter.

At *p*H 2.7 the charge difference between Ap and Cp is 0.06 charge units. The resolution of the DEAE-Sephadex column described above is approximately 0.2 charge units. In a pancreatic ribonuclease digest no oligonucleotide is related to another by a change of Ap to Cp solely. But in a T1 ribonuclease digest such oligonucleotides are likely to occur and these will be chromatographed as a single peak on DEAE-Sephadex at *p*H 2.7 in 7 M urea. This has been observed by Rushizky et al. (1965).

5.2.2.2. DEAE-cellulose at pH 3.4

Sinha et al. (1965a, b) have used columns (0.8 × 40 cm) of DEAE-cellulose and gradients of NaCl in 0.1 M formic acid, 7 M urea at *p*H 3.4. At this *p*H the charge difference between Up and Cp is less than at *p*H 2.7 which would be expected to reduce the resolution; but any increased affinity of the DEAE-cellulose for Gp over Ap might be expected to increase the resolution. In practice, the fractionation of oligonucleotides under these conditions requires considerable care in column preparation and the use of *p*H control and slowly rising salt gradients. The above authors have used the method to fractionate the octanucleotides from pancreatic ribonuclease digests of R17 and

M12 viral RNAs, respectively. The nucleotide composition measurements that they give suggest that their fractionation is directly comparable with the fractionation of the octanucleotides in the pancreatic ribonuclease digest of $\mu 2$ viral RNA. The resolution obtained using DEAE-Sephadex at *p*H 2.7 ($\mu 2$ octanucleotides; Matthews 1968d) is better than that obtained using DEAE-cellulose at *p*H 3.4 (M12 octanucleotides; Sinha et al. 1965). More recently, Thirion and Kaesberg (1968) have used DEAE-cellulose at *p*H 3.3 in 7 M urea for extensive fractionation of pancreatic ribonuclease digests of M12 and R17 viral RNAs. The few details they give suggest that the resolution and recovery of these columns are worse than those of DEAE-Sephadex columns (Matthews 1968d).

DEAE-cellulose at *p*H 3 has been used for oligodeoxyribonucleotides (Ehrlich et al. 1972).

5.2.2.3. Dowex formate

Bayev et al. (1967) have used columns of Dowex-1 formate (4 × cross linked) for the fractionation of pancreatic ribonuclease isopliths from valine transfer RNA. The isopliths were obtained by column chromatography on DEAE-cellulose in 7 M urea *p*H 7.5 (§ 5.2.1.2). Without drying, desalting or removal of urea, the di-, tri- and pentanucleotides were well separated on 3 Dowex columns, each eluted with a linear gradient from 0.0–4.0 M formic acid and then with a linear gradient from 0.0–0.6 M ammonium formate in 4.0 M formic acid. The fractionation is qualitatively comparable with that obtained on DEAE-Sephadex *p*H 2.7. No sequence isomers were present. Two pairs of oligonucleotides were incompletely resolved (ApUp + ApɄp and ApGpdi-HUp + ApGprTp) and these were separated by rechromatography of the whole of each peak on the same Dowex columns but using a constant eluant concentration.

5.2.2.4. DEAE-cellulose at pH 4.4

More work is needed on the fractionation of T1 ribonuclease digests. The procedure of Rushizky et al. (1965) is to fractionate the mixture according to chain length on DEAE-Sephadex at *p*H 7.6

Subject index p. 487

and then fractionate each isoplith according to the Up content of each component on DEAE-Sephadex at *p*H 2.7 all in 7 M urea as described above. Those fractions which contain components differing in Ap and Cp content and in nucleotide sequence, are then fractionated on DEAE-cellulose columns at *p*H 4.0 or 4.4 in 7 M urea. At this *p*H, Ap and Cp have different charges and the effect of this is enhanced by the higher affinity of DEAE-cellulose for purines than for pyrimidines. Accordingly, Rushizky et al. (1965) have succeeded in separating the components of four fractions from the *p*H 2.7 column into groups differing only in nucleotide sequence. They used large columns, 2.2×75 cm, and correspondingly large volumes of eluting buffer. The elution requires slowly rising salt gradients and *p*H control. As a typical example, the conditions used for fractionating the hexanucleotides (rAp, $(4-r)$Cp, Up)Gp, $r = 1, 2, 3, 4$ were: 200 A_{260} units load; 2.2×75 cm column of DEAE-cellulose eluted with a linear gradient of total volume 8 l from 0.2 M ammonium acetate 0.05 M NaCl *p*H 4.4 to 0.2 M ammonium acetate 0.15 M NaCl at a flow rate of 56 ml/hr. The decision to use *p*H 4.4 seems to have been based on Stockx and Vandendriessche's (1963) measurements of mononucleotide p*K*s in 7 M urea. It is possible that *p*H 4.0 and DEAE-Sephadex would give slightly better resolution in view of the doubts about the applicability of Stockx and Vandendriessche's measurements discussed above (§ 5.2.2.1), since the charge differences between Ap and Cp are 0.22 at *p*H 4.4 and 0.28 at *p*H 4.0 calculated on the basis given above.

Several of the peaks obtained by Rushizky et al. (1965) during chromatography of oligonucleotides on DEAE-cellulose at *p*H 4.4 in 7 M urea were split into poorly resolved components which were presumably oligonucleotides differing only in nucleotide sequence. In some respects this is a disadvantage and experience with DEAE-Sephadex columns at *p*H 2.7 suggests that DEAE-Sephadex columns might have adequate resolving power at *p*H 4.0 but would not fractionate the nucleotide sequence isomers. This would give sharper, more easily identified peaks, especially in complex mixtures.

However, such partially resolved peaks can often be adequately and conveniently purified after desalting by dialysis or dilution followed by rerunning in the same chromatographic system (Penswick and Holly 1965). Sometimes even better results are obtained by re-running in the same chromatographic system but with a constant eluent concentration (Cantor and Tinoco 1965), or at a different temperature (Apgar, Everett and Holley 1966).

5.2.3. Large oligonucleotides

Before further discussing the fractionation of nucleotide sequence isomers, it is appropriate to consider the fractionation of oligonucleotides in the size range 10–100 nucleotides. Such oligonucleotides have usually occurred in partial T1 ribonuclease digests of transfer RNAs, or in mixtures of undigested transfer RNAs. For many purposes, the methods described above are applicable. Holley et al. (Apgar et al. 1965; Penswick and Holley 1965; Forget and Weissman, 1969) used columns of DEAE-cellulose eluted with gradients of sodium chloride in 0.02 M Tris 7 M urea *p*H 8.0 at both room temperature and 55°C. Their highest resolution was obtained in 0.35×220 cm columns which were obtained by joining two 110 cm columns with a small piece of Tygon tubing. Relatively small volumes of eluent are required with such long thin columns. Dutting et al. (1966) have used similar columns as well as columns of DEAE-Sephadex A-25 at *p*H 7.5 and *p*H 3 at both room temperature and 55°C. Very high resolving power was obtained. The principles of fractionation are similar to those discussed above, but even in 7 M urea (which is used partly to ensure high recoveries) the influence of nucleotide sequence can be seen with these long oligonucleotides and on DEAE-Sephadex A-25 the effect of exclusion should begin to show.

Miyazaki et al. (1966, 1967; Miyazaki and Takemura 1966) have used column chromatography on DEAE-Sephadex A-25 to fractionate tRNA from *Torulopsis utilis*. They were able to purify an alanine, a valine and an isoleucine tRNA using 3 elution systems: 1) Linear gradient of ammonium sulphate in 0.02 M potassium acetate, 1% dimethylformamide, *p*H 5.3; 2) Linear gradient of KCl in 1 M potassium phosphate + 5% dimethylformamide, *p*H 6.1 or 6.2 at 30°C;

Subject index p. 487

3) Linear gradient of KCl in 0.5 M sodium borate, *p*H 6.8 to 7.2 at 30°C. The buffers for this stage were stored above 20°C.

Mirzabekov et al. (1966) used a combined temperature and ionic concentration gradient to fractionate tRNA mixtures on DEAE-cellulose. DEAE-cellulose has also been used by Kaiser (1969) and by Zapisek et al. (1969) for tRNA and larger RNAs.

More recently, DEAE-Sephadex A-50 has been used for preliminary fractionation followed by benzoylated DEAE-cellulose (BD-cellulose) which gives a greater resolution (Gillam et al. 1967; Takeishi and Ukita 1968; RajBhandary and Ghosh 1969; Smith and Marcker 1970; Hunter and Jackson 1971; Ghysen and Cellis 1974). The BD-cellulose columns are eluted with 10 mM sodium acetate *p*H 5, 10 mM $MgCl_2$, 2 mM β-mercaptoethanol containing up to 1 M NaCl and possibly 10% ethanol. These systems can be used to separate charged tRNAs and if the tRNA of interest is charged, *in vitro*, with a radioactive amino acid this provides a convenient label for tRNA for that amino acid.

Another approach has been to use reverse phase chromatography. The system is, basically, anion exchange chromatography with the active exchange sites, a quaternary ammonium chloride, present as a thin film on the surface of small beads of an inert support, polychlorotrifluoroethylene. These beads are available ready for use as RPC5 or RPC6, which give different separations, from e.g. Miles Laboratories Ltd. The elution conditions are similar to those used with BD-cellulose. The practical aspects have been covered in a series of articles in Methods in Enzymology (Grossman and Moldave 1971; Kelmers and Heatherly 1971; Pearson et al. 1971).

5.2.4. Sequence isomers

The final stage of the complete fractionation of the complex mixtures of oligonucleotides we have been considering has not been fully worked out. However, the following considerations are important in the fractionation of sequence isomers.

Differences in nucleotide sequence can give rise to differences in: a) secondary structure or shape of the oligonucleotide; b) overall charge of the oligonucleotide; and c) the distribution of charge over the oligonucleotide. In general, for a given oligonucleotide, these properties will be functions of the *p*H and ionic strength of the solution and of the temperature.

The effect of *p*H on oligonucleotide conformation has been shown, for example, in an interesting study of absorption and optical rotatory dispersion spectra by Warshaw and Tinoco, 1965 and Cantor and Tinoco, 1965. Their study also shows that the conformations of (Gp, Ap)U are very different at *p*H 7 and they suggest that optical rotatory dispersion measurements can distinguish between trinucleotide sequence isomers. They do not discuss the application of their work to oligonucleotide fractionation but this would seem to be an interesting field for study.

Mirzabekov et al. (1966) have pointed out that as the temperature of an oligonucleotide solution rises, the oligonucleotide structure becomes 'looser' so that more sites on the molecule can 'reach' binding sites on the ion-exchanger and so binding becomes stronger. This should be a nucleotide sequence-dependent effect, and they have used it for the fractionation of mixed transfer RNAs on DEAE-cellulose.

A form of secondary structure of oligonucleotides arises from stacking of the bases which is stabilised by the hydrophobic interactions between the bases. This is largely destroyed by non-polar solvents such as 7 M urea. Sequence isomer separation is often carried out in the absence of urea. Separation is observed on DEAE-cellulose columns in ammonium carbonate, *p*H 8.6, where, for example, (Up, Cp)CpUpG are well separated (Zachau et al. 1966a). This is presumably due to differences in charge distribution in the oligonucleotide and the way in which this 'fits' the arrangement of binding sites on the DEAE-cellulose. It is interesting, however, to notice, for example, that (Ap, Gp)U are separated on DEAE-cellulose at *p*H 3 in 7 M urea, although (Ap, Gp)C are not separated (Cantor and Tinoco 1965). Possibly, the large positive charge on C 'masks' the effect of the positions of the purine nucleotides.

Sequence isomer separation of the products of pancreatic ribonuclease digestion poses a special problem when G-rich oligonucleotides appear. These tend to aggregate in aqueous solution and become difficult to handle.

Electrophoresis is a possible procedure for fractionating sequence isomers since the resistance to motion will be affected by secondary structure and charge distribution as well as by any effect due to differences in total charge. This can be seen on cellulose acetate at *p*H 3.5 by the separation of the tetranucleotides Gp(Gp, Ap)Up for example (Sanger et al. 1965). Electrophoresis on DEAE-paper in 7% formic acid is particularly powerful, and admirably complements electrophoresis on cellulose acetate at *p*H 3.5. For example, ApGpGpUp is separated from Gp(Gp, Ap)Up (Brownlee 1972).

Paper chromatography has also been successfully used for sequence isomer separation. For example, Fiers et al. (1965b) separated (Ap, Gp)Cp by paper chromatography on Whatman 40 paper eluted with isobutyric acid:0.5 N ammonium hydroxide (5:3 v/v), 5′-terminal Ap running faster in this system.

In conclusion, the methods described above should suffice to separate most mixtures of short oligonucleotides, $n=1$ to 10 nucleotides according to length and nucleotide composition. The fractionation of sequence isomers is less well documented but some successes have been reported. The methods can be extended to chain lengths up to about 100 nucleotides.

Desalting and concentrating oligonucleotide solutions

Having separated the complex mixture of oligonucleotides into fractions of constant chain length (isopliths), the next stage is to fractionate each isoplith on the basis of nucleotide composition. This may be achieved by paper methods or by further column chromatography (Rushizky et al. 1965). For both techniques it is usually necessary to remove the salts from the oligonucleotide solution and, for paper methods, to concentrate the solution before beginning the next stage.

The simplest method of desalting is dialysis (suitable for molecular weight >2000 dalton) and this can also be used for concentrating. A quicker alternative to dialysis is gel filtration which is available for molecular weight down to 1000 dalton. This produces a very efficient removal of salts and other low molecular weight substances such as urea but dilutes the solution to some extent and is difficult to apply to very large volumes (greater than a few hundred ml) or to viscous solutions. Very small volumes of solution can be conveniently desalted by paper chromatography. Volatile salts can be removed by rotary evaporation or freeze drying but these methods are not recommended unless the solution must be concentrated as well.

Solutions of oligonucleotides, particularly small ones, can be concentrated by column chromatography on DEAE-cellulose or charcoal. DEAE-cellulose is much more widely used. The concentrated solution contains 1 or 2 M ammonium bicarbonate or other

 Subject index p. 487

volatile substances which must be removed by repeated dilution and evaporation or freeze drying of the solution. This is an important disadvantage of the method and it is probably best used only for oligonucleotides up to 3 nucleotides long.

Larger oligonucleotide solutions can be desalted on DEAE-cellulose and the desalted solution concentrated by rotary evaporation, freeze drying, dialysis against Ficoll or gel filtration in a basket centrifuge depending on what apparatus is available. These methods are described below.

6.1. *DEAE-cellulose*

The classical method of desalting and concentrating oligonucleotide solutions consists of absorbing the oligonucleotides onto a small (1 × 10 cm) DEAE-cellulose column, washing off the salts and urea, and eluting the oligonucleotides with ammonium bicarbonate. The ammonium bicarbonate solution is then removed by rotary evaporation or freeze drying (Rushizky and Sober 1962a). This method must be applied with care. The resin should be well packed in a siliconised column and the flow rate should be 0.5–1.0 ml/min. The column should be equilibrated with dilute (1–10 mM) ammonium bicarbonate buffer *p*H 8.5 which will probably need degassing. The oligonucleotide solution will need diluting before loading and this may be done with 3 or more volumes water or 7 M urea. The column is loaded and then washed with 10 column volumes of water or 10 mM ammonium bicarbonate. The nucleotide material is eluted with 1 M ammonium bicarbonate, degassed, *p*H 8.5.

Care should be taken to see that the nucleotide material does indeed absorb during loading and is not washed off during washing (Matthews 1968a).

6.2. *Evaporation*

Evaporation of the concentrated ammonium bicarbonate solution is tedious as usually the residue must be redissolved and reevaporated several times to remove completely the ammonium bicarbonate. Freeze-drying suffers from the same disadvantage and it is also advisable to use only a partial vacuum to prevent oligonucleotide material being sucked into the pump. If small quantities are involved carrier nucleotides should be added and the evaporating or drying vessels should be siliconised (§ 4.3.3). Triethylamine bicarbonate may be used instead of ammonium bicarbonate.

6.3. Activated charcoal

Adsorption onto activated charcoal (Norit A) has been used for small oligonucleotides, up to tetranucleotides (Crane and Lipman 1953; Mandeles and Kammen 1966). The method is quicker and more convenient than DEAE-cellulose chromatography. Mandeles and Kammen (1966) used Norit A suspended in 1 mM phosphate 1 mM pyrophosphate buffer at *p*H 6.0 at a concentration of 100 mg/ml. The nucleotide solution is adjusted to *p*H 3 and 5 mg Norit for every optical density unit ($\sim$40 μg) of nucleotides is added. The charcoal is collected on a filter paper and washed with water. (A good quantitative measure of ^{32}P or ^{14}C radio-activity may be obtained by counting the dry filter paper in a Geiger–Muller thin window counter.) The nucleotide material is eluted with a small volume of a mixture of ethanol, water and ammonia (600:400:6.5; v/v/v) which is then removed by drying under reduced pressure at 40°C.

Zachau et al. (1966a) used charcoal columns (Carboraffin C treated with 95% ethanol – 8% *sec.* octanol, dried and degassed) at 4°C. The oligonucleotides were adsorbed, the column washed with water, and the oligonucleotides eluted with 8% aqueous phenol, *p*H 7. The phenol was removed with ether extraction. However, in later experiments they preferred dialysis at least for penta- and higher oligonucleotides.

6.4. Paper chromatography

Small volumes may be conveniently desalted by paper chromatography. The solution, $\not>$ 50 μl/cm is loaded as a small spot or line on a strip of filter paper. The salts are eluted with a solvent in which the mobility of the oligonucleotide material is zero such as 95% ethanol. The oligonucleotides are then eluted with water. Very small volumes of eluent can be dried for concentration or storage under a partial vacuum as spots on a sheet of polythene or Parafilm.

6.5. *Dialysis*

This is an extremely valuable method for large molecules. In an experiment with the hexanucleotide ($n=6$) peak from a pancreatic ribonuclease digest of μ2 phage RNA it was found that 1% of the nucleotide radio-activity was lost through the dialysis bag per hour at 4°C with stirring. Dialysis is thus feasible for oligonucleotides of degree of polymerisation $n \geqslant 6$ (molecular weight $\geqslant$ 2000 dalton). Dialysis has been used for tetranucleotides ($n=4$) but considerable losses are experienced (Vanderbussche and Fiers 1966; Lee and Deniset 1967).

Dialysis tubing should be pre-treated by boiling in 0.1 M EDTA or bicarbonate solutions or both successively, and thoroughly rinsed in distilled water. The tubing and washing solutions should be kept scrupulously clean and free of nucleases. Gloves must be worn to avoid contamination with nucleases secreted through the skin. Washing the dialysis bags, particularly the inside, removes the plasticiser which would otherwise contaminate the oligonucleotides, and boiling reduces the pore size.

The simplest dialysis procedure is to tie a double knot firmly in one end of treated dialysis tubing, add the solution to be dialysed and then tie another double knot above the solution. The bag is then placed in a large (usually 1–5 l) beaker of the solution to be dialysed against. The solution is stirred for at least 8 hr at 4°C. Some space for expansion should be left in the top of the tube because it is difficult to empty an overfilled bag and in extreme cases of expansion during dialysis the bag could burst.

The time to reach equilibrium can be approximately halved by using a rocking dialyser arranged so that an air bubble in the dialysis tube moves up and down the tube as the apparatus rocks so providing very good mixing.

In principle the time could be reduced further by forcing the solution through an ultrafiltration membrane under pressure but we have no experience of the application of this method to oligonucleotides. Ultrafiltration could also be used for concentrating oligonucleotide solutions.

Oligonucleotide solutions can be concentrated using ordinary dialysis tubing if a high concentration of a high molecular weight solute is introduced into the water outside the dialysis bag. Polyvinylpyrolidone (PVP) can be used, but Ficoll, a dextran polymer, sold by Pharmacia Fine Chemicals AB, gives generally cleaner solutions. The oligonucleotide solution is dialysed against 20% Ficoll in water. Care is necessary to see that the volume of oligonucleotide solution does not get so low that major losses are incurred in the knot of the dialysis tubing. Alternatively, the oligonucleotide solution can be placed in a measuring cylinder, and dry Ficoll in a dialysis bag lowered in so that the final volume of the oligonucleotide solution is below the end of the bag (Fig. 6.1).

6.6. *Gel filtration*

Oligonucleotide solutions with molecular weight $\geqslant 1000$ dalton can be desalted on Sephadex G-10 or Biogel P-2. Larger oligonucleotides (m.w. > 5000 dalton) are usually desalted on Sephadex G-25; other gels can also be used. The gels are examples of cross-linked dextran or poly-acrylamide gels respectively, formed into beads which act as molecular sieves. Their use in gel chromatography or molecular sieve chromatography or gel filtration, has been fully discussed in this series (Fischer 1969), so only an outline appears here and at other places in this manual (§ 1.1).

The gel beads ('fine' grade: 200–400 mesh) are pre-swollen by soaking in buffer overnight and then packed into a 30–40 cm long column whose volume is at least 3 times the volume of the sample

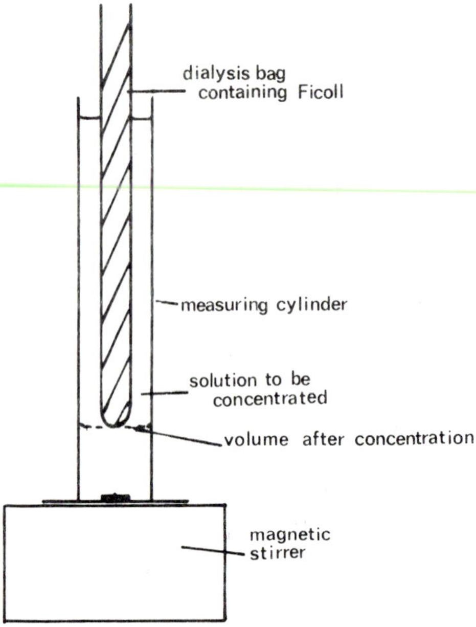

Fig. 6.1. Concentration of macromolecules by dialysis against Ficoll.

to be desalted. The columns are packed and operated at relatively low pressures, a few tenths of a metre of water, otherwise the column techniques are similar to those described previously. The column is eluted with 0.01 M ammonium carbonate or other very dilute volatile buffer at 10–20 ml cm^{-2} hr^{-1}. It may be possible, particularly with polyacrylamide gels like Biogel P-2 to elute with water but secondary binding effects may occur (§ 2.3.3). Such dilute buffer solutions can be easily removed by freeze drying or rotary evaporation.

The oligonucleotide solution is loaded carefully on the top of the column. If it contains, for example, 7 M urea it can easily be layered on the top of the column under the eluting buffer. The top of the column can be protected by a filter paper. If there is no density difference the top of the column is allowed to run almost dry and then the solution carefully allowed to soak in followed by elution buffer. If a specially designed column end piece is used the sample can be introduced through it but no air bubbles must be introduced in the process. The column effluent is monitored and the oligonucleotide solution, which emerges first, is collected. These columns are very reproducible, in volume terms, and it is not necessary to monitor a column once it has been calibrated. When at least one column volume of eluting buffer has been fed into the column it may be used again immediately without further regeneration provided no secondary binding has taken place.

Concentration can be achieved by gel filtration but this method does not appear to be widely used (Fischer 1969). Basically, dry gel is added to the dilute solution and in swelling the gel takes up solvent leaving high molecular weight solute outside the beads. The solution outside the beads is recovered by centrifugation in a basket centrifuge (from MSE Ltd.) or a swing out rotor fitted with filtration tubes. The centrifuge conditions are important.

Essentials of gel electrophoresis

Zone electrophoresis in stabilised media has been used for many years for the fractionation of protein mixtures. Until the introduction of starch gels by Smithies in 1955, electrophoretic separations depended entirely on the existence of differences in effective charge between protein species. In general, the electrophoretic mobility is determined by the net electrostatic force acting on the particle, and this depends on the potential gradient, the effective charge (taking account of counter-ion binding, and shielded charges) and the frictional resistance. In nucleic acids, the constancy of the charge:mass ratio limits the possibility of separation by purely electrophoretic means, for each added unit of charge brings with it an additional unit of frictional resistance. This compensation is clearly shown by the experiments of Olivera et al. (1964), in which constant mobility in free zone electrophoresis is maintained over a wide range of molecular weights. It is true that this law may break down in extreme cases, and Shack and Bynum (1964) showed that native and denatured DNA could be separated in such a system. The reasons are two-fold: on the one hand the frictional properties of native and denatured DNA differ grossly, and on the other hand their electrostatic free energies are widely disparate, and are reflected in the extents of charge neutralisation by counter-ions.

The possibilities of more general application of electrophoresis to the separation of nucleic acids arose with the advent of gels of controlled pore size for zone electrophoresis. Although agar gels were first used for electrophoresis of proteins by Gordon and his associates in 1948, and retardation effects were shown by the variation of gel concentration, the use of 'molecular sieving' in electrophoresis was not really exploited until the advent of starch gels. Smithies (1955) showed that the electrophoretic mobility of proteins in high-concentration gels of partly hydrolysed potato starch was controlled by their molecular weights as much as by their charge.

Polyacrylamide gels, containing covalent cross-links, were first used by Raymond and Weintraub (1959) and represented a considerable advance over starch, because stable gels could be prepared over a very much wider range of matrix concentration, because other aspects of the composition, such as the cross-linker concentration, could be controlled, and because charged impurities, which give rise to adsorption and electro-osmotic effects, could be almost wholly eliminated; moreover, the high transparency of the gels rendered them ideal for densitometry. The potential of polyacrylamide gel electrophoresis for separation of nucleic acids was not demonstrated until 1964, but since then the method has shown itself to possess unsurpassed resolution over an enormous range of molecular weights, and its possibilities are still far from exhausted. For analytical work it would be no exaggeration to claim that the method has largely superceded sucrose gradient centrifugaion.

Simultaneously with the exploitation of polyacrylamide gels, as applied to RNA, other workers, primarily in Bulgaria, were developing the use of agar and agarose gels. These are less versatile than polyacrylamide, in that the practicable range of agar concentration is only about 0.5–4%, whereas polyacrylamide can be used between about 2.2 and 30%. However, in the high-molecular weight range, agar gels are just as effective, and the upper molecular-weight limit is higher. They have, as we shall see, some other advantages. Recently, ways have been developed of combining both media for the study of high-molecular weight materials.

Starch gels were also shown (Beney and Székely 1966) to permit good fractionation of RNA, but it now seems unlikely that they would offer any advantage over polyacrylamide, agar or agarose.

Subject index p. 487

7.1. General principles of gel electrophoresis

In gel chromatography (using Sephadex, Sepharose or Bio-gel, which consist respectively of cross-linked dextran, agarose or cross-linked polyacrylamide), the solution of macromolecules is passed through a column of beads of the given material, and the solute molecules penetrate the solvated matrix to an extent which depends on their Stokes radii. The separation will depend then on a partition coefficient for the distribution of the solutes between the inside of the bead and the free solvent outside. The molecules which are least able to penetrate will be excluded from the beads and will emerge from the column without retardation. Smaller molecules will be progressively retarded by restricted diffusion within the beads and will emerge only at higher volumes of eluate (see Fischer, Vol. 1, Part 2 of this series). In gel electrophoresis, the solute molecules are impelled towards the electrode by a force equal to the product of the potential gradient and their charge. They will be retarded by the inherent hydrodynamic drag, that is to say the product of the velocity and the frictional coefficient, and in particular by the size-dependent probability that they will collide with a matrix molecule. The essentially similar natures of chromatographic gel filtration and gel electrophoretic fractionation has been noted (Rodbard and Chrambach 1970), and will be briefly discussed (§ 7.3).

An important feature of gel electrophoresis is that diffusion is restricted in the matrix, and remarkably sharp zones are consequently obtained. This is discussed in a paper by Richards and Lecanidou (1971), which should be consulted for a quantitative treatment.

The electrophoretic mobility of a species in agarose or poly-acrylamide gel is determined by the Stokes radius, the effective charge, the nature of the counter-ions, the potential gradient, the concentration of agarose or polyacrylamide and, to a lesser extent, by the number of cross-links. For a solute molecule of appreciable size there will be a gel concentration at which the mobility is so diminished that the molecules do not enter the gel. The mobility in fact is a smooth function of the gel concentration, which must therefore be selected to suit the molecular-weight range of interest.

The mechanical properties of the gel change with acrylamide concentration, and can be modified within limits by adjusting the relative number of cross-links. Most workers use a commercial 20:1 mixture of acrylamide and methylene *bis*acrylamide, called 'Cyanogum 41,' which is satisfactory over a wide range, but not at very low or at very high concentration of polymer.

One of the advantages, as we have noted, of transparent media, such as agar or polyacrylamide, is that they are suitable for densitometry. The densitometry of stained nucleic acid zones presents no difficulties, but the possibility also exists of direct recording of zones by scanning in the ultraviolet. This has considerable advantages for purposes of quantitation, but raises technical problems. Agar and agarose, being polysaccharides, are transparent in the ultraviolet, and the background at 260 nm in gels of good quality arises almost entirely from scattering. This largely vanishes when the gel is dried, and the ensuing transparent films are very suitable for scanning and for spectrophotometry in general. Polyacrylamide contains the amide chromophore, which absorbs below about 245 nm. There are clearly, however, other impurities of unknown character, for gels begin to absorb markedly below about 280 nm. The absorption can be diminished by recrystallisation of the monomer before polymerisation, or by prolonged pre-electrophoresis. Scanning at 260 nm is then feasible, especially in gels of low concentration. Densitometry at 280 nm is satisfactory even in concentrated gels, and the loss in sensitivity relative to 260 nm is only a factor of about two. It will be clear that ultraviolet densitometry of nucleic acids is advantageous, in consequence of their high absorption. Moreover all RNA species at normal ionic strengths and temperatures have a similar molar absorptivity (in the range of 7200–7800 per phosphorus at 260 nm) so that the integrated absorbance at 260 nm will be proportional to concentration to within about 10%.

One of the most felicitous features of electrophoresis of nucleic acids in gels is the dependence of the mobility on size. Consequently, if a calibration can be set up in terms of known species, gel electrophoresis can be used for the rapid determination of molecular weights of unknown samples. Clearly this cannot be carried too far, for if there are gross conformational differences – for example in comparing a fully helical rod-like species with one that is only partly base-paired the method will be no more applicable than similar empirical determinations based on parameters such as the sedimentation coefficient or viscosity. To nullify such limitations, methods must be used in which all species are reduced to true homologues, most feasibly by complete elimination of base-pairing.

7.2. The chemistry of gel formation

Agar is a polysaccharide extracted from various red algae. The algae are boiled in water, acidified with acetic acid, and the extract is filtered and allowed to gel. An exudate containing impurities is removed on repeated freezing and thawing. The product is however impure, since it contains, in addition to the polymers agarose and agaropectin, various low molecular weight compounds and inorganic ions. On acetylation agarose acetate and agaropectin acetate are

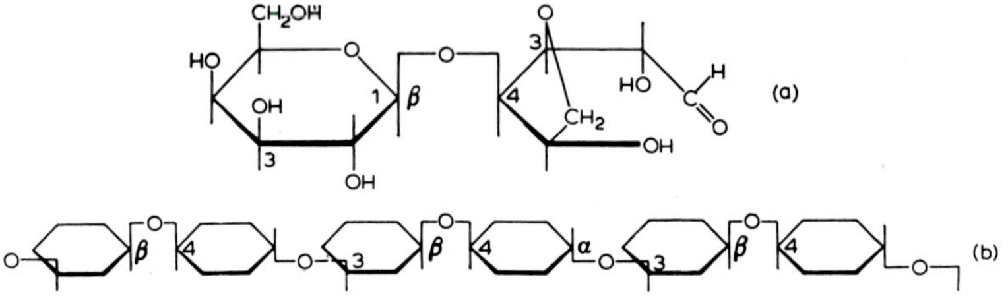

Fig. 7.1. Structure of agarose L: a) repeating unit; b) section of polymer.

formed. These may be separated and the former is reconverted to agarose by saponification. The agarose polymer consists of repeating disaccharide units composed of β-D-galactopyranose and 3,6-anhydro-L-galactose termed agarobiose (Fig. 7.1). Interchain hydrogen bonds are presumed to form the cross-links which lead to the formation of gels.

In contrast to agarose, polyacrylamide is a synthetic polymer, and gel formation depends on chemical cross-linking. The bifunctional acrylamide derivative, N,N′-methylene-*bis*-acrylamide is included in the polymerisation mixture to insert cross-links between chains of

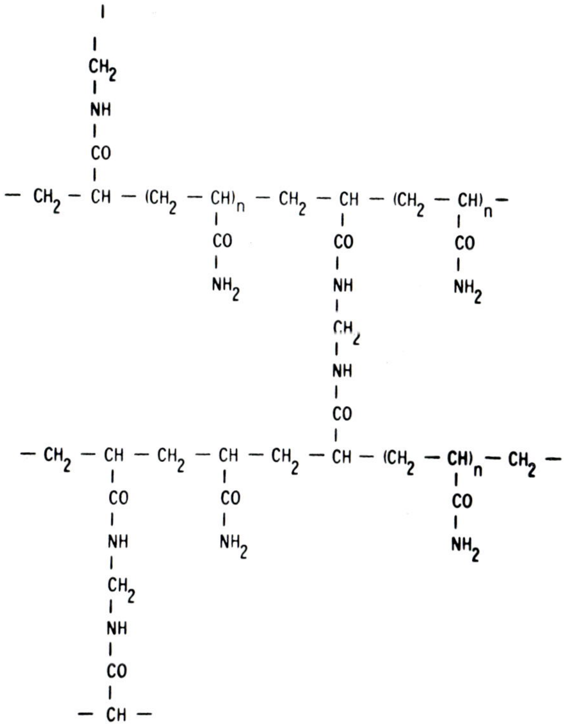

Fig. 7.2. Structure of polyacrylamide cross linked by N,N′-methylene-*bis*acrylamide.

polyacrylamide (Fig. 7.2). However cross-links may also be introduced with other types of bifunctional reagent. Diacrylate or tartarimide cross-links (Fig. 8.1) are particularly useful because they are readily hydrolysed, and the gels can consequently be dissolved in alkali or acid respectively after electrophoresis for recovery of the RNA fractions, e.g. for radioactivity measurements.

The proportion of cross-linking reagent may be varied to generate gels with different mechanical properties. The lower the cross-linker concentration the more deformable the gel. Polymerisation in the absence of cross-linking reagent produces a viscous solution of high molecular-weight polyacrylamide. A higher percentage of cross-linker is required in dilute acrylamide gels to provide mechanical strength. Conversely, concentrated gels require a low cross-linker concentration if they are not to be brittle and unmanageable. Gels with a relatively low number of cross-links swell to a greater extent on immersion in fixative solutions after electrophoresis. The percentage of cross-linker will alter the relative mobility of RNA molecules to some extent, in accordance with change in pore size (Fawcett and Morris 1966). Richards et al. (1965) give the following equation as a guide for the selection of cross-linker concentrations:

$$100R - 6.5 = 0.3C \qquad (7.1)$$

where C is the total acrylamide concentration and R is the fraction by weight of cross-linker in the monomer mixture. Cyanogum 41, the mixture of acrylamide and N,N′-methylene-*bis*-acrylamide in the proportions 95:5 by weight, is commercially available from a variety of suppliers, and can be used to form gels over a wide concentration range. It has been shown that the effective pore size is apparently minimised by this proportion of cross-linking agent (Fawcett and Morris 1966). Moreover the resulting gels have the highest optical clarity, because the scattering is also minimal. These effects will be further considered later (§ 7.5.4).

Polymerisation is initiated by free radicals which can be generated in a number of ways. The most commonly used reagents for this purpose are riboflavin and ammonium persulfate, or Fenton's reagent for acidic gels down to *p*H 1 (Jordan and Raymond 1969). Free radicals are generated from riboflavin by irradiation with near-ultraviolet light, the most convenient source of which is an ordinary fluorescent strip-light. Small concentrations of amines such as tetramethyl ethylenediamine (TEMED) or dimethylaminoethyl cyanide (DMAEC) are included as catalysts. The rate at which the gel forms is proportional to the product of the concentrations of the free radical generator and the catalyst, and also depends on the temperature. The polymerisation is effectively inhibited by oxygen, so that the acrylamide solution is best degassed under suction, and contact of the surface with air must be prevented.

7.3. *Theory of molecular sieving*

No comprehensive theory of molecular sieving processes as yet exists. A number of semi-quantitative treatments have however been evolved, and in general take as their starting point Ogston's model, in which the gel is represented as a random arrangement of rods or strings of beads (Ogston 1958; Ogston and Phelps 1961); from the dimensions of these, the volume fraction available to a spherical molecule as it migrates through the matrix can be derived. The theory may be simply applied to gel filtration by assuming with Laurent and Killander (1964) that Ogston's fractional volume for a given molecular species, which is given by

$$f_V = e^{-ls/4} \tag{7.2}$$

(where l is the length of matrix fibre per unit volume, and s the surface area of the molecule) can be equated with partition coefficient f for distribution of that species between the matrix and the free solvent. Morris (1966) first suggested the analogous assumption for gel electrophoresis, that f could be equated with the ratio f_0 of the electrophoretic mobility (u) in the gel to that at zero gel concentration, i.e.

$$f = u/u_0 \tag{7.3}$$

In other words, the mobility of an assemblage of identical molecules through the gel is proportional to the volume fraction from which they are not excluded by the gel matrix material. The predictions according to this scheme for the dependence of mobility on gel concentration and Stokes radius are in good qualitative accord with observation for a series of native proteins (Morris 1966). This moreover provides a rational link between the mobility of a given

Subject index p. 487

molecular species in gel electrophoresis and its elution volume in gel filtration.

This approach has been elaborated by Rodbard and Chrambach (1970). They consider the volumes available to the migrating molecule both in the Ogston model of a matrix of long thin rods, and in case of a matrix composed of randomly disposed planes. These two extreme cases (infinite rods and rods of zero length, i.e. points) lead to different expressions for f, and consequently for the average pore size. The average pore radius is proportional respectively to $T^{-\frac{1}{2}}$ and $T^{-\frac{1}{3}}$ in the two cases, where T is the total concentration of gel matrix in monomer units. These expectations are borne out for gels of very low and very high cross-linker concentrations, which correspond closely to the two ideal situations (Fawcett and Morris 1966).

Further, Rodbard and Chrambach define a 'retardation coefficient', K_R, such that

$$\log u/u_0 = K_R T, \tag{7.4}$$

a relation that is known to hold good for a variety of molecules in various systems, the cross-linker concentration being held constant. The retardation coefficient is clearly related to the mean pore radius, and the effective radius, R, of the migrating molecule. In the two limiting cases, as before:

$$K_R^{\frac{1}{2}} = c_1(R+r) \quad \text{and} \quad K_R^{\frac{1}{3}} = c_2(R+r) \tag{7.5}$$

c_1 and c_2 being constants, and r the fibre radius. From experimental data on proteins Rodbard and Chrambach obtain the reasonable value of 7 Å for r, in remarkable agreement with 8 Å value derived from gel filtration on beads of the same material. With RNA, the effective value of R, and its physical significance, is less easily defined and different values for r are obtained (Richards and Lecanidou 1971).

7.4. *Theoretical aspects of factors affecting resolution*

This problem has been considered by a number of workers, but the most pertinent study, which moreover is directed towards electrophoresis of RNA, comes from Richards and Lecanidou (1971). They consider in the first place the effect of diffusion, and make the assumption that the free-solution diffusion coefficient, D_0, of a migrating molecule is attenuated to the same degree by the gel as is the free solution mobility, that is

$$D/D_0 = u/u_0 = f \tag{7.6}$$

Since both these transport processes depend on the frictional coefficient of the molecule in the same way, this is a very reasonable assumption, and explains why under conditions of severe retardation zones remain extremely sharp. By application of Fick's laws, Richards and Lecanidou determine the evolution of the zone half-width with time, and derive the important result, confirmed by experiment, that the zone-width, provided the ratio of diffusion coefficient to retardation factor is of the right order, depends to only a slight extent on the width of the starting zone applied at one end of the gel. For typical conditions there is no detectable loss in resolution for an initial zone width of up to 2 mm, and even for a 1 cm column of RNA solution applied to the gel there is only a 25% increase in band width.

When the total mass of sample is increased beyond a critical value, conductivity disturbances within the zones lead to spreading and asymmetry. The point at which this effect becomes obtrusive will depend, in a manner that has been theoretically derived, on the ionic strength of the buffer and the mobility of its ions: Richards and Lecanidou suggest for a typical system, such as they use (see also below), a loading of 0.5 μg in cylindrical gels of 0.5 cm diameter in 0.05 M ionic strength buffer. At higher ionic strength higher loadings can be tolerated without loss of resolution.

7.4.1. Gel concentration for best resolution

Rodbard and Chrambach (1970) evaluate T_{max}, the gel concentration corresponding to maximisation of $\delta u/u$, by differentiation, and obtain K_R between 1/e and $1/e^2$, an expression which leads to the result that maximal separation is to be expected when the gel concentration,

Subject index p. 487

T_{max}, is $2/(K_1+K_2)$, where K_1 and K_2 are the value of K_R (see eqs. 7.4 and 7.5) for the two species to be separated. However, because of diffusion, the conditions for maximal separation (of the zone peaks) do not correspond to optimal resolution. Instead the optimal gel concentration, T_{opt}, is given by $4/(K_1+K_2)$. Moreover in the case of a set of homologues of identical free solution mobilities, the mobility at T_{max} is about 1/e, or 0.37 of the free solution mobility, and that at T_{opt} $1/e^2$ or 0.135 of the same. This relationship

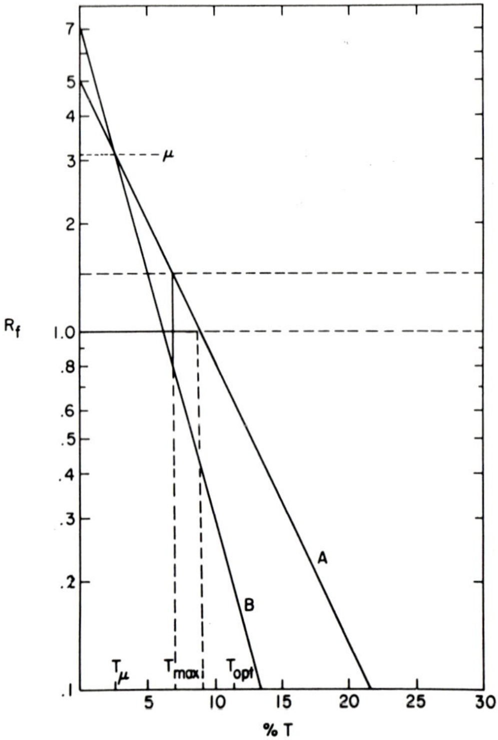

Fig. 7.3. Gel concentration for optimal separation (after Rodbard et al. 1974). The situation (mobilities of components A and B converging at zero concentration) is the 'size isomerism' case of Rodbard et al. T is the total acrylamide concentration. T_{max} is the gel concentration corresponding to maximum resolution, regardless of zone width, and T_{opt} that for optimal separation of the two components. μ is the mobility of RNA.

in terms of 'Ferguson plots', is illustrated in Fig. 7.3 (Rodbard et al. 1974).

It has to be recognised that there is thus far no full and satisfactory theory of gel electrophoresis and in general the best that can be expected of theoretical analyses is the rationalisation of observed effects. Their practical impact is therefore slight, and workers in the field have preferred to avail themselves of empirically derived rules in designing fractionation experiments. As to the choice of gel concentration, which is the most important experimental variable, Peacock and Dingman (1968) have suggested that optimum resolution is obtained when the mean molecular weight is approximately half the molecular weight corresponding to zero mobility, M_0, obtained by extrapolation (Fig. 7.4). From this figure an optimum (or at least satisfactory) gel concentration can be chosen for determination of molecular weights of RNA in any given range. It can be seen that at high acrylamide concentrations the change in M_0 with gel concentration approaches a limiting value. Thus for oligonucleotides it should be advantageous to choose a gel of the highest workable concentration.

Results on oligodeoxynucleotides (§ 10.1) show the clear resolution of successive oligomers of $(dAT)_n$ differing by only one base pair. Calculations by Richards and Lecanidou (1971) suggest that for larger species under optimal conditions comparable resolution may be obtained. The relation (Boedtker 1960) between $s^0_{20,w}$ measured at sufficiently high ionic strength (say 0.1–0.2) and molecular weight for typical single stranded RNAs is

$$s^0_{20,w} = 0.02\ M^{0.5} \tag{7.7}$$

The more concentrated the polyacrylamide the more slowly the RNA molecules will migrate. Typical curves of mobility against gel concentration are shown in Fig. 7.4b. Beyond a certain concentration the mobility will become so low that within any reasonable time the distance of migration is insufficient to permit satisfactory separation. Indeed, gradients of polyacrylamide concentration have been used, in which the electrophoretic mobility of each species diminishes with

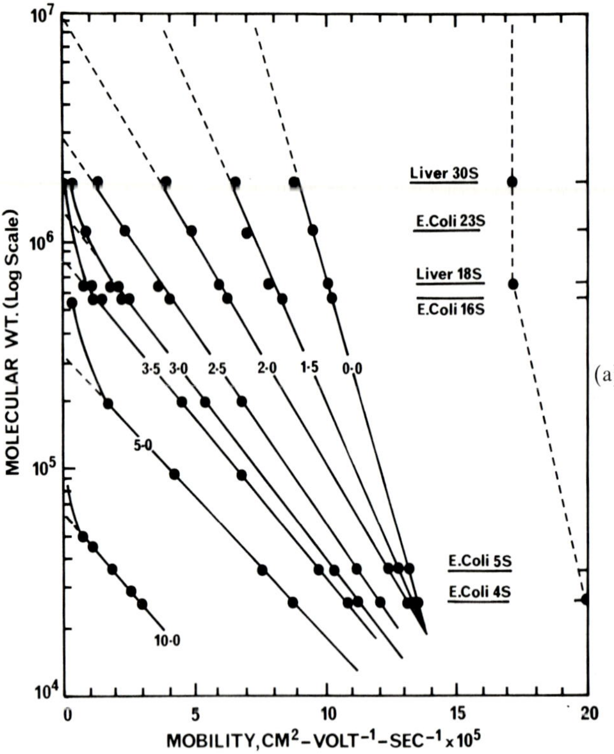

(a)

---

distance of migration, until in principle it becomes essentially stationary at a position in the gradient depending only on its Stokes radius. This is referred to as pore-limit electrophoresis. Since diffusion is strongly restricted in concentrated gels, a relatively high gel concentration is advantageous for good resolution (see Richards and Lecanidou 1971). In practice the gel concentration is selected to be a compromise between resolution and time of experiment. Spectacular fractionations have been achieved in very long runs in polyacrylamide gels of high concentration, as will be seen later (§ 9.2.2).

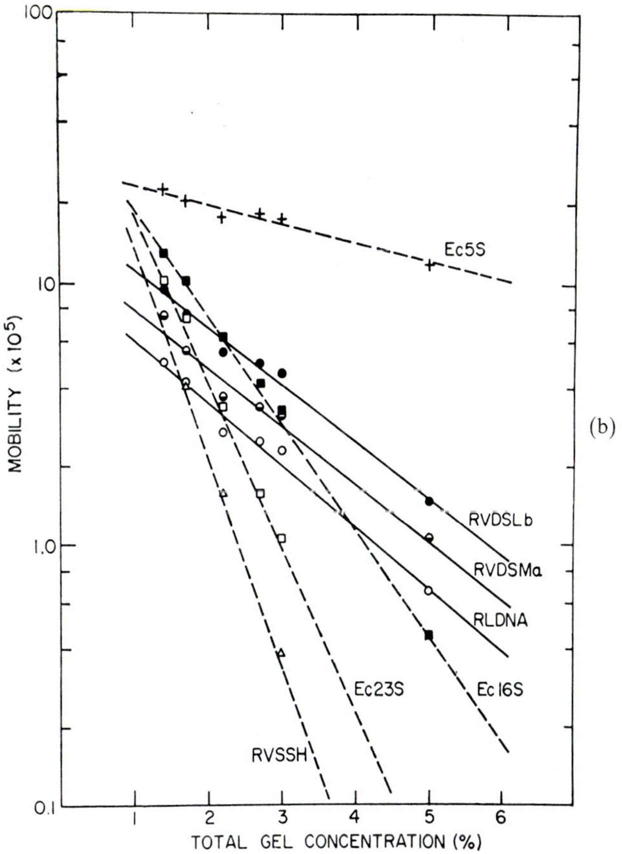

Fig. 7.4. a) Molecular weight-mobility relationships for electrophoresis of RNA in composite polyacrylamide-agarose gels of the stated acrylamide concentration (%) (adapted from Peacock and Dingman 1968). b) Dependence of mobility on gel concentration for single-stranded (dotted lines), and double-helical (rod-like) RNAs (full lines) (Fisher and Dingman 1971).

7.5. Experimental methods

Gel electrophoresis is variously used to identify and characterise species in a mixture, to determine their relative concentrations, to measure their radioactivity, and to isolate them in modest bulk.

Microelectrophoresis, for such purposes as the analysis of RNA from a single cell (say 10^{-9} g), clearly provides a special challenge. We consider these aspects in turn. The same general principles apply to electrophoresis in tubes or rectangular slabs of polyacrylamide, agar or agarose or their mixtures. The most important manipulative factor determining the regularity of zones in the electrophoretic pattern is the evenness of the gel surface at the point at which the sample is applied. A flat meniscus prior to setting is obtained in tubes by layering the liquid acrylamide monomer solution with buffer. An even surface in flat gels is ensured by layering (in the case of vertical gels) or by using a plastic mould which forms the sample slots (either vertical or horizontal gels).

7.5.1. Apparatus for basic methods

7.5.1.1. Disc gels

A common scheme for polyacrylamide gel electrophoresis in tubes is the 'disc' method. This was so named because of a sharpening procedure (Kohlrausch regulation), which was introduced by Ornstein (1964) and Davis (1964) with the object of causing the components to stack up in contiguous discs in a cylindrical gel of low concentration before entering the higher concentration gel, in which the separation actually occurs. This procedure, which is still often used, depends on the use of discontinuous buffer systems, in which an ion front from the reservoir buffer moves through the sample and causes macromolecules to migrate into an increasing potential gradient, and so accelerate and collect into a very thin zone. It is now recognised (Hjertén et al. 1965) that sharpening of the sample zone can be achieved in other ways: applying the sample in a medium of low ionic strength compared with the gel buffer leads to an increased voltage drop across the volume element containing the sample which leads again to an acceleration within this volume, with consequent zone sharpening. In any case, however, there is always a discontinuity in mobility at the solution/gel interface because of retardation by the gel, and the sample therefore tends to accumulate in a narrow band at the top of the gel before entering. For this

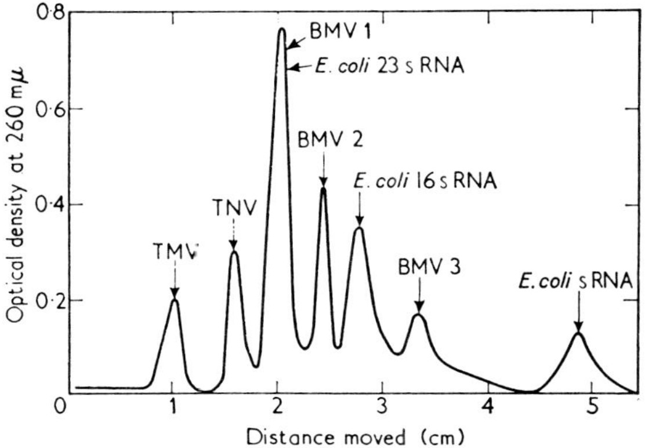

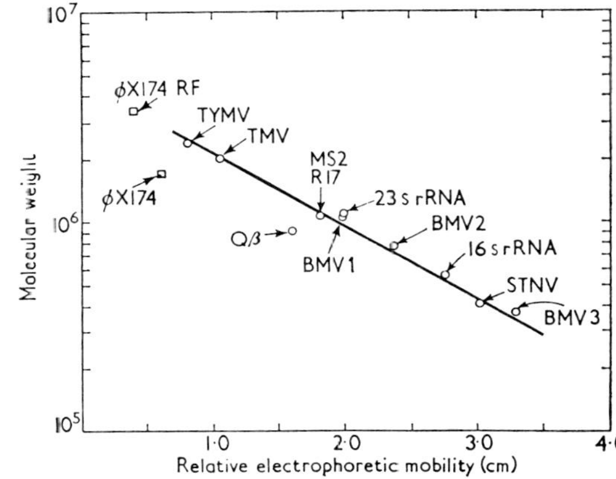

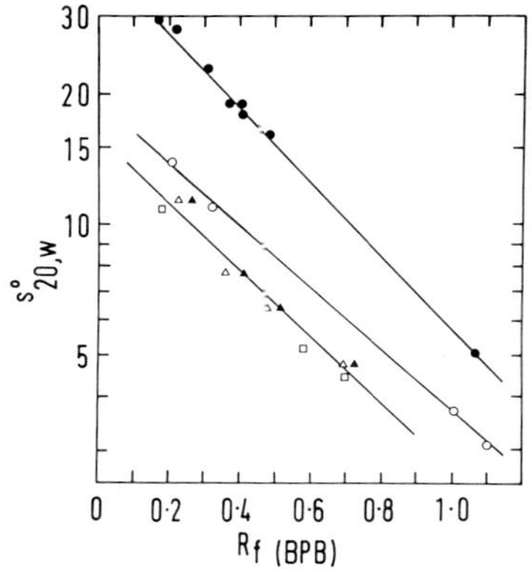

Fig. 7.5. Some typical molecular weight-mobility (or sedimentation coefficient) relationships for electrophoresis of RNA in polyacrylamide gels, showing conformational effects: a) set of single-stranded viral and ribosomal RNAs in 2.4% gel (Bishop et al. 1967). b) shows a typical separation of different species on a single gel, displayed as a densitometric trace; c) native single-stranded RNAs (●), formaldehyde treated RNAs (○), polyriboadenylic acid fractions with (△) and without (▲) formaldehyde treatment, and polyriboruridylic acid fractions (□) treated with formaldehyde. These data show that the mobilities are little affected by single-stranded stacking, but substantially by partial base pairing, and that formaldehyde treatment is inadequate to reduce RNA to the conformation of a single-stranded unpaired polynucleotide (from Pinder et al., 1974).

reason the discontinuous system, with matching of ionic mobilities, has been discarded by most workers, and so especially has the use of 'spacer gel'. We do not believe that it offers significant advantages in routine use and its elimination certainly halves the labour involved in setting up an experiment (see however Gordon, this series Vol. 1 supplement where disc electrophoresis of proteins is discussed).

However, the configuration of the apparatus devised by Ornstein and Davis has been retained in many laboratories, and it is available in several commercial versions. It is shown in Fig. 7.6. Glass tubes approximately 0.6 (i.d.) × 8 cm are convenient and are retained in the upper reservoir by grommets. The electrodes are generally of platinum wire. The reservoir volume should be no less than about 0.5 l, for otherwise serious contamination with electrode products in the time of an average run is hard to avoid. External cooling, say with an electric fan, is often desirable. This apparatus can be improved by arranging for the tubes of gel to be immersed in buffer for the greater part of their length, to provide a heat sink (cf. Fig. 7.7). A considerable number of tubes (often 6–10) can be accommodated in such an apparatus. It is moderately convenient in use, will take large sample volumes, and is almost foolproof.

One of the disadvantages of the type of apparatus of circular design shown is the absence of any barrier to prevent the diffusion of electrode products through the buffer and into the gel. If this is allowed to happen, in the course of a long run, the *p*H will change, alien ions, including protons, may migrate into the gel and frequently react with the polyacrylamide matrix, and precipitate the RNA. This can be avoided by changing the buffer at intervals (when the *p*H has changed detectably to *p*H-paper), and using a good buffer at sufficient concentration. An alternative solution is to use an apparatus of rectangular design, incorporating a barrier, such as a screen containing holes with porous plugs between an electrode chamber, and the bulk of the buffer compartments (Fig. 7.7). Alternatively, one may use external electrodes, e.g. reversible calomel electrodes, consisting of a paste of mercury and calomel under a saturated potassium chloride solution. Contact with the buffer compartments is best made

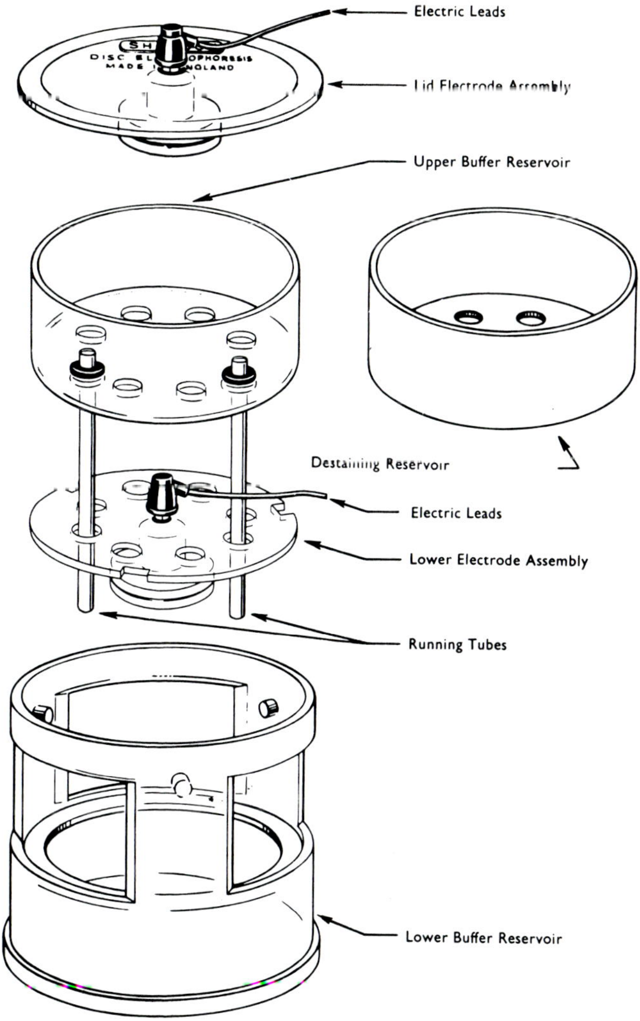

Fig. 7.6. Basic design, after Davis (1964), of analytical electrophoresis apparatus for cylindrical gels. The tubes are held in the upper compartment by liquid-tight silicone-rubber grommets. The electrodes are platinum wire (by courtesy of Shandon Instrument Co. Ltd.).

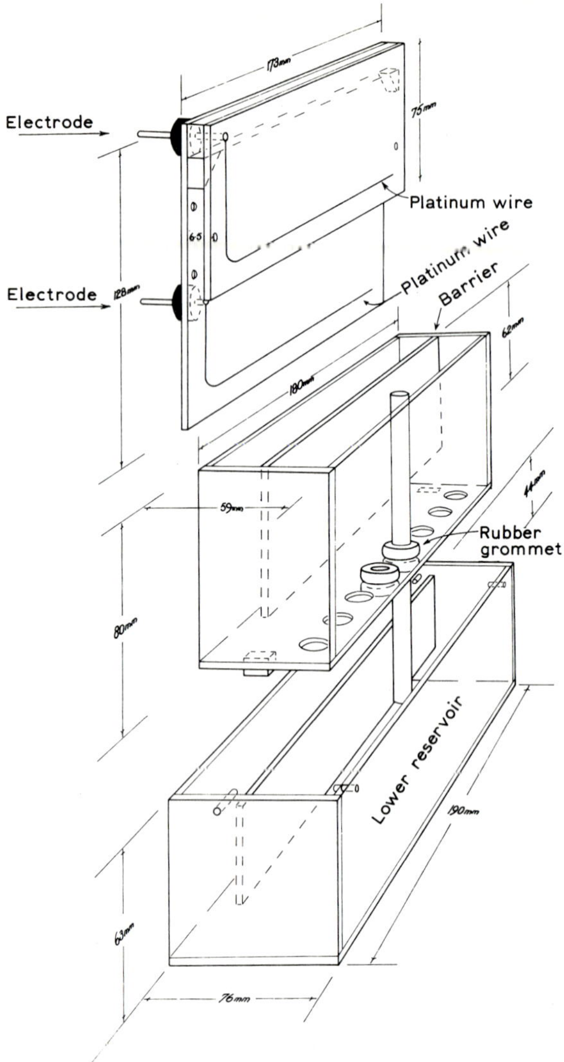

Fig. 7.7. Modified design of cylindrical gel analytical electrophoresis apparatus. One of the design features, which may also be embodied in the circular layout (Fig. 7.6) is that the tubes are immersed in the lower reservoir buffer for better heat dissipation. A further advantage in this system is the presence of a barrier which impedes the diffusion of electrode products into the buffer solution.

by means of agar or polyacrylamide bridges containing potassium chloride solution, about 1 M. These survive for many runs, and do not leak much salt into the buffer. There is of course an appreciable voltage drop across the bridges so that a greater voltage will be required from the power supply than in the conventional arrangement. In one electrode, mercury is oxidised to calomel; in the other, calomel is reduced to mercury. Consequently if the electrode connections are interchanged between successive runs, the electrodes will maintain themselves indefinitely, so long as the platinum wires remain immersed in the paste at the bottom (Fig. 7.8).

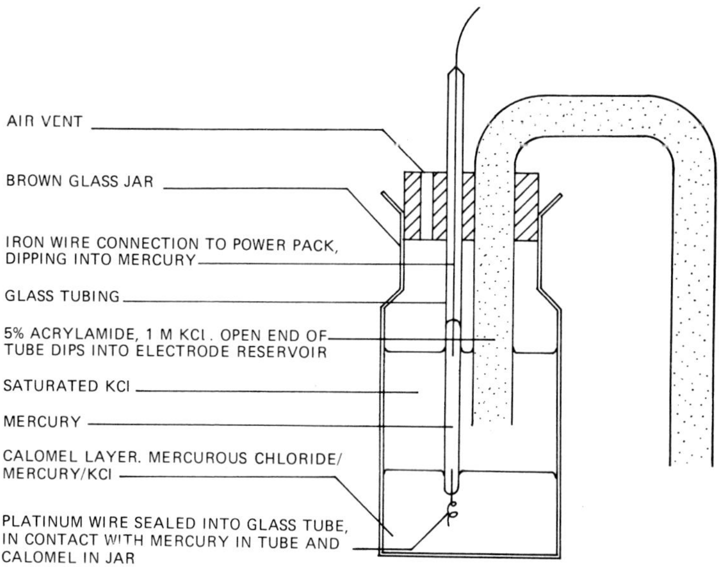

Fig. 7.8. Reversible mercury-calomel electrode with the parts consisting of a 250 ml wide-mouthed reagent bottle, a vented and drilled rubber stopper, a soft glass tube with platinum wire sealed into the end, mercury, a wire to the output of the power supply, saturated KCl, and a glass tube containing 5% polyacrylamide gel made up in 1 M KCl. The tube dips into the buffer reservoir of the electrophoresis apparatus. The anode and cathode should be interchanged after each run. This arrangement will prevent all contamination of the buffer with electrode products even in very long runs (J. C. Pinder, Ph.D. Thesis, London University, 1974).

Subject index p. 487

It requires a measure of skill and practice to achieve an equal voltage drop in all tubes. The tubes themselves should be of high quality to ensure an even bore, and must all be filled to precisely the same level, using scratch marks on the glass. The apparatus must be such that the tubes are symmetrically distributed around the electrode or bridge, and blank gels should be used rather than blocking the holes for tubes if it is not required to run the full complement of gels (unless of course a symmetrical arrangement can be maintained). Even so, comparison of zones by dead-reckoning is difficult (though not impossible: see Lewicki and Sinskey, 1970), and the split-gel technique (Clarke, 1964; Leboy et al. 1964), where two samples are applied to a single tube, usually with a dividing strip, extending, say, 1 cm down from the top, may be useful.

Materials Cylindrical gels of acrylamide may be cast in glass or Perspex (Lucite, Plexiglass) tubes; gels containing agarose do not adhere and tend to slide out, so tubes cannot be used. Gels adhere less readily to Perspex, which is consequently often recommended for concentrated gels. The replacement of gels into Perspex tubes (which can be desirable when it is required to equilibrate the gel with a buffer different from that used for the setting reaction) is easier. However very dilute (eg. 2.5% or below) gels tend to slip even out of glass tubes (and more especially Perspex), and may have to be supported by a rim of plastic tubing the external diameter of which is such that it fits tightly in the tube at the bottom, or by wrapping a layer of surgical gauze around the bottom of the tube, to which it can be secured by a rubber band. Very concentrated gels present their own problems, and in particular are difficult to remove from the tubes without breaking. A disadvantage of Perspex is inferior heat dissipation.

Gel dimensions The length and diameter of the tubes can be varied within limits. Tubes 6–10 cm long and 5–7 mm internal diameter are in common use. The diameter of the gel is limited by the need for adequate heat dissipation. The commonly observed occurrence of curved zones may usually be attributed to heating effects; molecules migrate faster in the centre of the gel, where temperature is higher, than near the circumference. Richards and Lecanidou (1971) have demonstrated these effects under controlled conditions. Efficient cooling or the use of lower currents permits the use of thicker gels which may be useful for running relatively large samples. If the diameter of the gels is small, increased difficulty may be experienced in removing them from the tubes, especially at high acrylamide concentrations. Longer gels may be useful for increasing the distance between the separated zones by running for longer times at a given voltage drop per unit length of gel. The increased resolution so obtained may be particularly desirable for excising single zones for preparative purposes or for radioactive counting. Gels of up to 40 cm length have proved of value for preparative separations. At the same time it must be borne in mind that the longer the run, the greater the diffusional broadening of the zones. It is advantageous to use gel slabs (see below) rather than tubes for large migration distances because of the intractable nature of long cylindrical gels.

7.5.1.2. Flat gel beds: general considerations

For direct comparison of samples, and many other convenient features, including better densitometric analysis, flat gels with samples applied in slots, are to be preferred. With agar and agarose the tubes do not, in any case work, since these gels do not adhere satisfactorily to the glass and tend to slide out. Gel slabs may be horizontal or vertical. Horizontal methods are alleged to suffer from electrodecantation effects: sample molecules in the application slot concentrate at the boundary of the gel, and the concentrated solution, being denser than the solvent, falls to the bottom of the slot. The result is an uneven distribution from top to bottom of the sample area, which leads to some loss of definition, since at all but very low concentration, the mobility is somewhat affected by concentration. Be this as it may, horizontal gels have been used in many laboratories, with excellent success. They lend themselves well moreover to the use of an efficient cooling system: e.g. the gel can be placed over a hollow metal plate, through which water is circulated (Vasu 1969). The reader's attention may be drawn at this point to the application illustrated in Fig. 10.8. Here, despite theoretical reasons for preferring apparatus of vertical design, in practice equally good resolution may be obtained with horizontal gels which may be more convenient to handle.

Perhaps the most rational geometry for polyacrylamide electrophoresis is that of vertical flat-bed systems (Akroyd 1968; De Wachter and Fiers 1972).

The system was devised to allow the reproducible production of acrylamide slabs containing an acrylamide concentration gradient, but is altogether suitable for conventional use. Forms of all the systems mentioned here have been used in the authors' laboratory and give good results. Vertical, flat beds, however, offer nearly all the advantages of the disc system with none of its limitations, and is particularly recommended.

Few issues of the analytical journals go by without the appearance of a new design for gel electrophoresis apparatus, and there are no doubt many satisfactory alternatives to the three versions that we have discussed. Microelectrophoresis and preparative electrophoresis pose special problems, and will be considered separately (§ 7.5.2.2; § 7.5.2.3; ch. 9).

7.5.1.3. Horizontal flat gels

A convenient apparatus for horizontal electrophoresis can be made from Perspex sheet and a glass plate as shown in Fig. 7.9, designed by Vasu (1969). The gel is poured into the space between the plastic mould carrying the sample slots and the bottom glass plate separated by rectangular Perspex spacers and closed off. After polymerisation, the gel is inverted onto the glass plate which serves as a support during electrophoresis and the plastic mould is peeled away carefully, so as not to damage the sample slots. The gel can be soaked in buffer to remove contaminating chemicals or to introduce a different solvent.

For electrophoresis, connections are made to reservoir buffer

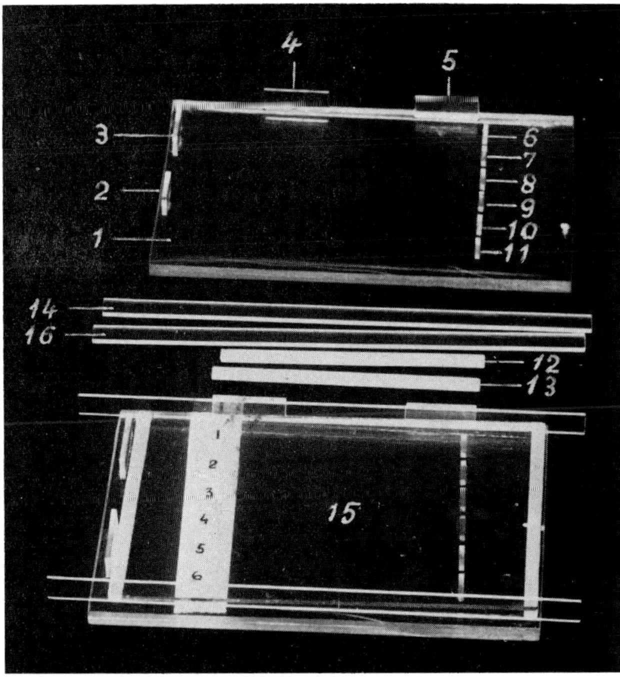

Fig. 7.9. Flat-gel horizontal electrophoresis apparatus. Design of Vasu (1969), and reproduced here with details supplied by him. The apparatus is made of Perspex and the base plate (1) is $18.6 \times 13.0 \times 0.5$ cm. The vertical pieces (2, 3, 4, 5) are all $3 \times 1 \times 0.2$ mm, and the sides are defined by slats, 12 and 13, respectively $10.8 \times 0.5 \times 0.3$ cm and $11.2 \times 0.5 \times 0.3$ cm, and 14 and 16, which are $20 \times 1 \times 0.2$ cm. The glass upper plate, 15, is $16 \times 11 \times 0.2$ cm. This is placed on top of the base plate, resting on the slats (except the side piece 16) mounted as shown, 14 supported by 4 and 5, which are sealed to the plate. Likewise at the ends, are slats 12 and 13, the former supported by 2 and 3. The slot formers stick to the lower plate, and measure $1.2 \times 0.2 \times 0.2$ cm. The acrylamide solution is poured down an inclined glass plate into the gap, and slat 16 is put in place. After polymerisation, the side slats are eased out with a razor blade and the device is inverted. The end pieces are likewise removed, and sheets of Whatman 6 MM paper are used to make contact with the reservoir, one layer above, another below the gel. After loading, and during the run, the gel is covered with a thin plastic sheet.

compartments with filter paper or plastic sponge wicks, cut to the width of the gels, and impregnated with buffer. Alternatively, one may cast a longer gel, which overlaps the supporting plate at both ends, and dips directly into the buffer compartments. During electrophoresis evaporation is prevented by covering the gel with polyethylene film or Saran, which is applied after the run has commenced and the sample has entered the gel. Alternatively (or additionally), the gel is enclosed in a humidity chamber. The Shandon Universal Electrophoresis tank is convenient for this purpose, though for long runs larger buffer compartments are desirable. The covering prevents drops of condensation which form on the lid of the apparatus from dropping onto the gel. In the absence of a humidity chamber it is probably best to spread a layer of paraffin oil on the surface of the plastic sheet in contact with the gel. If the plate carrying the gel is placed on a hollow brass block with an inlet and outlet for circulating tap water, good heat transfer is achieved and shorter runs at higher voltages are possible.

7.5.1.4. Vertical flat gels

The simple apparatus for vertical flat bed electrophoresis (Fig. 7.10), described by Akroyd (1968), consists of two thin glass plates taped together and separated by spacers, which also form the sides of the compartment, and to which the glass plates are clamped. The gel sits between the glass plates and this sandwich is mounted vertically with the aid of plastic gaskets in a reservoir of ample volume. The cell stands in the lower reservoir, while the upper reservoir is placed behind the top of the cell and is connected to it by a filter paper wick. The height of the buffer over the gel should be the same as that in the buffer reservoirs to prevent siphoning. The electrodes are in the buffer compartments, and excessive trouble from contamination with electrolysis products is avoided by circulating buffer continuously between the upper and lower reservoir with a small pump (e.g. an aquarium pump). Alternatively, the buffer reservoir may contain baffles to prevent electrode products from diffusing into the gel. A variant, also described by Akroyd (1968) employs water cooling which permits the current to be doubled. The home-made apparatus is as satisfactory as many which are commercially available. It can be modified to meet individual requirements; for example, 40 cm long glass plates have been used to increase the distance of the separations for the isolation of nucleic acids for sequence determination.

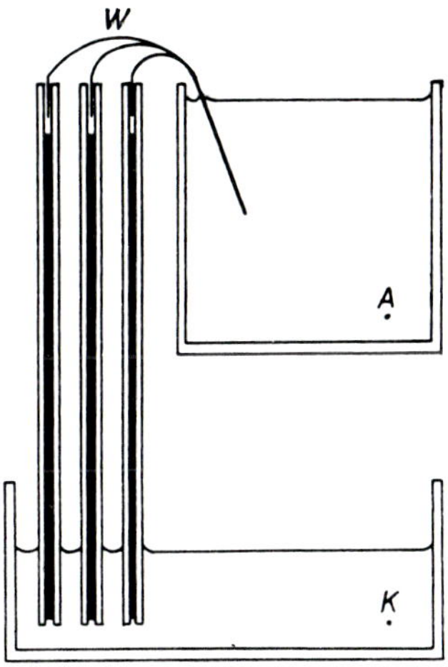

Fig. 7.10. Flat-gel vertical electrophoresis apparatus of the Akroyd type, showing three gels being run in parallel (De Wachter and Fiers 1971).

For filling, Akroyd supports his apparatus in a block of plasticine, to close the end of the gel compartment, and fills to within a few cm of the top of the glass and then overlayers with water. If tall gels are required and, because of the hydrostatic pressure, or for any other reason, there is leakage at the bottom, the gel can be set in two layers, a shallow layer at the bottom and, after this has set and the water layer been removed, the remainder of the gel solution is poured in. Sample compartments are made by thrusting tightly fitting pieces of rubber cut from rubber tubing between the plates. Using the same apparatus, a number of workers have preferred to construct a sample slot former from Perspex sheet which fits into the top of the cell, and around which the gel may set. This has the appearance of a wide-toothed comb and may be designed to permit one or several

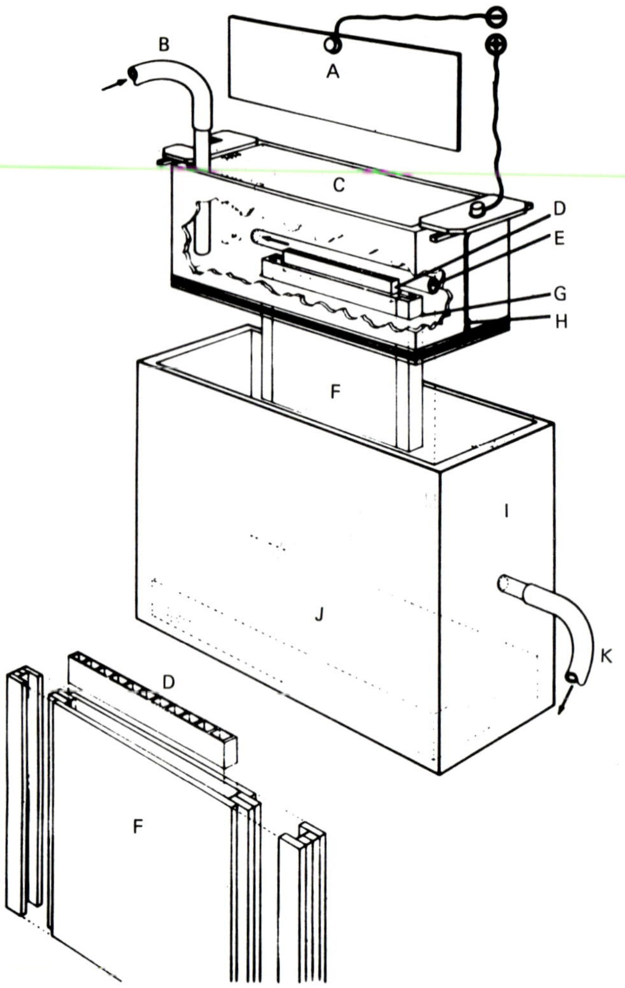

Fig. 7.11. Flat-gel vertical electrophoresis apparatus: a more complex design, adaptable for the utilisation of several flat gels simultaneously. A is the anode, B an inlet for circulation of buffer in the upper reservoir, C, D the sample slot former, E the electrode, F the gel, H a silicone rubber gasket, J the lower reservoir and K the outlet for buffer circulation from the lower reservoir (by courtesy of Universal Scientific Co.).

samples to be run. The width of the teeth from front to back may be slightly less than the width of the gel, thus presenting barriers to migration along the glass faces. For preparative purposes a single broad band of sample can be applied.

A number of manufacturers have marketed apparatuses for vertical starch gel electrophoresis, which can equally well be used for poly acrylamide gels. A good design is that of Fig. 7.11. A commercial apparatus with water-cooled plates manufactured according to the design of Raymond (1964) by E-C Apparatus Corporation (Fig. 7.12) has been successfully used, notably by Peacock and Dingman (1968) for the separation of high molecular weight RNA in gels containing down to 3.5% acrylamide, or less, when agarose is included. An apparatus allowing multiple flat gels to be run in parallel is made by Universal Scientific Co.

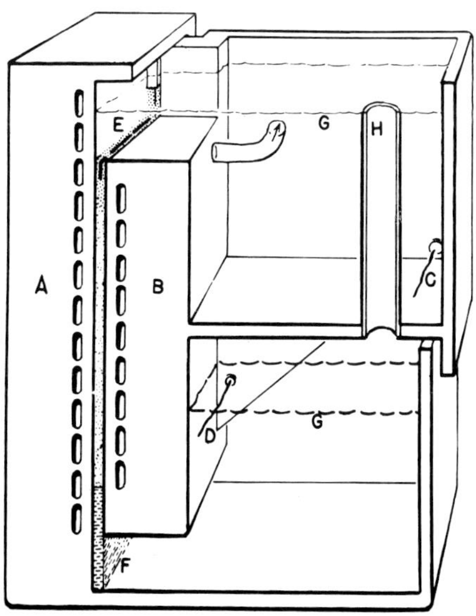

Fig. 7.12. Flat-gel vertical electrophoresis apparatus after Raymond (1962), and manufactured by E-C Apparatus Co. The gel is supported on a sponge strip, F, and is confined between two cooling plates A and B. The samples are applied in slots, E, C and D are electrodes. G the reservoir buffer levels, and H a constant-level tube.

7.5.2. Elaborations of basic methods

7.5.2.1. Two-dimensional gel electrophoresis

Two-dimensional gel electrophoresis of RNA has been used for two purposes. One general problem has been to identify RNA species migrating in the form of nucleoprotein particles, e.g. ribosomes and viruses. In this case, the buffer used in the second dimension is one in which the RNA and protein components are dissociated. RNA species of known size can be run in parallel with the sample in the second dimension.

The strategy is simply to combine two analytical separations. A sample may first be run in a cylindrical gel, which is either sliced longitudinally to generate a flat strip or applied whole to a slab. It must then be embedded in new gel at the surface of the pre-formed slab to provide good contact. Again, the first dimension may be run in a flat gel, and a strip cut off for application to the second gel, which may be horizontal or vertical. In general it is advantageous to make the acrylamide concentration in the second dimension higher than in the first to bring about zone sharpening at the interface before the second separation begins.

The second dimension may serve simply to improve separations. Enhanced resolution may be necessary because there is a wide range in the size of RNA species present in a mixture, in which case a low polyacrylamide gel concentration separates the high molecular weight RNA species and may be followed by electrophoresis at a higher concentration gel to optimise separation of the low molecular weight species (the magnitude of this type of effect is illustrated in Fig. 7.13). Alternatively, for the same purpose, a gel gradient may be used. The mobility of RNA species may be differently affected by the use of a denaturing solvent in the second dimension. This may occur by reason of the loss of secondary structure *per se*, or because of the dissociation of two or more strands in a base-paired complex in an enzymically 'nicked' molecule. In principle, compositional differences may be used to separate nucleic acid species of the same size and conformation, and therefore mobility at *p*H 7, by performing, in the second dimension, zone electrophoresis at a *p*H in the ionisation range of the bases. Excellent results have been obtained using a neutral gel in one dimension, and either acid *p*H, or 6 M urea (or both) in the other (see Fig. 7.14) (De Wachter and Fiers 1972).

7.5.2.2. Microelectrophoresis

The methods which have been discussed allow considerable scope for reduction of scale. There is now a sizeable literature of research on proteins involving electrophoretic analysis of the contents of single cells. The earliest successful results were obtained with fibres pulled from polyacrylamide gel, and subsequently two good procedures have been evolved, one based on cylindrical gels in glass capillaries, the other on very thin leaflets of gel (or microslabs). The capillary technique is probably the more generally tractable, and for protein work has been adapted for acrylamide gradients and for isoelectric focusing, as well as molecular weight determination by electrophoresis in sodium dodecyl sulfate. It has been successfully applied to the fractionation of RNA. The first application was that of Ringborg et al. (1968) and Egyhazi et al. (1969), who used composite agarose-polyacrylamide gels to fractionate the RNA of salivary glands of *Chironomus* larvae. The acrylamide solution is introduced by capillarity into 5 μl glass capillaries. The samples are loaded with a hand-pulled microcapillary, and in most respects the technique is similar to the conventional procedure already described. Naturally the manipulative techniques are much more exacting, and ingenious methods have been devised for loading known volumes of sample in the microlitre range, for microdensitometry of stained gels and for isolating components from a mixture by electrophoretic extraction. The diameter of the capillary is about 0.5 mm and separations may cover, say, 3 cm. Samples down to the nanogram level can be analysed. Results of remarkable quality have been obtained. We do not propose to deal here with the manipulative details of this specialised aspect of gel electrophoresis, since they have been described in full detail by one of the innovators in the field, in a book devoted to a considerable extent to microelectrophoresis (Neuhoff 1973), and to which reference should be made.

Subject index p. 487

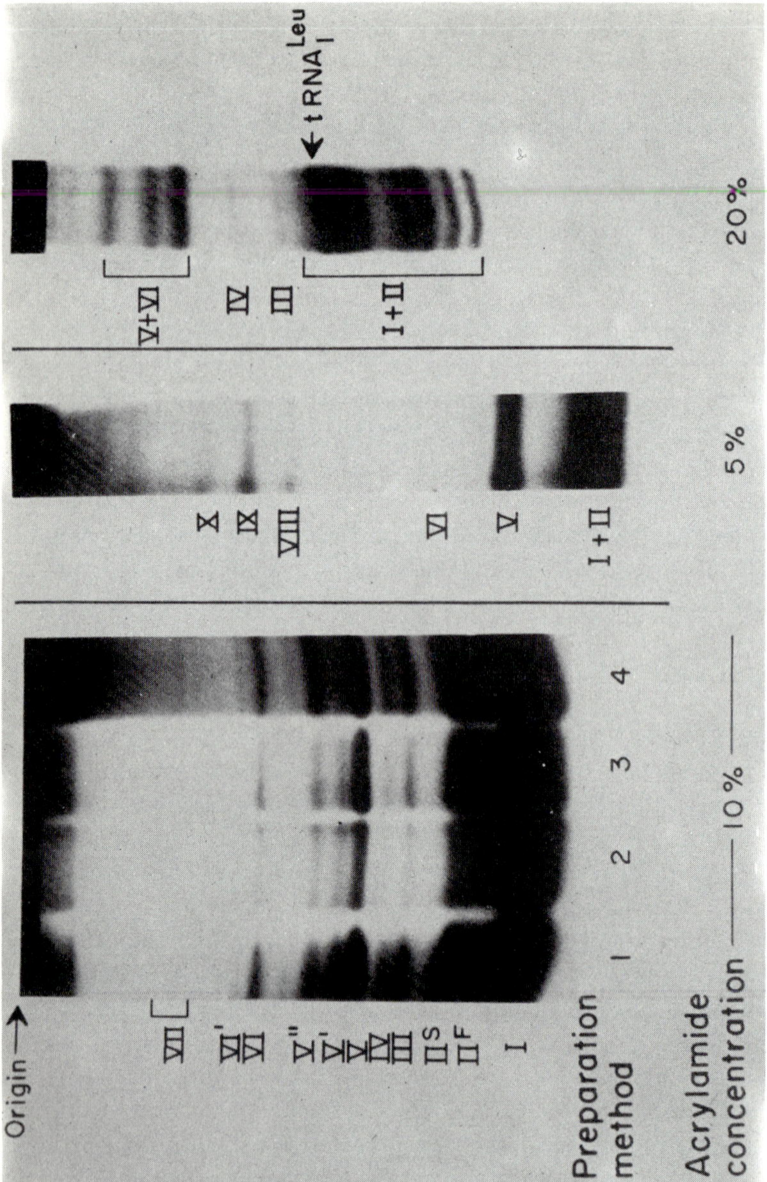
Origin
tRNA Leu I
V+VI
IV
III
I+II
X
IX
VIII
VI
V
I+II
VII
VI'
VI
V''
V'
V
IV
III
II S
II F
I
Preparation method
1
2
3
4
Acrylamide concentration
10%
5%
20%

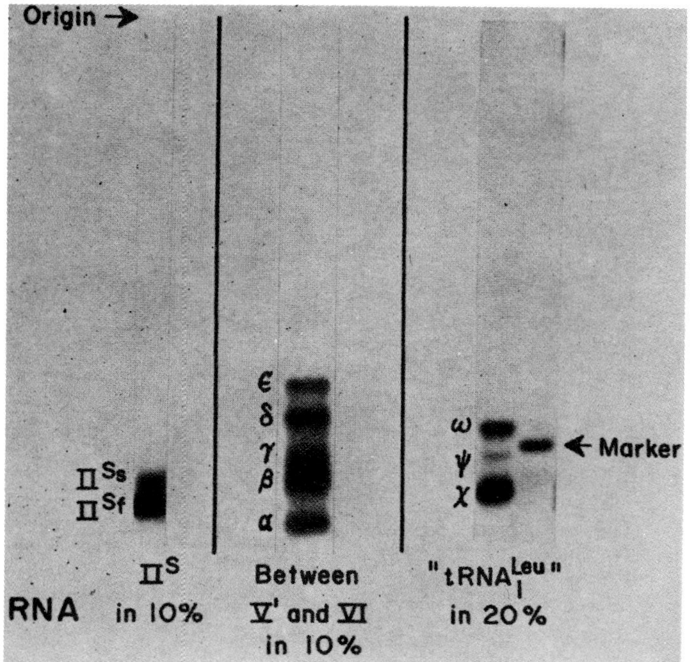

Fig. 7.13. A) Autoradiograph of ^{32}P-labelled tRNA mixture on flat gels, of 10, 5 and 20% acrylamide. B) Re-electrophoresis of 3 selected slices of these gels. The first two slices were run at 10% in the second gel. The third slice at 20% (Ikemura and Dahlberg 1973).

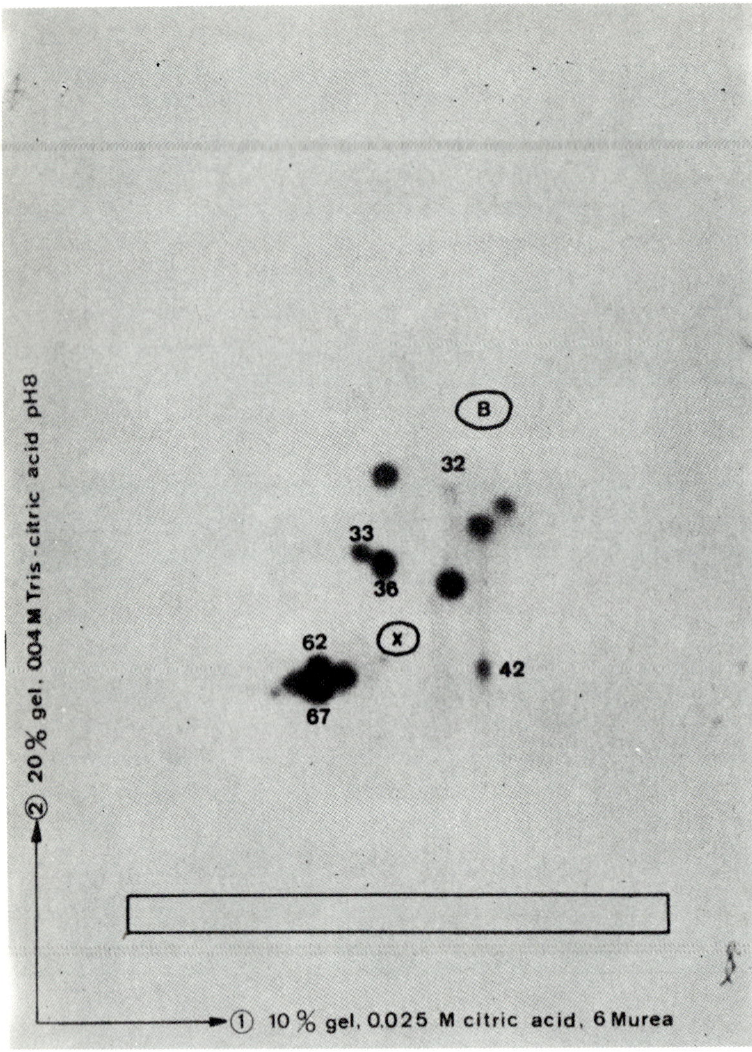

B
32
33
36
X
62
42
67
② 20 % gel, 0.04 M Tris-citric acid pH8
① 10 % gel, 0.025 M citric acid, 6 M urea

(a)

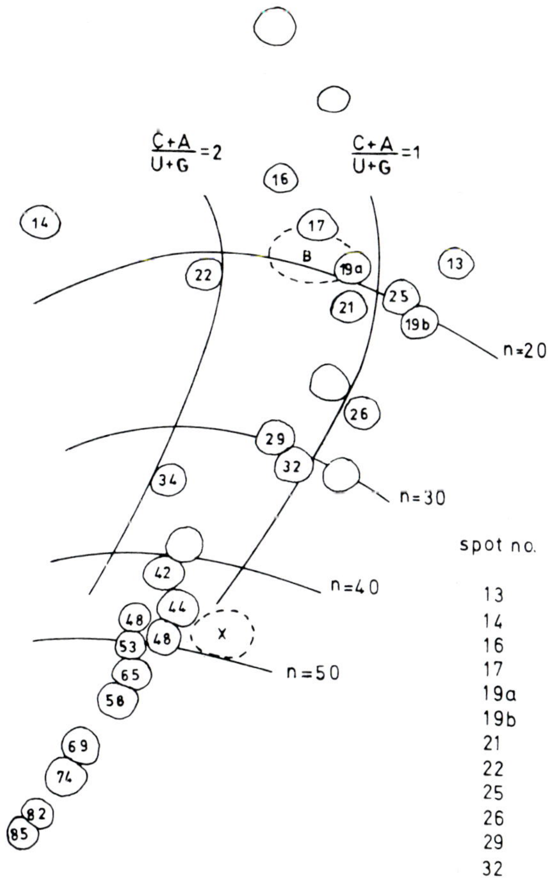

spot no.	(C + A)/(U + G)
13	0.62
14	2.75
16	1.29
17	1.12
19a	1.11
19b	1.11
21	0.91
22	2.14
25	0.79
26	0.86
29	0.93
32	1.00
34	1.86

b

Fig. 7.14. a) Autoradiograph of two dimensional gel showing resolution of low-molecular weight RNA species. Note that zones on a common ordinate would be unresolved in the first dimension. The rectangle shows the position of embedding of the first-dimension gel. b) Map showing the dependence of migration rates in the two-dimensional system on base-composition. The effect of base composition depends on the fraction of bases present that have a p*K* in the acid range, which pertains to the second dimension (De Wachter and Fiers 1972).

Subject index p. 487

7.5.2.3. Preparative techniques

Fairly wide use has been made of preparative gel electrophoresis in protein chemistry, and in principle there is no reason why the same procedures should not be adopted for use with nucleic acids which have the advantage that much may be accomplished with very small quantities of purified material. Thus, it is relatively easy in many situations to introduce radioactive label at very high levels and specific activity, and the use of ^{32}P for this purpose offers a degree of sensitivity that cannot be matched in work on proteins. The extinction coefficients of nucleic acids are also very high in the ultraviolet, so that with say 20 μg in 1 ml or less it is possible to measure optical properties, thermal melting profiles, sedimentation coefficients, and even molecular weights by sedimentation equilibrium in an instrument equipped with scanner optics. Consequently, the sacrifice of resolution that, by a malign law of nature, always accompanies any attempt to scale up an analytical fractionation method is often at least partly avoided.

There are two general strategies open to one: a) after electrophoresis, zones may be individually excised and the nucleic acid extracted, i) by diffusion into a buffer in which the slices are bathed, or by macerating or pulverising the gel by hand or in a commercial apparatus; ii) by using a gel with hydrolysable cross-links, or iii) by causing the zone to migrate out of the gel and into a confined volume of buffer by electrophoresis. The alternative approach is: b) direct electrophoretic elution from the bottom of a column of gel. The first approach (a) is used in sequencing work, usually allied to extraction by course (i): method (ii) is not generally satisfactory if the nucleic acid has to be recovered undamaged, for the hydrolysis conditions are rigorous. Before the zones can be extracted they must be located. This may be done by staining, although here again covalent damage is hard to avoid with any certainty; alternatively, an identical gel (or strip of the sample pattern from a flat gel) may be stained and matched against the unstained gel; or if the sample is radioactive, a rapid autoradiogram may often be obtained, which will locate the zones. Alternatively, the gel may be sliced into equal pieces along its entire length, each one extracted and the nucleic acid determined by ultraviolet absorption or radioactivity. A distance-nucleic acid concentration profile can then be constructed. This of course is relatively arduous.

Direct elution techniques involve the collection of the eluate by a continuous stream of buffer, which is then fed to a fraction collector, by way of an ultraviolet monitor if desired. Some examples of successful applications will be given in ch. 9. In principle this type of technique can be scaled up considerably, to the milligram level, but great care in the design of the apparatus is required if the separations are not to be vitiated by heating in the thick gels that are used, and if there is not to be distortion of the zones. Some loss of resolution, as we have remarked, appears inescapable.

7.5.3. Detection and quantitation of separated components

The simplest procedure for detection of RNA is to scan the gel, directly after the run, in the ultraviolet. Using recrystallised acrylamide, gels or subjecting the gel to pre-electrophoresis before sample application, scanning at 260 nm is possible. For gels of high concentration it will be necessary to operate at longer wavelength, with considerable loss of sensitivity. With agar and agarose there are no such problems, and scanning of the wet gel is possible, though prior drying gives the best results. If for one reason or another direct densitometry does not appear possible or desirable, then the gels may be stained.

A further painless method of detection is due to Eisinger (1971): slab gels are cast between two plates, one of quartz and one of a fluorescent glass, such as uranium glass. When the gel is viewed under illumination from an ultraviolet lamp, the fluorescent glass gives rise to a yellow–green background on which the nucleic acid zones stand out as black bands. The progress of a run can be monitored in this way, and photographically recorded.

7.5.3.1. Staining

Staining has a number of obvious advantages: in the first place it produces a permanent visual record of the experiment. Secondly, the eye is always better able to detect partly resolved zones than the densitometer. There are a number of reasons for this, one of which is the 'stepped wedge' illusion, whereby an inflexion in an intensity profile is perceived as a minimum (Holiday 1937). Thirdly, a densitometer cannot cope with the same enormous range of absorbance (optical densities) that the eye can discriminate, so that very weak or very strong bands will not be faithfully recorded relative to the remainder. Fourthly, zones in visible light can be recorded without interference from ultraviolet background absorption, and very much less obtrusion from scattering. Finally, many dyes can apparently be taken up in a ratio of one dye molecule per nucleotide (Stone and Bradley 1961), and since the molar residue absorptivity of an RNA is of the order of 7500 and that of a typical acridine dye is 50,000 or more, a gain in sensitivity of up to about ten can in principle result. On the other hand, using the familiar 'stacking' dyes, considerable deviations from Beer's law would not be surprising (Steiner and Beers 1960; Stone and Bradley 1961), and not all RNA species will necessarily give rise to the same colour values in consequence of differences in stacking coefficients. Claims in the literature of linear response must be treated with caution: many possibilities exist of compensating errors, and, if precise quantitation is important, it is necessary to ensure that under the experimental conditions a linear law is indeed obeyed.

The choice of stains is wide: acridine orange, pyronine Y, toluidine blue, methylene blue, gallocyanine, and 'Stains-all' (a carbocyanine dye, described in § 8.3.1.3) have all been used. Acridine orange gives a somewhat lower sensitivity – though a large gain is possible by making use of its fluorescence – but at the same time it binds very strongly and is least easily removed by over-vigorous electrophoretic destaining. With agar gels, staining is best done after drying, using the same dye solution.

Although it has been shown that diffusion of RNA in gels is a relatively slow process (Richards and Lecanidou 1971), it is considered highly advisable to precipitate the RNA when staining. Experience now shows that if the stain is made up in a sufficiently acidic solution RNA will precipitate, and probably nothing is to be gained by including heavy metals in the staining solution.

Destaining may be accomplished simply by soaking in the staining solvent, preferably in a dish attached to a rocking mechanism. For the impatient, electrophoretic destaining is recommended. Many apparatuses have been devised, and in general the dye is caused to migrate out across the shortest dimension of the gel. The tubes or slabs may be confined between porous plastic plates (Richards and Gratzer 1968) (Fig. 7.15 Shandon Scientific Co.), placed on a grid over charcoal (Stanton 1965) or simply contained in a plastic frame

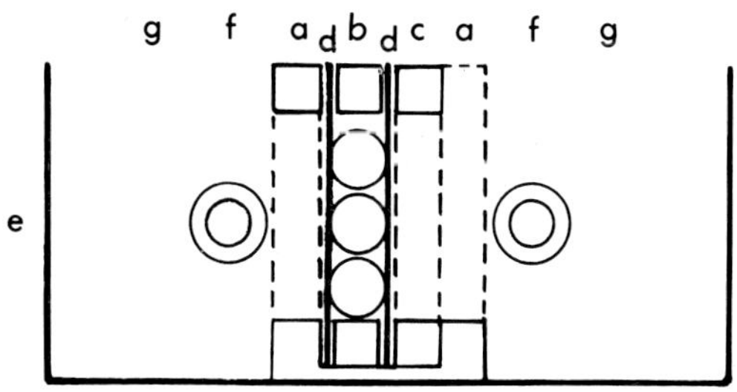

Fig. 7.15. Electrophoretic destaining apparatus (Richards and Gratzer 1968): cross sectional diagram of electrolytic destainer. Three gels are shown in the gel compartment (b) composed of a perspex (lucite) frame bounded by two sheets of Vyon porous plastic (d). This compartment rests in a holder made of two further perspex frames (a) joined along their bottom and sides. The gel compartment and the porous plastic are held in the holder by a fourth removable perspex frame (c). The holder fits tightly into a perspex tank (e) and thus separates the two buffer compartments (g), which are normally filled with 10% acetic acid. The potential is applied through two $\frac{1}{4}$ in carbon rods (f) which are mounted in the tank through rubber grommets.

with electrodes of large area on either side (Fig. 7.16). For flat gels a good apparatus is available from Gradipore, in which 5% acetic acid is circulated by means of a pump, through cotton pellets which absorb the dye and are replaced when saturated. The danger in electrophoretic destaining is that the dye will be removed from the RNA zones as well as the background, and it is therefore important not to use too high a voltage. Patience at this stage is advised.

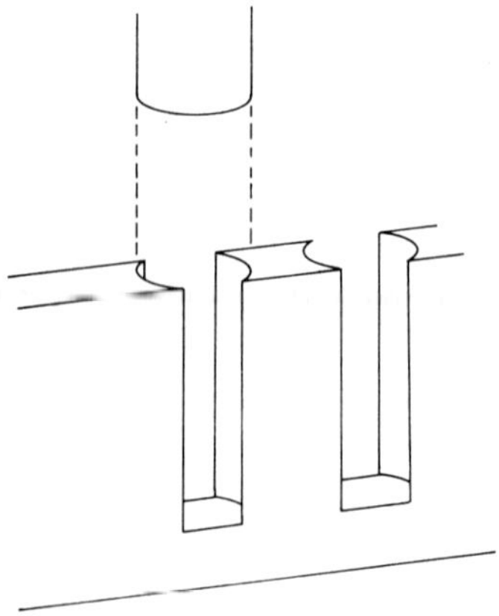

Fig. 7.16. An alternative design for a destainer. The cylindrical holes contain the gels, the sides of which are left exposed. This frame is placed in a vessel containing destaining solution, with an electrode on either side (B. Tiplady, personal communication).

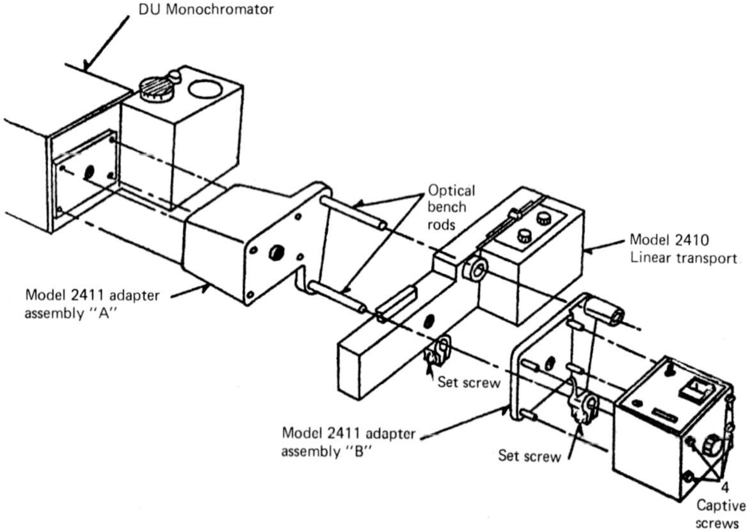

Fig. 7.17. The Gilford gel scanning attachment for spectrophotometer. The gel (cylindrical) is seated horizontally in a rectangular silica tray, which is driven across the beam in the linear transport assembly (by courtesy Gilford Instrument Co.).

7.5.3.2. Densitometry

Many densitometers are available, the best ones for the present purpose operating on monochromatic light. Instruments, such as the many designed for scanning of X-ray diffraction patterns or spectrographic plates (best known amongst which is the Joyce–Loebl microdensitometer), use white light, or at best a broad band glass filter, and these must in principle give rise to erroneous results, for the unabsorbed part of the light, outside the absorption band of the dye, will appear as an apparently too high transmittance of the sample. Ideally in such an instrument, which operates by null-balance with an optical wedge, a wedge with the same spectral characteristics as the zones should be used, and can in fact be constructed to a good approximation. Such problems are obviated, however, if an instrument based on a monochromator is used, such as the Gilford 222 photometer fitted with the Model 2410-S Linear Transport System and 2411 Adaptor (Fig. 7.17), or the Unicam SP1800 double-beam spectrophotometer with an excellent scanning accessory. There are a number of other desirable characteristics of a densitometer for gels: a deep focus helps to sample the whole depth of a zone; the gel should be fairly near the detector to minimise scattering losses; and the stray light characteristics of the monochromator should be good enough to make it possible to cover a wide range of absorbances. Clearly the width of the slit image at the gel should be narrow enough to resolve close-lying zones.

The zones as recorded (if on an absorbance, rather than a transmittance basis) can be quantitated by measuring the area under the peaks by planimetry, triangulation, cutting out and weighing or simply counting squares; or the densitometer may have an integrating facility.

Many home-made and other commercial instruments have been constructed. Excellent results in the ultraviolet and visible have been obtained with an instrument designed and described by Tsanev and Staynov (1964) and Staynov and Stainov (1969).

The gel may be laid on a silica plate (or glass for visible scanning), or it may, as in the Gilford design, be confined in a narrow silica cell with flat walls. This is narrower than the gel which is compressed when introduced, and so does not present a curved gel surface to the beam. This is advantageous in that it minimises both adventitious lens effects due to curvature, and errors due to surface aberrations. In favourable conditions, and with a good monochromator, linearity of optical response up to an absorbance of 3 can be achieved. A number of cheaper densitometers utilising filters in place of monochromatic light are available. The Joyce–Loebl 'Chromoscan' has been fairly widely used. This and the larger Joyce–Loebl microdensitometer employ optical wedges to balance the sample absorbance. A glass filter can (and should) also be inserted so as to limit the wavelength-sensitivity. The use of an optical wedge with the absorption spectrum of the RNA-dye complex in such an instrument has been alluded to (Staynov, personal communication, has constructed such wedges by making up a dye-RNA solution with agarose and letting the gel set in a wedge-shaped container. The gel is then dried down on a glass plate). For any given densitometer and experimental circumstances, where the quantitation of the relative amounts of RNA (by staining intensity) is required, it should be stressed that it is prudent to check the linearity of the measured absorbance with RNA concentration, using known concentration increments of nucleic acid. The procedures for reducing the ultraviolet background of polyacrylamide gels to increase sensitivity for ultraviolet measurements are dealt with in § 8.2.1.

7.5.3.3. Recording and storage

Instead of densitometric evaluation gels may readily be photographed by transmitted light. The simplest method is to make contact photographs, by placing the gel on a suitable photographic plate, and exposing it to light. This is not however always satisfactory, especially for cylindrical gels, and more versatile procedures are described in the experimental section (§ 8.3.1.4).

The gels can be stored indefinitely in dilute acetic acid; cylindrical gels can be sealed into Perspex boxes of dimensions just sufficient to hold all the gels from a run, using chloroform, or a solution of

Perspex in chloroform to make the boxes watertight. Another convenient storage procedure is to put the gels in their dilute acetic acid wash into small flat-bottomed tubes (e.g. sample storage sets made by R. P. Cargille Laboratories, Inc.), and store them in the accompanying boxes which have an indexing list. Alternatively, the gels can be allowed to dry in air, when they become small, hard and transparent, the size of matchsticks. The zones are visible in such dried gels, but the gels can also be re-hydrated by immersing in water. An advantage of agar or agarose gels is that after drying on a glass plate they can be detached as a tough pliable film, ideal for densitometry, photography and storage. Unstained gels can be illuminated by an ultraviolet lamp (Woods glass filter) and if placed over a sheet of white paper the RNA components become clearly visible as dark zones on the yellow fluorescent background from the paper. The RNA does not diffuse during drying, and is suitable for all manner of spectroscopic studies.

7.5.3.4. Radioactivity

Where radioactive components are being fractionated, there are two ways of recording the radioactivity of separated components in a gel. These are autoradiography and extraction followed by counting. The label may be tritium, carbon or phosphorus isotopes. The direct counting method is in many respects preferable to autoradiography. It is more suitable for tritium, is generally quicker to give results (except for a very high level of radioactivity), and is quantitative. A prerequisite is an efficient and accurate means of slicing the gels. Several good designs of gel slicers exist. The gel may either be sectioned with a row of blades or wires all at once, or it may be dealt with by a device of the bacon-slicer principle. Alternatively the gel macerator can be used in which the acrylamide is forced through a small orifice and pulped as it goes. Before transfer to the scintillation vials the RNA can be extracted by diffusion, alternatively the gel may be dissolved by chemical brute force, or more gently if a hydrolysable cross-linking reagent is used in its preparation. For plaque counting, the gel slices can be simply dried onto paper.

Autoradiography is rapid and simple with ^{32}P, less so with the other available radioisotopes. Highly efficient techniques have been developed for use in sequencing, though these always demand strong labelling with ^{32}P. Flat gels give best results in autoradiography, but cylindrical gels can be sliced longitudinally to give flat strips. Practical details for the exploitation of a selection of the more widely interesting methods are given in § 8.3.1.5.

7.5.4. Gel composition

As already noted (§ 7.4) there are some empirical and semi-empirical guidelines to the choice of gel concentrations and composition. The concentration of bisacrylamide giving mechanically tractable gels is given by Eq. 7.1 (§ 7.8), though a fixed concentration of 5% of the total acylamide is used by many workers, as in the mixture Cyanogum 41. Gels of very high concentration are stiff and very difficult to remove from the tubes, and fragment easily. The practical higher limit is probably 25–30%. At the opposite extreme, gels of less than about 3% acrylamide are soft, and almost fluid below, perhaps, 2.2%. To obtain a gel of equivalent pore size which is more manageable, one may choose a somewhat lower concentration of acrylamide and raise the proportion of *bis*acrylamide, within limits (but see below). Peacock and Dingman (1968) introduced the addition of agarose (say 0.5%) as a mechanical stiffener where it is desired to operate at still lower acrylamide concentration. It may then of course be asked what advantage remains over agarose alone, which, as we have observed, gives excellent results in the high-molecular weight range, considering especially the greater effort involved in setting up an experiment (since the agarose has to be dissolved separately and maintained at a narrowly defined temperature for mixing with the acrylamide and other components). The chief advantage does appear to be great flexibility in the selection of effective pore size. Moreover at, say, 3% acrylamide which has a smaller pore size than agarose gels, the addition of agarose is still helpful if the gel is to be sectioned or sliced since these operations are very difficult with soft gels.

The effect of acrylamide concentration on the gel characteristics must be considered, and is capable of theoretical analysis. Richards and Temple (1971) have considered in terms of the theory of rubbery elasticity the concentration-dependent properties of polyacrylamide gels. They introduce the concept of an ideal gel, defined by the relative values of the total monomer concentration T_0, and that of the cross-linker C. When $T > T_0$, where T_0 is the value of T for an ideal gel, one has a 'crumpled gel', in which there is too much acrylamide, so that the polymer molecules are less extended than they would be in the unperturbed free solution state. Conversely, when $T < T_0$, there is not enough acrylamide polymer to link the ends of the *bis* molecules to polyacrylamide neighbours in the solution. This is a 'clustered gel', and if the polyacrylamide strands are not to be stretched beyond their normal solution end-to-end distance into extended chains, rather than coils, there must be clustering of molecules. A crumpled gel if soaked in water will reach equilibrium ($T = T_0$), corresponding to the natural extension of polyacrylamide chains, by swelling, as is commonly observed in practice, when cylindrical gels are removed from the tube and soaked in staining and clearing solutions. Clustered gels will not swell and will have the characteristic property of turbidity, brought about by a non-uniform distribution of matrix molecules (clustering). This too has been often remarked on, in relation to gels of low acrylamide concentration. Richards and Temple show that gels which swell are not turbid, and turbid gels do not swell. In practice they confirm that the constant proportion of 5% bisacrylamide (as in Cyanogum 41) leads to satisfactory gels over a wide range of concentration.

In agar and agarose, where there are no covalent cross-links, highly clustered gels do not form. At the same time the pore size for 0.5% or even higher concentrations is large, satisfactory for example for electrophoresis of ribosomal RNA (Tsanev et al. 1969). The upper limit of manageability on the other hand is about 5%, so that gels of agar or agarose cannot be used to separate species of low-molecular weight. They are however convenient for high-molecular weight molecules because of their good mechanical properties, and optical characteristics. Most workers use approximately the acrylamide concentrations shown in Table 7.1 for different molecular weight ranges of RNA (the concentration is rarely critical since gels of all concentrations separate nucleic acids over a wide molecular weight range as illustrated for example in Fig. 7.4b). Nevertheless a change of gel concentration can reveal heterogeneity not otherwise obvious. Advantage can be taken of this effect on two-dimensional gels. Fig. 7.13 shows another approach: slices are cut from a 10% gel and subjected to re-electrophoresis at higher concentration and zones are then resolved which are not visible in the first dimension alone.

TABLE 7.1

Acrylamide concentration appropriate to different molecular-weight ranges of RNA for satisfactory electrophoretic separations.

Molecular weight	Percent acrylamide
Oligomers–10,000	15–20
10,000–50,000	10
50,000–200,000	5
200,000–2,000,000	2.2–3

7.5.5. Choice of buffer

Since, as we have indicated, there is in general little to be gained by the use of complex discontinuous buffer systems, almost any buffer functioning between about *p*H 5 and 9 can be used. Not all buffers give equivalent results however, for there are without doubt interactions between the nucleic acids and the counterions, which in some degree influence the patterns that are obtained. Some scope also exists in the choice of ionic strength. This can be varied within quite wide limits. Low ionic strength (as well as buffer ions of low mobility, such as Tris and similar large organic ions) makes for a large voltage drop across the tubes at a low current; this will minimise heating, and be favourable for rapid separations. Note that the voltage drop across the buffer compartments can also be appreciable under such circumstances, and it should not be assumed that all the applied potential is dropped across the tubes, as would to a first approximation be true in more concentrated buffers). The obverse of these advantages is that the buffering capacity is low, and changes in *p*H, with migration of ion fronts due to electrode products into the gels, will occur the more readily. Irrespective of concentration, it is desirable to operate at a *p*H giving maximum buffering capacity for the buffer in question.

For reasons that are not entirely apparent, slow runs at high ionic strengths often lead to better separations, a particularly striking example being in the separation of $d(AT)_n$ oligomers by Elson and Jovin (1969), discussed in § 9.2.2.

It would be generally considered ill-advised to use a *p*H at either extreme for, in both acid and alkali, slow hydrolysis of the phosphodiester chain must be anticipated, and especially in acid, depurination will also occur. It may be noted however that by entering the *p*H range of ionisation of bases the possibility arises of creating differences in charge:mass ratio between different species, depending on their composition, which could in principle form the basis of otherwise impossible separations. This strategy has only recently been attempted, and has met with some success, especially when used in conjunction with a conventional *p*H in two-dimensional electrophoresis (Fig. 7.14b). Composition-dependent change of charge due to partial ionisation of bases supposedly leads also to fractionation in gel isoelectric focussing (Drysdale and Righetti 1972). Of course the true isoelectric point of a nucleic acid would be at very low *p*H, since to reach it a proportion of the backbone phosphate groups would have to become protonated. The basis of the effects seen in the 'Ampholine'-containing systems is therefore uncertain, and very possibly involves the formation of complexes between the RNA and the polyampholytes, rather than a result of the *p*H gradient *per se*.

A further restriction arises when it is required to scan gels directly in the ultraviolet, for then buffers with absorption in this region may not be used. The most common example of such buffers are barbiturate derivatives. It may also be noted that some buffers may liberate particularly damaging, noxious and even toxic gaseous products at the electrodes: one such is cacodylate, from which free cacodyl appears to form.

Buffers which have been widely employed are Tris acetate, *p*H 7.8 and Tris phosphate, *p*H 7.7 (Loening 1968). (Tris hydrochloride should be avoided because of hypochlorite formation at the anode.) Buffers may be made up as concentrated stock solutions and mixed in the correct proportions with acrylamide, agarose, initiator and catalyst.

7.6. Gel electrophoresis and conformation of nucleic acids

7.6.1. Homology and variability in RNA conformation

The use of electrophoretic mobility as a measure of molecular weight is predicated on the assumption that all molecular species involved, both the calibration standards and the unknown, form part of a hydrodynamically homologous series. Such a situation appears to have been substantially achieved for proteins complexed with the detergent SDS (Reynolds and Tanford 1970a): the weight ratio of SDS: protein is a constant for nearly all proteins, and according to the data of Reynolds and Tanford (1970b) the particles of complex can be regarded as ellipsoids in which the minor axis is constant, and the major axis increases smoothly with molecular weight. Thus the retardation by a polyacrylamide gel, that is to say, the mobility, depends only on the molecular weight. A similar result could be achieved in nucleic acids, since the charge:mass ratio is always essentially constant, if conformational differences could be eliminated. That significant frictional differences exist between different RNA species (excluding even the self-evidently different double-stranded molecules that behave more or less as rods) and are reflected in electrophoretic mobility anomalies, is obvious from the results of several workers, in particular Loening (1969) who found that not all RNAs adhered to the same molecular weight calibration, and that their apparent molecular weights interpolated from such calibration changed significantly with ionic strength. Subsequently Groot et al.

(1970) and Grivell et al. (1971) showed that when attempts were made to measure the molecular weight of mitochondrial RNAs by their electrophoretic mobility relative to a calibration set of cytoplasmic ribosomal species, a change in the running temperature from 2° to 28°C led to a 40% increase in the apparent molecular weight. Similar effects were observed in the agarose-acrylamide mixed system by Fisher and Dingman (1971). This must be presumed to be a consequence of a greater temperature effect on the hydrodynamic coil characteristics of mitochondrial than of cytoplasmic RNA, because of differences in the extent and/or stability of their secondary structure. At the other extreme, attempts to use the gel method to measure the molecular weights of temperature-insensitive unpaired species, such as the poly(rA) tracts at the ends of messenger RNAs, would be grossly in error in the opposite sense if the usual RNA mixtures were used for calibration purposes.

Thus, although the electrophoretic mobility in aqueous solvents should always give at least a reasonable rough estimate of molecular weight, and in most cases a fairly accurate value, several workers realised that a more reliable approach would be to eliminate conformational differences by destruction of base-pairing and so reduce all polynucleotide chains to something approaching hydrodynamic homologues. It has of course to be remembered that even a chain devoid of base-pairing is not entirely structureless, since it retains the non-cooperative local stacking interactions between adjoining bases. The work of Eisenberg and Felsenfeld (1967) has clearly shown however that the frictional properties of a single-stranded chain are not greatly affected by stacking until this approaches completion at low temperature, when rod-like behaviour supervenes. Indeed it has been found that fractions of the highly stacked poly(rA) and the totally unstacked poly(rU) fall on the same mobility–molecular weight calibration in aqueous gels at room temperature (Pinder and Gratzer 1974). Thus, within the precision of gel electrophoresis experiments, we are entitled to disregard factors of single-strand stacking, as well as composition-dependent differences in coil flexibility, solvation or counterion fixation.

7.6.2. Electrophoresis in denaturing media

An attempt to destroy all base-pairing in RNA by treatment with formaldehyde was made by Boedtker (1971). This appeared to give good results but the apparent promise has not been borne out (Staynov et al. 1972; Boedtker, personal communication) apparently because of partial reversal of the reaction of the formaldehyde with the bases when the reaction mixture is cooled down to the running conditions. Aberrations may also result from the formation of covalent cross-links by this reagent. Reagents such as 8 M urea have also been used to destroy secondary structure, but at neutral *p*H and room temperature this may not be sufficiently powerful. De Wachter and Fiers (1972) have used 8 M urea in acid solution as a denaturant for RNA in two-dimensional work. This is probably effective, and indeed extremes of *p*H are in themselves sufficient to break down base-pairs, but in these conditions there are also composition-dependent changes in net charge due to ionisation of the bases. Neutral 8 M urea at elevated temperatures has also been tried (Reijnders et al. 1973) but the procedure is cumbersome and difficult, and produces zones of poor quality.

An apparently successful method, which has a number of advantages, and seems to allow unequivocal determination of molecular weights with considerable accuracy was developed by Staynov et al. (1972), and consists in running gels in the non-aqueous solvent, formamide. In this medium both base-pairing and single-stranded stacking are eliminated and electrophoretic separations of high quality are obtained, often, in our hands, better than in aqueous systems. Because of the chemical characteristics of formamide which is an ionising solvent, high activities of hydrogen or hydroxyl ions must be avoided and ionic impurities must first be removed from the solvent by ion-exchange. Formamide thus treated will serve as a medium for polymerisation of the acrylamide, and the gels can therefore be prepared directly in this solvent. Despite the hygroscopic nature of the formamide it does not appear necessary to use formamide rather than water in the reservoirs. In the original formulation of Staynov et al. the supporting electrolyte was sodium chloride with no buffer, and external electrodes were used to maintain neutrality and guard against contamination with electrode products. Subsequently the system was redesigned, barbital being used as a buffer. It should be noted that the efficacy of a buffer in a non-aqueous solvent cannot be inferred from its behaviour in water, and that its titration curve must be determined in formamide to establish appropriate conditions for its use.

The molecular weight-mobility relations shown in Fig. 7.18 indicate that all RNA species do indeed behave as homologues in formamide. Most strikingly, poly(rA) and poly(rU) fractions conform to the same law. Two-stranded viral RNAs do not necessarily melt spontaneously at room temperature, but remain in the fully melted state after heating to 40 or 50°C (Pinder et al. 1974a). The formamide method has been successfully used for molecular-weight determination of such species (Bevan et al. 1973).

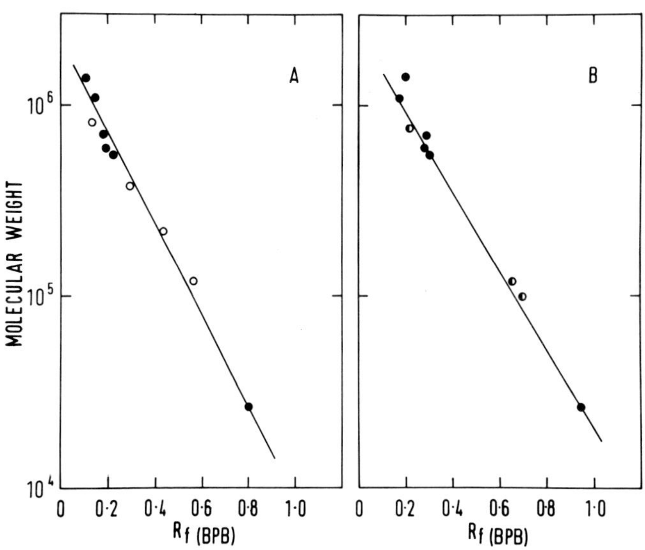

Fig. 7.18. Molecular weight-mobility relationships for a series of RNA species (●) polyriboadenylic acid fractions (○) and polyribouridylic acid fractions (◐) in formamide gels (Pinder, Staynov and Gratzer).

Subject index p. 487

It seems likely that both the accuracy and precision of formamide gel electrophoresis as a method for determination of molecular weights is limited by the uncertainty in the molecular weights of RNA standards (Duesberg and Vogt 1973; Pinder et al. 1974b). With the advent of improvements in ultracentrifuge technique, and particularly a recent method of determination of partial specific volumes (published values of which are startlingly varied), it may be hoped that enough definitive standards will soon become available to cover the entire molecular-weight range, and allow a more exact evaluation of the limits of accuracy of formamide gel electrophoresis. For characteristics of RNA in formamide and a demonstration of its denaturing efficacy, reference should be made to the work of Pinder et al. (1974a). It may be noted that the ultraviolet transparency of good quality formamide allows the scanning of gels directly at 280 nm, but the absorbance rises rapidly below 265–270 nm, and the medium is effectively opaque at 260 nm.

7.6.3. Double-helical nucleic acids

Takahashi et al. (1969) showed that native high-molecular weight DNA was capable of migrating electrophoretically in agarose gels, and that the mobility was related to the molecular weight in much the same way as for single-stranded RNA species. Given the availability of suitable molecular-weight standards, this seems therefore to offer at once a means of analytical fractionation and molecular weight determination for native DNA. Later Zeiger et al. (1972) showed that DNA would migrate in 2.5% composite polyacrylamide-agarose gels, but that in this medium the mobility was more or less independent of molecular weight, though there was a marked dependence on base composition. That molecules in the 10^7 molecular weight range should migrate at all in such a medium is in itself remarkable, for they have contour lengths many times the effective pore size, which is in the range of only a few nm (Fawcett and Morris 1966). As to the molecular weight dependence of mobility, it soon transpired that this depended on the size range of the molecules under study.

The first systematic study of double-stranded RNA was that of Shatkin et al. (1968) who examined reovirus RNA on 2.5 and 5% polyacrylamide gels, and resolved ten bands, which, based on calibrations by sedimentation analysis, spanned the molecular-weight range $0.8–7.5 \times 10^6$. In both gel concentrations these components evinced a log-linear molecular weight-mobility relationship. Using these same calibrated reovirus RNA components, Wood and Streissle (1970) found that eight double-stranded RNA species present in wound tumour virus lay with great precision on the same calibration line. Similar data were obtained for a set of two-stranded viral RNAs by Kawata et al. (1970). The absence of a molecular-weight dependence in the mobility of DNA relates only to molecules of very high molecular weight, and can then be circumvented by irreversible denaturation: Hayward and Smith (1973) working with phage DNAs of $2–30 \times 10^6$ molecular weight per strand found that, whereas no fractionation occurred when the native molecules were run, prior denaturation in alkali gave rise to single strands, which could be well separated and yielded excellent molecular weight calibrations – notably better in fact than obtained for a wide range of single-stranded RNA species. With two-stranded DNA the log (molecular weight) *vs* R_f relation is a smooth concave curve (a good example occurs in the work of Danna et al. (1973) on fragments of SV40 DNA), or in the conditions of other workers (Pettersson et al. 1973), a straight line which curves steeply upward in a critical molecular weight range. Up to a molecular weight of about $1–2 \times 10^6$ there is good resolution, and the calibration curve is satisfactory for molecular weight determination, but above this the curvature increases rapidly and resolution vanishes, even though in a gel of sufficiently low concentration the molecules still migrate well enough. Some further unusual features in the electrophoresis of two-stranded species were brought to light by Fisher and Dingman (1971). In the first place, at molecular weights above a critical region, near 4×10^5, the rate of migration, by contrast with that of the corresponding single-stranded species, became essentially independent of gel concentration over a wide range (at least 1–3% total gel concentration

Subject index p. 487

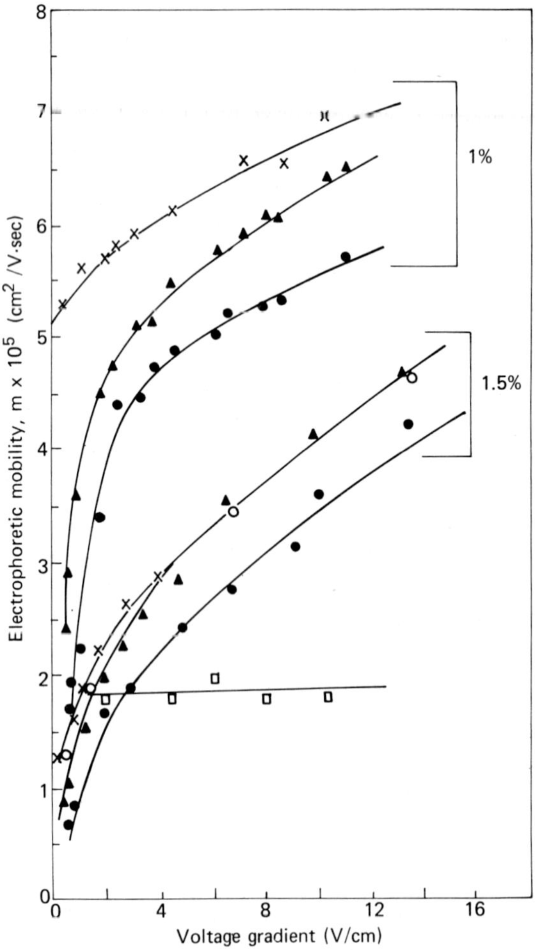

Fig. 7.19. Dependence of electrophoretic mobility of native DNA on the applied voltage in polyacrylamide-agarose composite gels, of the indicated acrylamide concentrations. The samples are T2 (●), T1 (▲) and PBSX (×) DNA, and fragments of T2 (○) and T1 (□) DNA (Lishanskaya and Mosevitsky 1973).

in mixed polyacrylamide-agarose gels). Secondly, the relative mobilities show a marked dependence on the voltage (Lishanskaya and Mosevitsky 1973). These effects are shown in Fig. 7.19 reflecting the way in which this remarkable effect of gel concentration acts in only at a sharply defined value of the molecular weight. The retardation coefficient, K_R merely expresses the slope of the mobility-gel concentration plot, ie. $\log M = \log M_0 - K_R T$, where T is the total gel concentration and $\log M_0$ the intercept on the ordinate.

The only obvious explanations of these effects is that the native DNA migrates by virtue of orientation along the direction of the potential gradient, and in effect threads its way through the interstices of the gel. The anomalously low retardation in the electrophoretic gels stands in dramatic contrast to the exclusion of similar molecules from molecular sieves in chromatography. The degree of orientation is evidently governed by the magnitude of the voltage gradient, i.e. the orienting force up to some limit, dependent, no doubt, on the rate of rotational relaxation (cf. orientation by flow or electrostatic fields). Moreover at a molecular weight above the critical limit, it is not surprising that the gel concentration has little effect on the mobility, if this really depends only on the ability of the molecule to orient. The dependence of mobility on composition could be related to the degree of flexibility of native DNA (which is generally taken to have a segment length of about 200 Å), or on the helix dimensions, which, it has been averred, vary with composition (Bram 1971).

According to Dingman et al. (1972b) conditions of voltage gradient and gel concentration can be found (specified in their paper), in which double-stranded species, be they DNA or RNA, in the molecular-weight range $0.02–2 \times 10^6$ fall on the same mobility calibration as single-stranded (i.e. partly paired RNAs), whereas denatured single strands derived from the two-stranded molecules lie on a different curve, most probably because of a low content of the type of internal complementarity that is evidently built into most naturally single-stranded RNAs. The coincidence of the calibrations for the single and double-stranded species has no significance in itself, but is only a chance event for a particular gel concentration, as will be seen. It is not surprising that in staining with a metachromatic dye (in this case 'Stains-All') the response of single and double-stranded species is different (Dingman et al. 1970). By densitometric scanning at two wavelengths (corresponding presumably to the aggregated and unaggregated forms of the bound dye), it is possible in principle to distinguish between the two types of conformation. A similar observation, with a visually detectable difference in colour is reported for toluidine blue by Bevan et al. (1973).

The conformation dependence of the mobilities of nucleic acids in polyacrylamide gels has been taken a stage further by Dingman et al. (1972a), who have looked also into the effects of cyclic structure. They find that circular single-stranded DNA (which, as has been shown theoretically and experimentally, has a markedly lower frictional coefficient than linear) can be separated from linear DNA of the same molecular weight. Moreover circular duplexes may similarly be resolved from linear duplexes of the same molecular weight. (Why circular duplexes migrate at all is not clear in terms of the orientation concept. It is of course possible that the molecule assumes a compact disymmetric form, double helices lying parallel to the long axis, which again is able to penetrate the gel by orientation – a mechanism denied to species of random-coil like character.) Again a single-strand break in a double-helical supercoiled circular DNA, which is known to cause relaxation of the supercoil, changes the mobility sufficiently to permit separation from the intact circular form. According to Dingman et al. it is not only the linear duplex DNA, but also single-stranded linear DNA that (unlike single-stranded RNA) displays a voltage dependence of mobility (Fig. 7.19).

Aaij and Borst (1972) have also demonstrated the separation of closed circular DNA double helices from their linear counterparts in polyacrylamide gels, and have found that log-linear calibrations of molecular weight against relative mobility can be set up. A conspectus of the differences in electrophoretic behaviour between three conformational types – linear single-stranded, linear double-stranded and circular double-stranded – is available from the curve relating mobility and gel concentration obtained by Harley et al. (1973). These profiles depend strikingly on the conformation type and Harley et al. suggest that they could be used to discriminate between them. This claim would seem to be justified if the molecular weight is defined, at least within fairly broad limits. It might be rendered wholly unambiguous by comparing the mobility-gel concentration profile of the native material with that observed after alkaline denaturation (Hayward and Smith 1973), the latter form serving for molecular weight determination, relative to standards in the same state. Harley et al. find that the mobility-gel concentration curves can in all cases be faithfully represented by a second-order polynomial, the coefficients being determined by a standard least-squares curve-fitting routine, i.e. in the form $u = \mathrm{a} + \mathrm{b}T + \mathrm{c}T^2$, where u is the mobility and T the gel concentration. Examples of the characteristics profiles are shown in Figs. 7.20 and 7.21.

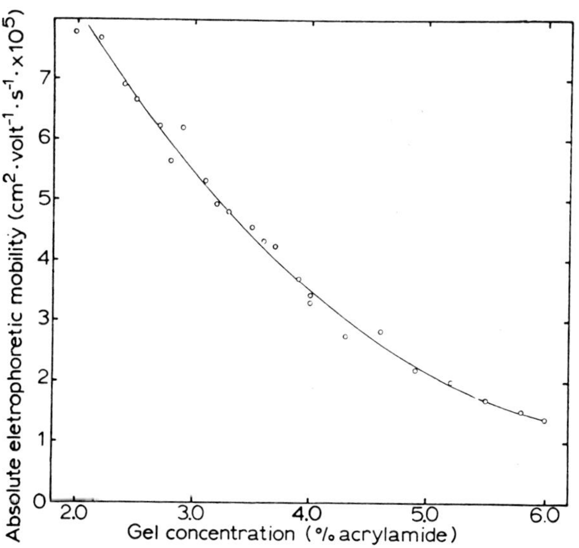

Fig. 7.20. Plot of absolute electrophoretic mobility versus gel concentration for a typical data set, derived here from 23 separate analyses of Mycophage PS_1-III, a double-stranded linear RNA. The curve represents the second-order polynomial curve derived from this data set by regression analysis.

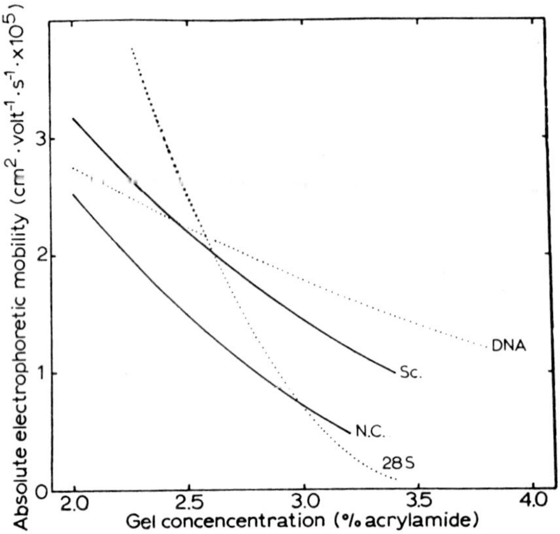

Fig. 7.21. Dependence of mobility-gel concentration profiles of DNA on conformation. Samples are supercoiled SV40 DNA (sc), nicked circular SV40 DNA (NC) and HeLa cell linear double-stranded DNA. A single-stranded species, 28 S HeLa cell ribosomal RNA is also shown (Harley et al. 1973).

To summarise the salient points: two-stranded nucleic acids migrate in gels and, up to a molecular weight of $1–3 \times 10^6$, depending somewhat on the system, can be separated by molecular weight. Above this the mobility depends appreciably on composition but hardly at all on molecular weight, regardless of gel concentration. Single and double-stranded species may be distinguished by measuring mobility as a function of gel concentration, as well as by differences in colour response to the stain. After alkaline denaturation excellent molecular weight-mobility calibrations can be obtained for all molecular weights. Different conformational forms (single and double-stranded, linear, circular and super-coiled) of identical molecular weight can all be separated by gel electrophoresis, and possibly uniquely identified. One may anticipate that some pretty applications of these basic findings will emerge in many branches of nucleic acid research.

The practice of analytical gel electrophoresis of nucleic acids

In this chapter the experimental practice of analytical polyacrylamide gel electrophoresis will be set out. Analytical methods have been evolved to operate on a scale of say 1–10 μg or 1000 counts per minute per component, though this can often be appreciably reduced. We shall not concern ourselves here with true micro-techniques, which function down to the level of the contents of a single cell in some cases, since these are of specialised interest, and have been fully dealt with in a recent and authoritative monograph on micro-methods in molecular biology (Neuhoff 1973).

Analytical polyacrylamide gel electrophoresis at the present stage of technology can be made to serve a number of useful purposes. The object may be simply to reveal polydispersity (say degradation) in a sample of RNA. The patterns obtained, however, may be analysed to yield the relative amounts, the kinetics of labelling with radioactive metabolic precursors, and a number of physical properties of the separated species, notably the molecular weights, but touch possibly also on the conformation and effective charge properties of individual nucleic acid species. Gel electrophoresis may also help in the study of molecular structure by controlled degradation or study of the mechanism of action of a nuclease, and of course it is required in the first step of sequencing operations. Selected examples of such applications will be described in ch. 10. We shall aim here to cover such aspects of the technique as are relevant to its utilisation in these various senses.

8.1. Preparation of RNA

Thorough deproteinisation of the RNA is essential for gel electrophoresis; otherwise streaking or even accumulation of material at the origin may be observed. Two procedures described by Loening (1967), and based on earlier work of Kirby and co-workers, appear to be satisfactory. The tissue homogenate containing the RNA to be extracted is first shaken at room temperature with detergent, either 0.5% sodium dodecyl sulphate and 5% sodium 4-aminosalicylate or 2–5% sodium tri*iso*propylnaphthalene-sulphonate. In the first case the suspension is shaken at 0–5°C with phenol containing 0.1% w/v 8-hydroxyquinoline, and, in the second case, the same solution with 10% *m*-cresol added. The phases are separated by centrifugation at 1000 g for 10 min and the phenol extraction of the aqueous phase is repeated once or twice. The RNA is precipitated at −20°C from the aqueous phase by the addition of 2% w/v sodium acetate and 2.5 vol of ethanol or 3% w/v NaCl and 2 vol ethanol. To remove DNA, the precipitate is dissolved in buffer (0.2 M Tris, *p*H 7.5)+1.5 M NaCl and a good quality deoxyribonuclease at 10 μg/ml is added. The solution is incubated at 5°C for 30 min, followed by the addition of sodium dodecyl sulfate and deproteinisation with phenol as above. The final RNA is reprecipitated from 0.3 M sodium acetate twice, washed once with ethanol and dried *in vacuo* before dissolving in electrophoresis buffer.

8.2. Gel components

The usual combination of components in the polymerisation mixture, and the only one for which we shall give experimental details comprises buffer salts acrylamide monomer, methylene N,N′-bisacrylamide (Bis), tetramethyl ethylenediamine (TEMED) as catalyst and ammonium persulfate as initiator. Variants are possible as mentioned in the previous chapter: other catalysts may be used and also there may in some cases be advantages in eschewing the use of the persulfate, for example, when it is important to avoid too rapid setting of the gel in the course of more than usually complex pouring operations. In such circumstances, photo-initiation by riboflavin is an entirely satisfactory alternative, though, as normally used, it appears to give rise to softer gels, presumably by initiating more, and therefore shorter, chains. Polymerisation ensues only after the solution is irradiated, most simply by a small fluorescent strip-lamp placed a few centimetres away. Details are to be found in Smith (1968). Neither ammonium persulfate nor riboflavin are satisfactory for setting gels in buffer of very low *p*H, and here Fenton's reagent can be used (Jordan and Raymond 1969).

Another variation of the above procedure is the introduction of hydrolysable cross-linkers in place of the methylene bisacrylamide, when it is desired to dissolve gel slices after the experiment to

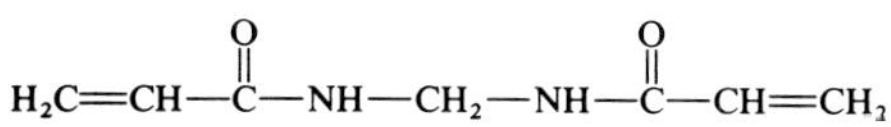

(I)

and

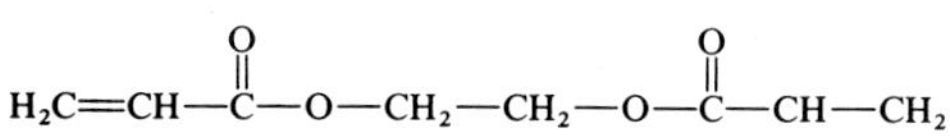

(II)

Fig. 8.1. Hydrolysable cross-linking agents. Exposure of gels prepared with these reagents as cross-linkers to mildly alkaline conditions leads to dissolution. I is diallyltartardiamide (Anker 1970) and II is ethylenediacrylate (Choules and Zimm 1965).

release the RNA, e.g. for radioactive counting. Two such have been employed, one being hydrolysable at alkaline *p*H (too high to allow any hopes that the RNA will not be to a greater or lesser extent covalently damaged) and the other in 2% periodic acid. These are, respectively, ethylenediacrylate (Choules and Zimm 1965) and N,N′-diallyltartardiamide (Anker 1970) (Fig. 8.1). They are used in the same way as Bis, but give gels of somewhat different mechanical properties. For the preparation and use of these reagents see the references cited. Both preparations are simple, but ethylene diacrylate is now available from Bordon Chemical Co.

Gels from the natural polysaccharide polymers, agar and agarose, can give good results with nucleic acids. They provide satisfactory molecular sieving in the high-molecular weight range, but are poor media for separating low-molecular weight species, since the highest manageable concentration of gel is not much greater than 4%. We have already noted, and will consider in practical terms, the use of agarose in composite gels to add mechanical rigidity to polyacrylamide of very low concentrations. Agarose is in principle better than agar, since the latter contains sulfate groups, the charge of which leads to a large and undesirable electro-osmotic flow, and the possibility of adsorption effects (Staynov 1972). Not all agarose samples gives good results; satisfactory preparations are those from BDH (British Drug Houses); L'Industrie Biologique Française, and Marine Colloids (called Scakem Agarose).

Agarose gels are transparent to ultraviolet light, so the problem of poor UV transmission is eliminated, especially in dried gels in which the scattering characteristic of the gel state, is absent. Beyond the advantages for scanning, Tsanev (personal communication) has described the use of air-dried agarose gels as a matrix for such operations as spectrophotometric titrations. The ionisation state of a species such as RNA in the gel is always that corresponding to the *p*H of the solution from which it was dried. Thus by immersion in buffers of chosen *p*H, the agarose film quickly re-equilibrates with the new *p*H. It is possible by this means to examine, for instance, intact ribosomes in *p*H ranges in which they would precipitate from free solution.

8.2.1. Purification of gel components

Some samples of acrylamide apparently contain large quantities of acrylic acid as an impurity, as well as ultraviolet-absorbing matter, which is apt to vitiate attempts at direct ultraviolet scanning. Some companies (e.g. BDH) now provide a more highly purified acrylamide, which is preferable in this respect. Loening (1967) advocates recrystallisation of both acrylamide and Bis, and this undoubtedly leads to a great improvement in the ultraviolet transparency of the gels. A less demanding, and equally effective procedure is simply to subject the gel to pre-electrophoresis (in the absence of a sample) for a sufficient time; say 2 hr, with the standard disc gel system. The reservoir buffer is then changed, and samples are applied as usual. It should be borne in mind that the problem of transparency increases with the acrylamide concentration and in low-concentration gels it is often possible to avoid any purification procedure. If desired a substantial improvement in gel transparency can be obtained by soaking the gel in buffer before use. In the case of cylindrical gels this would involve removal from the tube and subsequent replacement – an impossibly tricky operation except for dilute gels. With flat gels there is no problem.

We have found pre-electrophoresis to be in general the most satisfactory procedure. Not only do absorbing impurities, which are evidently predominately charged, migrate out of the gel but pre-electrophoresis also has the advantage of eliminating the residual ammonium persulfate, which being a strong oxidising agent, is not usually a desirable component of the system. Damage to proteins by ammonium persulfate has been reported, and one could conceive of similar effects when labile minor bases are present, for example, in a tRNA. In discontinuous buffer systems pre-electrophoresis might present problems.

The procedure for recrystallisation of monomers follows Loening (1967). 70 g acrylamide are dissolved in 1 l chloroform at 50°C. The solution is filtered hot without suction. Crystals separate at −20°C and may be recovered by filtration, washed with chilled chloroform, heptane or both, and dried in air.

10 g of N,N′-methylene bisacrylamide is dissolved in 1 l of acetone at 40–50°C and filtered hot. The solution is slowly cooled to −20°C, and the crystals are washed with cold acetone either by centrifugation or filtration.

Because both acrylamide and Bis are highly neurotoxic the hot filtrations should be performed in a fume chamber. Care should be taken to avoid skin contact, inhalation of light crystals or ingestion (e.g. by pipetting of monomer solutions). The catalysts TEMED and DMAEC are likewise very poisonous and additional care must be taken to prevent evaporation into the atmosphere, since they are

Subject index p. 487

volatile. Once polymerisation is complete it is supposed to be safe to handle the gels.

8.3. Procedures for cylindrical gel electrophoresis

8.3.1. Aqueous polyacrylamide gels

8.3.1.1. Preparation for electrophoresis

Preparing the sample Nucleic acids should be in the concentration range 0.01–1 mg/ml and the total loading for analytical purposes is generally of the order of 0.5 μg RNA species. Gels can be overloaded in order to focus attention on minor components sufficiently separated from the bulk material, when the gross spreading of the major zones is of no consequence. In general, however, one should aim to use close to the minimum sample size capable of detection. One of the commonest mistakes of novitiates to the method is to overload the gels. Richards and Lecanidou (1971) have shown that deterioration of resolution occurs in their standard conditions if loads greater than 0.5 μg of a single RNA species are employed in tubes of 0.475×7.5 cm. Minimisation of load *volume* is not, as we have noted (§ 7.5) important: Richards and Lecanidou (1971) have shown that resolution is maintained with a sample column of up to 1 cm in tubes of 6 mm i.d.

Into some or all the samples in a run a trace of bromophenol blue is introduced as a marker. Since the best way of applying the sample is by a layer which will remain under the buffer without mixing, sucrose (or glycerol) is added to a concentration of about 5%. Most conveniently 1 tenth of a sample volume of 50% sucrose + 0.002% bromophenol blue is added to the sample before application to the gel. Relatively strong zones can also be observed directly during migration by addition of a little stain, such as pyronine Y or acridine orange, but inasmuch as this may cause differential perturbations of mobilities this is probably not advisable in any but fully defined systems. For additional sensitivity acridine orange-stained zones can be observed by illumination with light from an ultraviolet lamp (Woods glass filter).

Nucleic acids may be protected from the ubiquitous nucleases in a number of ways. The inclusion of small amounts of bentonite (e.g. 100 μg) is not detrimental if firm gels are used. However, in the absence of agarose, with dilute gels, e.g. 2.4% acrylamide both the gels near the origin and the resulting RNA patterns can be deformed by the bentonite which is particulate and negatively charged. Nucleases can be inhibited also by including sodium dodecyl sulfate (0.1%) in the sample, gel and reservoir buffers, but the detergent must be thoroughly removed by soaking the gel after the run if the usual stains for RNA are to be used, since it interacts with and precipitates the dye. In practice it is difficult to obtain clear and colourless backgrounds, even after extensive soaking of the gel prior to staining. Sodium dodecyl sulfate is transparent in the ultraviolet and therefore does not interfere with ultraviolet scanning of nucleic acids. Hence it is preferable to monitor the distribution of nucleic acids in gels containing SDS by this method rather than by staining with the usual dyes.

Detection of a few tenths of a microgram of nucleic acid is possible if it is contained within a single narrow sharp zone in a cylindrical gel of 6 mm diameter cross section, using e.g. methylene or toluidine blue as stains. For adequate signal/noise ratio in ultraviolet densitometry (e.g. in the Gilford instrument) a minimum of approximately 0.1 μg RNA in each zone is desirable. Larger amounts allow the use of a lower instrument gain, however, and less noisy traces are obtained. If it is required only to observe the distribution of radioactivity with highly radioactive materials, as is often the case in sequencing operations, 'invisible' amounts of labelled RNA may be run. In this case very often carrier RNA is added to the sample at an earlier stage (e.g. before digestion) to assist precipitation; the concentration of carrier must be sufficiently low to keep resolution in the optimal range.

The sample may be dissolved in diluted electrophoresis buffer or in water so that, being in a medium of lower conductivity than the gel, it experiences a high field and is rapidly accelerated to form a sharp layer at the gel interface. The bromophenol blue marker runs in front of all but the smallest oligonucleotides at neutral *p*H and so serves to indicate the progress of the run. The mobilities of RNA species relative to bromophenol blue are commonly reported. The diffuseness of the bromophenol after it has migrated 2/3 or 3/4 of the length of the gel is an unfortunate aspect of this procedure for comparing samples run in different gels. An RNA marker (e.g. tRNA) provides greater accuracy in determinations of relative mobility (R_f). During staining some swelling of the gel may occur. Bromophenol blue distance is measured before staining (in the course of which it diffuses out of the gel), whereas the RNA distance is measured after staining. Thus measurement of the total gel length before and after staining and correction for swelling is necessary for accurate determination of R_f relative to this marker.

For the precise location of trace amounts of radioactive RNA fragments in gels, De Wachter and Fiers (1971) advocate employing a dye mixture. R_f values of the individual dyes in several buffer systems have been published by these authors (Table 8.1).

Setting up the tubes Where cylindrical gels are used it is important that tubes should be scrupulously clean. It is recommended that after each run glass tubes should be soaked in chromic acid. They should then be scrubbed with a test-tube brush and detergent, rinsed and carefully dried with ethanol or in an oven.

Permanently siliconised tubes (prepared by dipping glass tubes in a 5% solution of dimethyldichlorosilane in chloroform) are said to facilitate cleaning as well as the removal of gels from the tubes immediately after electrophoresis (Smith 1968). Loening has advocated the use of Perspex tubes, as acrylamide gel adheres less firmly to Perspex than to glass. Adherence to glass is a problem with both very concentrated and very dilute gels which are apt to disintegrate during removal.

To set the tubes up for pouring gels, their ends must first be sealed, and they must be mounted vertically. For sealing, two small squares of parafilm may be separately stretched over the bottom and

TABLE 8.1

Electrophoresis conditions and migration distances in vertical slab gels (De Wachter and Fiers 1971).

Gel type[a]	1	2	3	4
Conditions				
Voltage[b] (V)	250	400	500	600
Current[c] (mA)	20	30	25	15
Time (hr)	16	16	18	18
Migration distance (cm)				
Trypan red	—	6.0	3.2	—
Xylene cyanol FF	—	13.0	7.6	20.0
Eosin	—	18.5	10.2	—
Bromophenol blue	31.0	23.0	13.5	—
Bromocresol purple	—	27.0	16.4	—
Fluorescein	—	32.0	20.5	—
Bacteriophage MS2 RNA	9.4	—	—	—
23 S ribosomal RNA (*E. coli*)	10.8	—	—	—
16 S ribosomal RNA (*E. coli*)	15.5	—	—	—
Transfer RNA (yeast)	32.5	13.8	4.5	—
Mononucleotides	Run off	35	28	—

[a] For the composition of the gels, see Table 8.2 (page 394).

[b] Voltage measured between the electrodes. The actual voltage on the gel is about 80% of this because of the resistance of the wick.

[c] Approximate current measured for a 2 mm gel.

twisted around the side of the tube. Plastic caps or rubber bungs may also be used, but the latter introduce a small cavity at the end of the gel, in which an air bubble is easily entrapped. If a ring of plastic tubing is inserted some distance into the bottom of the tube, it may then be closed off with a small glass rod. The removal of the bottom seal requires care, to avoid creating a vacuum which can damage the gel. Tubes are mounted vertically, most simply in a rack in which they are secured, either at the bottom, or near the top by pushing them through a hole in a stiff sheet of rubber or plastic.

will take longer to polymerise. Polymerisation is always attended by formation of a fine refractile boundary *almost* at the surface of the column. Elson and Jovin (1969) report the use of *iso*butanol for layering 20% polyacrylamide gels. The *iso*butanol must be removed soon after setting, otherwise it will dehydrate the gel.

Most of these difficulties can be eliminated and near-perfect interfaces between gel and buffer achieved, by the following procedure, recommended by Richards and Lecanidou (1971): the tubes are filled with acrylamide solution to a level about 1 cm above the mark corresponding to the required top of the gel, and overlayered with buffer. A hypodermic needle of the required length is fitted to a syringe and introduced vertically so that the syringe rests on the rim of the tube. The length of the needle should be such that its tip reaches the level required for the top of the gel. The liquid is then carefully sucked off including the original interface. This procedure minimises mixing of the gel and buffer solutions, and creates a very sharp boundary.

Gels should set in about 20 min, although longer times must often be allowed for dilute gels, and there is a strong temperature dependence: gels in the cold room will take much longer.

Photopolymerisation in riboflavin-containing solution is induced by placing a fluorescent strip light a few centimetres from the tubes, and is accompanied by bleaching of the yellow riboflavin colour.

It is customary to make up gels immediately prior to use, but experience shows that good results can be obtained with gels stored overnight, or even for several days or weeks. Some chemical manufacturers (e.g. Universal Scientific Co., Ltd.) indeed provide ready-made flat polyacrylamide gels which may be stored in contact with their buffer.

Immediately before applying the sample, the buffer layer is poured off and the tube above the gel is dried with tissue. The tubes are then inserted into the gel electrophoresis apparatus in symmetrical positions relative to the two electrodes. The tubes are mounted so that the ends project into the two buffer reservoirs. It should be checked that the upper compartment, where the sample is applied, is the cathode, otherwise disappointment will result.

Applying the sample Samples containing sucrose and bromophenol blue are carefully layered on the tops of the gels. The region above the top of the gel should be visible (i.e. above or below the grommets holding the tubes in place), so as to avoid blind layering operations. The tube above the sample is filled with reservoir buffer. Over-layering the sample with reservoir buffer to the top of the tube can be done with a Pasteur pipette with the tip drawn out to a fine point (preferably slightly bent) or with a syringe with a needle bent at right angles (in bending a syringe needle, a thick wire is first inserted into the hole: otherwise the needle will be blocked at the bend). The buffer is gently expelled against the wall of the tube. The presence of bromophenol blue in the sample helps to detect any mixing, or one may watch that the refractive index boundary between the sample solution and buffer remains sharp. Alternatively the sample may be layered under the reservoir buffer. The sample volume is not critical, as mentioned above, but should be no larger than necessary. For gels of 0.6 cm diameter, 0.05–0.15 ml is a convenient volume, but up to 0.5 ml may be used without great deterioration of the results if the ionic strength is substantially lower in the sample than in the reservoir and gel buffers.

After filling the tubes with buffer, the upper reservoir may be filled (e.g. through a funnel with its end directed away from the tops of the tubes) without fear of disturbing the sample. If air bubbles are lodged under the gels in the lower reservoir they should be dislodged with a bent Pasteur pipette.

8.3.1.2. Electrophoresis

In discontinuous buffer systems especially (Davis 1964; Ornstein 1964), the conductivity of the gel varies through the run. For this reason constant-current power supplies are always advocated. Though the resistance always varies somewhat, probably largely while the gel warms up to its equilibrium running temperature, it is not our experience that the use of constant voltage makes any appreciable difference to the appearance of the electrophoretic patterns. In any case, the voltage should be adjusted after perhaps 15 min, and thereafter, at least until serious chemical changes due to electrolysis occur, it will remain reasonably constant (typically at 5 mA per tube, for 8, 6 mm diameter tubes in the Tris-acetate buffer described above).

8.3.1.3. After electrophoresis

Removing the gel As the concentration of acrylamide increases, gels become increasingly difficult to remove from tubes. In general it is necessary to loosen the gel from the sides of the tube, and this can be accomplished by means of a long thin hypodermic needle or a water-filled syringe, taking care not to scratch the gel. The tube is rimmed with a needle, at both ends if necessary, while water is passed through the needle. Some pressure, depending on the gel concentration, is then necessary to expel the gel from the tube. In the case of dilute gels in Perspex it may be sufficient to remove the retainer (plastic ring or gauze), which it is prudent to attach to the bottom of tubes made from this material, and allow the gel to slide out. A rubber pipetting teat filled with water may be used to encourage the process. For stronger gels, the tube can be connected via rubber tubing to a water tap and the gel forced out by gentle water pressure. This requires practice. The junction of the rubber tubing and the gel tube is held firmly with one hand, and the water pressure is controlled with the other, being turned down when the gel begins to move. Application of a rubber bulb full of water is a good alternative. The gel should not be ejected too rapidly. It tends to break especially at the point passing the end of the tube (it is important that the end of the tube be smooth) and with insufficient care, the gel may emerge explosively and disintegrate. It is advisable to eject it into a beaker of water. For very stiff gels, Johns (1967) advocates cracking the tube in a vice, and peeling away the glass. Published photographs of gels pieced together from the fragments tell their own tale. It is worth mentioning that gels of very high acrylamide concentration become more manageable if say 15% glycerol is included in the gel buffer as a plasticiser.

Staining and clearing Dyes in common use for staining nucleic acids in polyacrylamide gels are acridine orange, methylene blue, toluidine blue and pyronine Y, although perusal of the literature on histochemical stains (Conn 1946; Gurr 1962) suggests that many others might be equally suitable. Even very small oligonucleotides (containing 10 nucleotide residues or even fewer) can be stained with acridine orange (Gould et al. 1969). The actual limiting factor may be the precipitability of the RNA rather than its ability to adsorb the various dyes. This may be expected to set in around 5 nucleotides in the conditions used (e.g. 15% acetic acid).

Dahlberg et al. (1969) made use of a dye which they termed 'Stains-all' (1-ethyl-2-[3-(1-ethylnaphtho[1,2d]thiazolin-2-ylidene)-2-methylpropenyl]naphtho[1,2d]thiazolium bromide from Eastman Organic Chemicals) because it stains RNA (bluish purple), DNA (blue) and protein (red).

In the procedure as used in the authors' laboratories the gels are immersed in a 2% solution of pyronine Y (or acridine orange) in 15% acetic acid for several hours; cylindrical gels are in test tubes, flat gels in developer trays. Background dye is removed by washing the gel in 5–10% acetic acid. Other workers using methylene blue and toluidine blue (Peacock and Dingman 1967) prefer the procedure of immersing the gel first in a solution of 1 N acetic acid for 15 min to precipitate the RNA, and then in a solution of 0.2% dye in 0.04 M acetate buffer at *p*H 4.7 (equal parts of 0.4 M sodium acetate and 0.4 M acetic acid) for 1 hr. Background dye is removed by several changes of water. It is best to stop short of complete destaining when there is still a trace of free dye in the bathing medium in equilibrium with the RNA, since otherwise the stain may also be stripped from the RNA. The RNA itself does not appear to redissolve and it is usually possible to restain it with fresh dye.

Several types of apparatus for electrophoretic destaining have been devised, and two designs have been shown in Figs. 7.15 and 7.16. In the first (Richards and Gratzer, 1968) (obtainable from Shandon Scientific Co.), the gels rest in a compartment bounded by porous plastic, e.g. 1/32″ thick Vyon (obtained from Porous Plastics, Ltd.). The plastic separates the gels from the electrode compartments containing carbon rod electrodes and 5–10% acetic acid. The rods are connected across a 50 V D.C. supply which passes about 0.5 A through the membranes and the gels. It is recommended to destain pyronine Y in a cold room. The second apparatus (Fig. 7.16) is rather simpler, since apart from depositing the gels in the slots provided there are no further assembly operations.

In electrophoretic destaining dye may be removed from RNA zones; too high a voltage must be avoided, and patience exercised. In fact, many workers prefer to avoid the risk of stripping dye from zones, and simply change the destaining fluid at intervals until the background is sufficiently clear. The process can be accelerated by placing the gels into slots in a Perspex frame in a dish in which they can be covered with liquid and mounting this on a rocking table, so that a gentle agitation can be maintained, alternatively a 'fish tank' water circulator can be used.

8.3.1.4. Evaluation of non-radioactive components

Stained gels can be kept for long periods in dilute acetic acid. Storage in the cold room with a drop of chloroform added to the medium discourages the growth of mould. The gels are best examined against a background of diffuse light. For this purpose a light box (e.g. Kodak 'Cold Light' illuminator) is appropriate.

Photography Gels are mounted on a uniform source of diffuse white light, e.g. a Kodak 'Cold Light' illuminator. Flat gels are placed in a clean Perspex dish over the light and tubes containing disc gels are mounted vertically on a frame against the light box which stands upright. The gels must be immersed in storage buffer. The camera is placed at a distance permitting the gels to be brought in focus. A viewing camera has the advantages that the gels can be seen clearly, and good development of the film is facilitated by virtue of the large size of the negative. Kodak Panchromatic film is recommended for gels stained with blue dyes (methylene or toluidine blue) in conjunction with a Kodak Wratten No. 58 filter (plus a No. 22 filter for increased contrast). The films are developed with Kodak DG10 Developer (diluted 1:4) for 4 min, or for lower contrast (when zones of widely varying intensities are to be recorded), May and Baker 'Qualitol' (diluted 1:9) for 4–5 min. Similar conditions are used for direct photography of unstained RNA in gels illuminated with UV light in a dark room. Polaroid film is also adequate for the photography of blue-stained gels and for UV photography, but not for gels stained with acridine orange or pyronine Y (magenta). In the latter case Ilford Orthoset film is recommended. If the zones are faint a No. 58 Wratten filter can be used. Otherwise no filter is needed. DG-10 Developer is used as described above. A rational approach to the choice of filters is to select one, for example from the Kodak Wratten Filter manual, with a window showing maximal transmission at the absorption maximum of the nucleic acid-dye complex. However the results obtained are probably not primarily dependent on the filter and, if a very exacting photographic record is required, extensive experimentation with film and development and exposure times is generally unavoidable.

Densitometry In preparing the sample for densitometry, it is essential to ensure that it lies at the beam focus, and in the case of cylindrical gels it is generally considered advisable that a flat surface is presented to the beam to prevent error from lens effects in the gel. This is best accomplished, as in the Gilford arrangement (Fig. 7.17) by slight compression of the cylinders between the walls of a silica trough. If the zones are distorted – for example by the 'funneling' effect that occurs when there is excessive heating during electrophoresis – errors may be expected. Moreover, surface imperfections, if the gel has been damaged during removal from the tube, or bubbles, can lead to artefacts. If there is any question of whether excursions in the densitometer trace are genuine, it is prudent to repeat the densitometry at a long wavelength, outside the absorption band of the dye, at which only the surface artefacts will be recorded.

Adherence to Beer's Law over considerable ranges of RNA concentration has been reported by various authors. It should be noted that stacking dyes, such as are usually used in staining, do not of themselves obey Beer's Law. It is reasonable to expect that at saturating concentrations of dye on a nucleic acid, Beer's Law will be obeyed, but there may be some degree of dependence on the composition of the nucleic acid. It is probably advisable for anyone concerned with precise measurements of relative concentrations in gels to check that under their experimental conditions, and with their materials, Beer's Law is in fact obeyed. Finally, it should be ensured that the scan rate is such that the recorder can follow the changes in absorbance without lag. Relative concentrations are obtained by integration of the areas under the peaks, e.g. by planimetry, or less exactly by cutting out and weighing.

Dye-elution The estimation of eluted dye constitutes an alternative method of quantitation. Zones, and samples of background (i.e. gel segments containing no zones) are cut out with a razor blade or scalpel. The pieces are macerated, for example in a Potter homogeniser, with a little salt solution, saturated with urea. The debris are separated by centrifugation, and are re-extracted. The extracts are bulked and either weighed or made up to a standard volume, and their absorbance is measured in a spectrophotometer. A good procedure (if RNA is not to be recovered) depending on the chemical stability of the dye, is to extract with 0.5 N alkali, when most dyes of the acridine type become detached from the nucleic acids, and elute readily from the gel matrix. The absorption maximum should be located in the spectrophotometer, and used for comparative concentration determination. At neutrality or in the absence of urea, it may be advisable to guard against deviation from Beer's Law by selecting a wavelength corresponding to the isosbestic point for the self-association of the dye (e.g. 492 nm for acridine orange).

8.3.1.5. Evaluation of radioactive components

As we have noted (§ 7.5.3.4), the two approaches are autoradiography and slicing, with or without extraction, followed by counting. For RNA the most usual isotopes are ^{32}P, ^{14}C and ^{3}H; ^{35}S can be incorporated into the minor thiolated bases, present in tRNA.

Autoradiography For autoradiography of ^{32}P-labelled RNA, wet gel slices may be used, since the high energy of the β-particles emitted enables them to penetrate the gel. Autoradiography of ^{14}C on the other hand requires a thin flat slice of dry gel. The following procedure is described by Fairbanks et al. (1965): the gel is placed in a specially constructed holder (Fig. 8.2) and sliced longitudinally into 4 slices by 3 taut wires in a frame, the two inner slices (1/16″ thick with flat faces) being suitable for autoradiography. The slice is

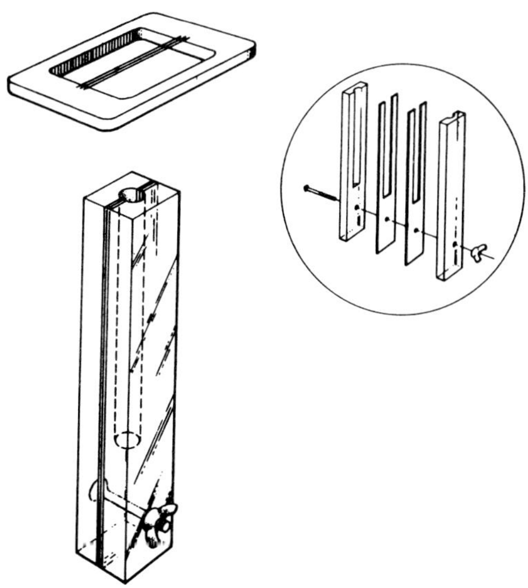

Fig. 8.2. Device for preparing flat longitudinal slices of cylindrical gels for autoradiography. The block (lower left) is made out of Perspex. The clearance between the walls and the spacers, and between the spacers themselves (expanded drawing at right) is sufficient to allow the framed taut steel wires (upper left) to be drawn through. This provides two flat sections of gel (Fairbanks et al. 1965).

Subject index p. 487

placed on Whatman 3 MM filter paper, which is then laid on a rigid piece of porous plastic, e.g. Vyon, fitting over the inverted top part of a small vacuum desiccator with the suction outlet at the bottom. While still wet the plastic with the gel slice(s) is covered with polyethylene sheet or Saran wrap, which is secured with a rubber band around the desiccator to make an air-tight seal. The water is removed from the gel by gently sucking air out through the bottom of the desiccator. An infrared lamp placed over the gel may help the process, but too rapid dehydration can lead to cracking of the polyacrylamide film. This procedure is applicable only to gels within a limited range of concentrations. Very dilute gels (3 or 4%) cannot be sectioned properly because they are not sufficiently rigid. The addition of agarose however overcomes this difficulty. Gels of 10% acrylamide or higher are brittle. Soaking the gel in glycerol solution as plasticiser has been suggested (Gordon 1969). The use of lower cross-linker concentrations, so that the gel swells on soaking may also help. A variant of the technique described by Adesnik (1973) entailing the use of an atmosphere of steam over the gel slice permits the drying of concentrated acrylamide without cracking. Fairbanks et al. suggest that drying should require a few hours. Radioactivity levels of 1000 dpm ^{14}C in a zone of 0.25×0.6 mm required a day's exposure to X-ray film to obtain a blackening sufficient for quantitation by densitometry.

Slicing the gel Three types of device have been used to obtain uniform horizontal sections of cylindrical polyacrylamide gels which can be used for measuring radioactivity. A frame containing wires at fixed intervals (e.g. 1 mm) can be used to cut the gel horizontally (Fig. 8.3). Secondly the gel may be sectioned with a microtome device, cutting at fixed intervals. Thirdly the gel may be extruded through a small orifice or wire mesh and fractions eluted into a fraction collector (or collected by hand).

A microtome is specially manufactured by Mickle Co., an adaptation of their tissue-slicing microtome, for slicing cylindrical polyacrylamide gels. It differs from the original microtome in having

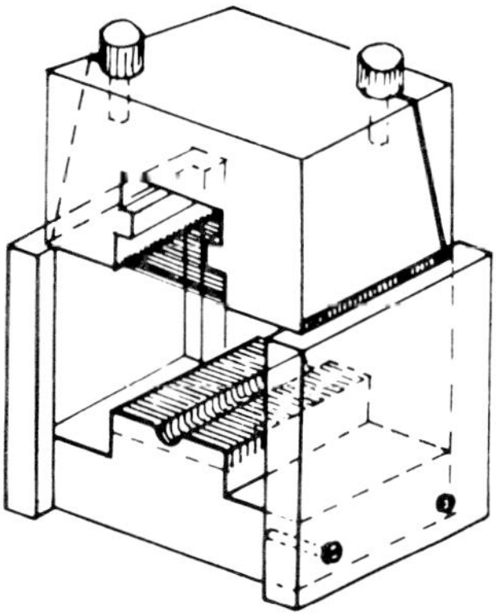

Fig. 8.3. Device for slicing cylindrical gels. The gel lies in the cylindrical groove in the brass block with grooves sawn at 1-mm intervals. The frame (above) has steel wire drawn round studs at both ends to give a separation equal to that of the grooves in the block. The wire grid so formed is drawn through the gel to give mm-thick discs (Chrambach 1966).

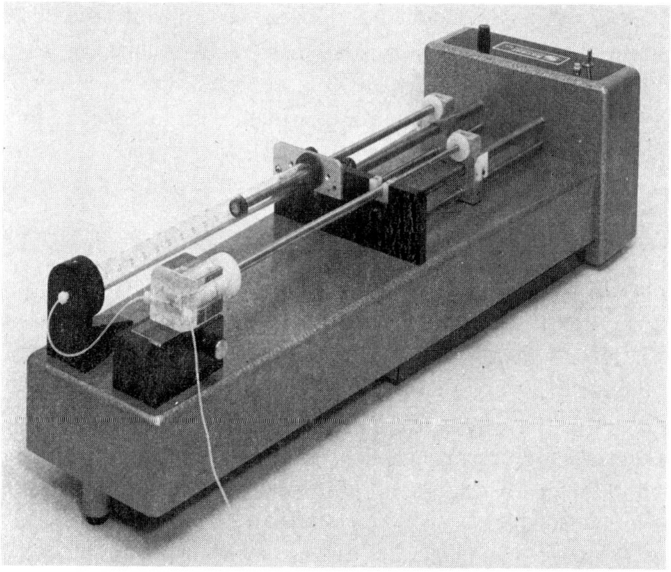

Fig. 8.4. Gel fractionator (Maizel 1966).

a stainless steel tray surrounded by troughs with an elevated platform in the middle for the gel. The troughs are filled with ground dry ice which hardens the gel, to allow cutting. Thus, very dilute and easily deformable gels may be sectioned with ease. The gel should be fixed between rubber stops since freezing is apt to cause expansion. This method of slicing is also applicable to very concentrated gels ($\geqslant 15\%$ acrylamide) without freezing, which is useful since other methods (e.g. Maizel's fractionator described below) are not suitable for such gels. Indian ink markers can be injected into the gel as an aid to relating migration distance and radioactivity.

The third type of device (Fig. 8.4) originated by Maizel (1966) in order to section cylindrical polyacrylamide gels, employs two motor-driven pistons which simultaneously force free buffer and the gel, contained in a stainless steel cartridge, through a narrow orifice (0.125 mm), or in the commercial version a wire mesh with the dimensions of an electron microscope grid, into a mixing chamber and out to a fraction collector. This device is specially convenient for radioactive samples, since the fractions can be collected directly into scintillation vials. A specially designed fraction collector to hold scintillation vials is manufactured to accompany the gel fractionator (Savant Instruments, Inc.). In an experiment with radioactive protein uniformly distributed through a 10 cm gel, Maizel reports collecting 60 fractions in which the radioactivity shows a variation of not more than 10%.

Radioactive counting Fractions containing ^{32}P or ^{14}C label may be counted either in a low-background gas-flow counter or in a scintillation counter. Only the latter method is sufficiently sensitive to deal with the weak β-emission of ^{3}H compounds.

Slices of gel can be dried on adhesive labels and transferred to planchets for counting in a gas-flow counter. Loening (1968) describes a method for processing a large number of samples. Slices are dried on 16 mm cine film, placing one slice on every other frame. The film is fed under a Geiger tube using a cine camera or projector mechanism and the counts for each slice are thus printed out.

Loening (1968) advocates counting ^{3}H-labelled RNA by putting slices of gel in 0.5 ml 6% piperidine base in open vials, and allowing them to dry in air. 0.5 ml water is added to each causing the gel to swell, followed by 12 ml of a water-soluble scintillation fluid. Some 90% of the RNA is extracted. Young and Fulhorst (1965) make use of the fact that polyacrylamide gels will dissolve in H_2O_2. Terman (1970) puts 1 mm slices of gel into tightly capped nylon scintillation vials with 0.3 ml NCS TM solubiliser (Amersham/Searle Corp.). The vials are shaken for 10–20 hr at 33–45°C. Swollen slices (about 4-fold increase in volume) could then be fully solubilised in toluene. 10 ml toluene containing 6 g/l Permablend (Packard) is added to each vial with swirling. Counting, performed with either a Nuclear Chicago Model 772 or Beckman 15-200 B Liquid Scintillation Spectrometer was achieved with an efficiency of 49% for ^{3}H.

Zaitlin (1970) reported low counting efficiency for concentrated gels by Terman's procedure and accordingly modified it to obtain higher efficiency. 1-mm slices of gel are placed in the bottom of glass scintillation vials; then 0.7 ml of a solution containing NCS diluted 1:9 v/v with water is added. Vials are tightly capped and heated overnight in an oven at 50°C, causing the gels to swell. The vials are tilted slightly during heating to ensure contact between the gel slice and liquid. To each vial is added 10 ml scintillation mixture containing 0.5% 2,5-diphenyloxazole and 0.01% 1,4-bis-2(5-phenyl-oxaxolyl)benzene (Packard Instrument Co.) in toluene. The vial is swirled to mix the contents and is then ready for counting.

Gels containing hydrolysable cross-links in place of N,N′-methyl-enebisacrylamide offer advantages for counting. To dissolve ethylene diacrylate cross-linked gels (Choules and Zimm 1965), 1-mm slices are placed in the bottom of 20 ml scintillation vials, and the digestion is started by adding 0.5 ml of a solution containing 9 vol of 1 M piperidine and 1 vol alcoholic Hyamine solution. The gel dissolves in 1–4 hr, depending on the acrylamide and diacrylate concentrations. The process is hastened by placing the vials on a shaker at 37°C. Following digestion, 10 ml Kinard's scintillation fluid is added and mixed to give a clear homogeneous solution. The piperidine concentration is sufficient to dissolve the equivalent of a 2 mm disc of gel.

Gels cross-linked with Anker's reagent, N,N′-diallyl-tartardiamide, dissolve in 2% periodic acid in 20–30 min at 37°C. Anker (1970) asserts that the gels take a somewhat longer time to set (1 hr for a 7% gel), but are otherwise equivalent to methylenebisacrylamide cross-linked gels, and that the periodic acid does not quench the scintillation.

8.3.2. Composite acrylamide/agarose gels

8.3.2.1. Preparation of the gel

The preparative procedure must take account of the fact that dissolved agarose sets to a gel at about 40°C, and that at this temperature the polymerisation of acrylamide is greatly accelerated. Therefore solutions must be warm before mixing but the agarose sets rapidly once the mixture is poured into the tubes at room temperature.

The following is the procedure for the preparation of gels containing 1.7% acrylamide, found to be optimal for the resolution for instance of the 45S precursor of mammalian rRNA into its components (Tiollais et al. 1972).

Acrylamide and bisacrylamide may be recrystallised if desired (§ 8.2.1.). The stock solution contains 19 g acrylamide and 1 g bisacrylamide in 100 ml water. The stock solution of catalyst contains 6.4 ml of DMAEC (Eastman Kodak) in 100 ml. It is reiterated that not all commercial agarose preparations give satisfactory results, and one of those listed in § 8.2 should be used to ensure success.

Tiollais et al. (1972) add 0.2% SDS to all solutions to inhibit nuclease activity. The 10× concentrated stock solution of borate buffer (Peacock and Dingman 1968) contains per litre: 108 g Tris base; 9.3 g EDTA (Na salt); 55 g boric acid; and 20 g SDS if required. This gives a *p*H of 8.3. It should be noted that sodium SDS is not soluble below about 15°C. The Li salt is soluble at 0°C.

Three solutions are prepared for each experiment. For 40 ml gel at 1.7% acrylamide: 1) 0.23 g agarose and 16 ml water are brought to boiling in a water bath with shaking (or by hand over a naked flame, or as described under slab gels, § 8.4.2.2 and advocated by Peacock and Dingman by boiling under reflux), and then placed in a water bath at 40–42°C. 2) 3.4 ml of the stock solution of acrylamide, 2.5 ml of the Stock Solution of DMAEC, 4 ml 10×concentrated Borate buffer and 14.9 ml water are mixed and placed in the water bath at 40–42°C. 3) 32 mg ammonium persulfate in 2 ml water is freshly made up.

14 ml solution (1) is mixed with solution (2) and then 1.25 ml of solution (3) is added. This mixture is then rapidly poured into the prepared tubes mounted in their rack. If Perspex tubes are used it is important with this mixture to retain the gel by means of a gauze or dialysis membrane attached to the bottoms of the tubes with a rubber band.

The agarose sets immediately at room temperature, while the acrylamide polymerises in about an hour. The gels may be used $1\frac{1}{2}$ hr after pouring. The quick setting of the agarose makes it difficult to achieve a flat gel surface by over-layering. Instead, the gel may be expelled cautiously from the tubes to a predetermined distance and the protruding portion trimmed off with a razor blade. This operation may be performed after removing the gauze or dialysis membrane (afterwards replaced) and applying pressure from a rubber teat at the bottom of the gel.

8.3.2.2. Electrophoresis and evaluation

Dingman and Peacock circulate cooling water to maintain the gels at 16–20°C, while running at 8 V/cm of gel, which with tubes of 7 mm i.d. led to 4.5 mA passed per tube. For wider gels the voltage must be reduced. Runs for the purpose of separating species of high molecular weight took 5–6 hr. After acid fixation of the RNA it can be stained by any of the usual dyes and cleared by washing (§ 8.3.1.3). For radioactivity counting, it is not necessary to freeze the gels before sectioning, as they are stiff. They may be sliced with a simple apparatus such as that shown in Fig. 8.3, and one may then proceed by one of the routines outlined in § 8.3.1.3 for dissolution and counting.

8.3.3. Formamide gels

Apart from the pre-treatment of the formamide, which is indispensable if the gel is to set, and for reproducible results, the method does not differ radically from that for aqueous gels.

8.3.3.1. Preparation for electrophoresis

Processing the formamide 2 g 'Amberlite monobed' mixed-bed ion-exchange resin MB-1 (BDH) is added to 60 ml formamide (BDH or Merck) and stirred vigorously to disperse the resin through the liquid for about 2 hr. In this time the specific conductance should have decreased from about 400 to some 5 μmho. The resin must not be left in the formamide for much longer than this. It is then filtered off and the solvent used within 3–4 days.

Preparation of acrylamide monomer solution Gels of acrylamide concentrations varying between 3 and 15% have been used. Formamide gels are somewhat softer than aqueous gels (with the same concentration of cross-linker), but their effective pore size is larger. Thus a 4% gel in formamide operates over about the same molecular weight range as a 2.5% gel in water. The procedure described is for 4% gels in 0.02 M barbital buffer, suitable for RNA in the molecular weight range 2×10^6–2×10^5. The following are dissolved in about 20 ml deionised formamide, and then adjusted with 1 N HCl with vigorous stirring to an apparent *p*H of 9.0 using a normal glass/calomel electrode pair with a *p*H meter previously standardised with an aqueous standard buffer; 0.85 g acrylamide, 0.092 g diethylbarbituric acid and 0.06 ml TEMED. Then 0.2 ml 18% aqueous ammonium persulfate is added and the volume made up to 25 ml with formamide. Degassing is not necessary, and the solution is poured into glass tubes.

Overlayering The solution columns are carefully layered with 70% formamide and left to set (about 30 min). The layered liquid is replaced with buffered formamide, prepared by dissolving 0.09 g diethylbarbituric acid in deionised formamide, adjusting the apparent *p*H to 9.0 with 1 N NaOH and making up the volume to 25 ml with formamide.

Applying the sample The sample is dissolved in buffered formamide containing 5% sucrose and a trace of bromophenol blue. In the case of two-stranded viral RNA it may be necessary to heat the sample to 50–60°C to effect complete denaturation. The sample (usually 10 μl at 1 mg/ml) is applied to the gel and overlaid with a 1-cm column of buffered formamide, and the tube is topped up with 0.02 M aqueous NaCl. The sample is thus only in contact with formamide.

8.3.3.2. Electrophoresis and evaluation

The best results have been obtained with 0.02 M aqueous NaCl in the reservoir buffer (1 l each). For 7 mm i.d. × 7 cm gels, electrophoresis is performed at 5 mA/gel and the rate of migration of the marker is similar to that in aqueous gels. In the course of one hour there is a considerable voltage drop. To maintain a neutral *p*H in the reservoir, it is necessary either to circulate the upper and lower reservoirs to provide constant mixing or to use external electrodes. The latter is the best method. Reversible calomel electrodes are conveniently used, and the polarity reversed after each run, so as to maintain long-term neutrality. The electrodes are connected to the buffer reservoir by means of a bridge of 5% polyacrylamide containing 1 M KCl in a glass U-tube. The design is shown in Fig. 7.8.

The following solution is used for staining: 0.5% acetic acid, 0.1% pyronine Y and 1 mM citric acid. The gels are stained overnight and destained by washing in 10% acetic acid. Formamide does not interfere with densitometry in the ultraviolet at 280 nm.

8.3.4. Polyacrylamide concentration gradients

8.3.4.1. Linear gradients

The following procedure giving a linear gradient of 2.5–12% acrylamide has been used by Caton and Goldstein (1971) to give uniformly good resolution for the whole molecular-weight range of total RNA preparations derived from ribosomes.

Buffer solutions for the procedure were as follows:

Gel buffer and electrode buffer: 0.02 M Tris, 0.02 M acetic acid, 0.01 M Na acetate, 0.001 M EDTA, adjusted to *p*H 7.5.

Buffered 60% sucrose solution: 15 g of sucrose and 0.75 ml of a buffer containing 1 M acetic acid, 1.4 M K acetate, and 0.001 M EDTA (*p*H 4.9), are made up to 25 ml.

Capping gel: 1 ml of melted agarose is added to 5 ml of 2–4 mM NaH_2PO_4, 1 mM Na_2HPO_4, 1 mM EDTA buffer (*p*H 6.6) also containing 0.001% bromophenol blue, and heated to 40°C. This solution is stored in the refrigerator, and remelted in a boiling water bath, and then cooled to 40°C before use.

Preparation of multiple gradient gels The preparation of the acrylamide gradient follows Margolis and Kenrick (1968), using the apparatus shown in Fig. 8.5a. The individual tubes (5 mm i.d. × 9 cm) are supported on a wire gauze in a polyethylene bottle, from which the bottom has been cut away. A 500-ml bottle will hold about 90 tubes. The bottle is connected to the gradient former with rubber tubing.

To prepare the gels, the rubber tubing is filled with gel buffer and the plastic bottle is filled to a level just above the bottom of the electrophoresis tubes. The gradient-forming device is packed in ice to prevent premature setting of the gel and filled as follows with 130 ml in each chamber:

	Chamber	
Per 100 ml buffer	1	2
Acrylamide	14.7 g	2.38 g
Bisacrylamide	0.3 g	0.12 g
TEMED	0.1 ml	0.1 ml
Ammonium persulfate	0.05 g	0.05 g

All components except the ammonium persulfate are dissolved and the solution is degassed. Ammonium persulfate is added last, always as the solid. The mixer of the gradient former is then started and the gel solution drained very slowly at first, into the packed plastic

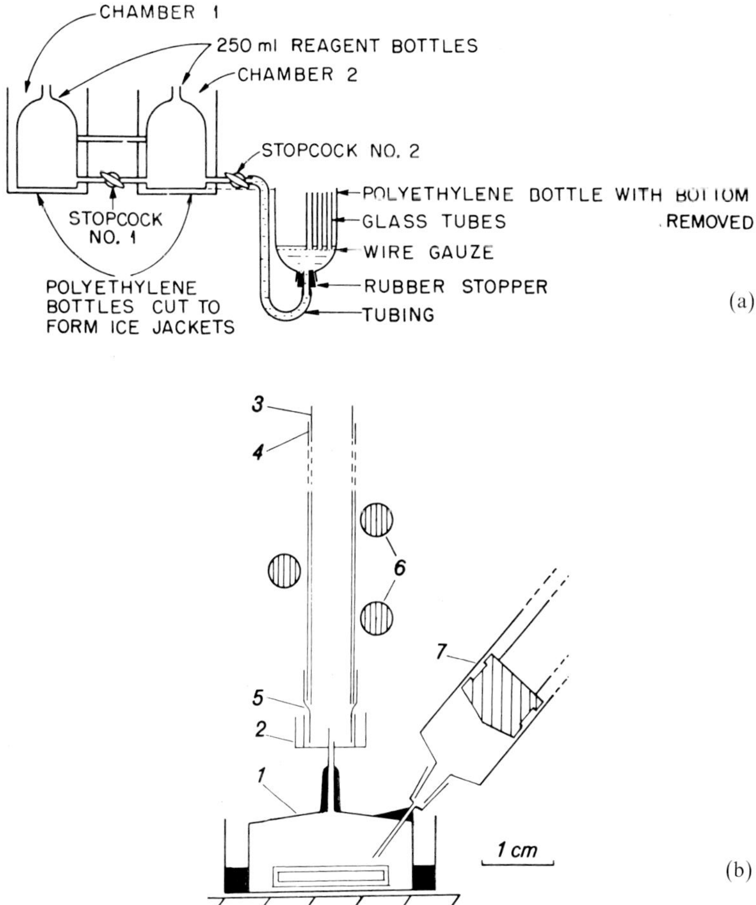

Fig. 8.5. a) Apparatus for preparing acrylamide gradients in tubes, which are packed vertically as shown into the chamber, consisting of an inverted plastic bottle, from which the bottom has been cut (Caton and Goldstein 1971). b) Simplified gradient generator for single tube gels made from a disposable hypodermic syringe (35 ml) sawn off as shown, with a needle cemented into the nozzle; (8) is a magnetic stirrer, (2) a serum cap and (5) thin tygon tubing, (3) thick-walled tygon tubing and (4) the electrophoresis tube, clamped (6). The needle of the syringe (7) is sealed into the larger syringe (Kidby 1970).

bottle until the tubes are filled to within 1 cm of the top. Gels are allowed to polymerise overnight and the tubes are then removed by cutting open the bottle, peeling off the excess gel, and trimming the gel off at the bottom of the tube. This procedure gives gels with a 2.5–12% polyacrylamide gradient and a 0.12–0.26% bisacrylamide gradient automatically buffer layered to give a flat surface. The bisacrylamide gradient provides optimum cross-linking through the whole length of the acrylamide gradient. Tubes prepared in this way can be stored under gel buffer in the refrigerator for long periods. Three precautions in particular should be observed, i) the tubes must be vertical during filling; ii) they must be filled very slowly at first to avoid mixing of the top of the gradient with gel buffer, and iii) they must not be pulled from the gel matrix after setting, for this is likely to break the gel inside the tube.

Preparation of the sample The gradient gels can be run in the usual way in the standard apparatus described in § 7.5.1.1, but we give here some details of the modification preferred by Caton and Goldstein. 4 OD units of an RNA mixture (or less of a single component) is added to 200 μl of buffered 60% sucrose solution and water is added to bring the volume to about 600 μl. About 150 μl of this solution is then layered on the dilute end of the gel. The sample is sealed in with 3 drops of the Capping Gel solution (kept at 40°C) which sets in a minute or two at room temperature.

Electrophoresis The buffer reservoirs are filled with cold (about 5°C) electrode buffer and any bubbles trapped at the top or bottom of the gel are removed. Electrophoresis is carried out at a constant current of 4 mA/tube (applied voltage about 90 V at the outset). Electrophoresis is continued until the bromophenol blue band migrates to about 1 cm from the bottom of the tube, usually about 70 min.

Some care should be taken in removing the gel since the top (2.5% end) is very soft. The gel is dislodged by rimming it at the 12% end and forcing water around the sides with a hypodermic syringe. Staining and destaining follow the usual way.

Simple device for a single gel A good simple design which can be quickly set up from available equipment is that of Kidby (1970). It is made from plastic disposable syringes, and is depicted in Fig. 8.5b. It will only of course fill a single gel tube at a time.

8.3.4.2. Exponential gradients

Because the relation between mobility and molecular weight is logarithmic, it might be supposed that a more even resolution over a wide range of molecular weight could be achieved with an exponential rather than a linear gradient. Good separations on a gel containing an exponential gradient of 2.5–20% acrylamide were obtained by Mirault and Scherrer (1971) of rRNA and ribosome precursors from HeLa cells. Gradient generators to produce a gradient of any desired shape can be constructed with appropriately shaped vessels, but a number of commercial models are available (e.g. from LKB Industries and Isco). A contrivance that will make a gradient of any desired shape, specially adapted to the needs of gel electrophoresis is made by Universal Scientific Co. ('Gradipore' apparatus), and consists of a flexible curve constrained between two glass plates. The curve divides a concentrated from a dilute solution, and can be manipulated to give the required gradient, the liquids from both compartments flowing from an outlet into tubes or slabs. The same firm provides pre-made flat gels containing a gradient from 4 to 25% acrylamide, ready for use.

The outlet from the mixing chamber of the gradient generator may be led into a device such as that of Caton and Goldstein (1971), (§ 8.3.4.1), or by way of a manifold into the tubes individually. Mirault and Scherrer, on the assumption that the polymerisation velocity is proportional to the acrylamide concentration on the one hand, and that of TEMED and persulfate on the other, arranged that both the latter components were added at a concentration inversely proportional to that of the acrylamide (e.g. for 10 ml of 2% acrylamide 50 μl each of 10% TEMED and 10% persulfate were added, but for 10 ml of 6% acrylamide 16.7 μl only of each). The gels were prepared at room temperature but the acrylamide mixtures were kept in ice and the TEMED and initiator were added just before mixing. The 30% acrylamide stock contained 0.5% *bis*-acrylamide to make gradients of high acrylamide concentrations, such as 8% upwards. This was found to lead to gels of uniform optical properties. Mirault and Scherrer tested the accuracy of the gradient by including bromophenol blue in the solution and measuring its concentration through the gel spectrophotometrically. They note that any apparatus design for casting gradient gels must meet the following conditions: rapid mixing; a small dead volume between mixing chamber and tubes; no mixing of the acrylamide gradient during flow, and no diffusion before polymerisation.

8.3.4.3. Pore limit electrophoresis

If the gel concentration at one end of the gradient is such as to bring the migrating RNA species completely to a standstill, one has 'pore-limit' electrophoresis, which is held by some workers to give particularly good results on mixtures containing a wide range of molecular weights. A sharpening process operates continuously in this system. Good results on RNA mixtures have been obtained by Grossbach and Weinstein (1968).

8.4. Procedures for slab-gel electrophoresis

Electrophoresis in slabs may be performed horizontally or vertically and three types of apparatus have already been described (ch. 7). The choice of slab gels rather than cylindrical gels may be dictated by any one of a number of considerations, e.g. simplified autoradiography, a better shape for densitometric evaluation, ease of obtaining a precise comparison of the mobilities of different electrophoretic species or, according to some views, greater simplicity of manipulation. Ultimately the choice remains primarily a matter of taste or prejudice, though it is hard to escape the feeling that the slab system is on balance the more rational. As already pointed out, the apparatus shown in Figs. 7.9 and 7.10 are easily constructed in Perspex in the laboratory workshop. The commercial apparatus shown in Fig. 7.11 for vertical gel electrophoresis is perhaps simpler to use than the basic design given in Fig. 7.10 and embodies water cooling. The latter apparatus however affords the advantage of flexibility in the choice of length and width of gels. Thickness of gels can be varied in either apparatus. Horizontal gels may be preferred for speed of assembly, and when gels are soft and difficult to handle. Because of the electrodecantation (see ch. 7), which operates in horizontal gels, it is generally supposed that vertical gels have the edge in resolution and uniformity of zones for densitometry. Procedures for electrophoresis of nucleic acids using the selected examples of types of apparatus will be given.

8.4.1. Horizontal gel electrophoresis

For the use of the apparatus shown in Fig. 7.9 (Vasu 1969), all but one of the plastic slats are mounted on the plastic base which contains the sample slots and are covered by the glass plate. The acrylamide or agarose solution is poured down a glass microscope slide into the open side and finally the space is closed with the fourth slat. The apparatus is unsuitable for dilute gels, e.g. 2.2% acrylamide, because setting at the periphery is inhibited by atmospheric oxygen. It has however proved to be convenient for example for 5% acrylamide gels in formamide. The addition of agarose (see § 8.3.2) permits the setting of gels of low acrylamide concentrations. After the gel is set the apparatus is inverted and the plastic moulds are removed. The gel resting on the original glass cover plate can then be immersed in electrophoresis buffer until use. With this apparatus it is a simple matter to introduce a new buffer at this stage or to remove impurities by soaking. Electrophoresis is carried out as described (§ 8.4.2.1).

8.4.2. Vertical gel electrophoresis

Many workers have used methods based on Akroyd's concept of vertical gel electrophoresis, to be described in detail below, but other methods are also in use such as that of Peacock and Dingman (1967) with the commercial apparatus depicted in Fig. 7.12, manufactured by E-C Apparatus Co. All the variants of the gel composition and buffer to be described lend themselves to use in this convenient apparatus. Many workers find that cooling is unnecessary if the applied voltage is not too high. Others circulate air from a fan over the slab, and others again do all runs in the cold room. In general the only detrimental effect of heating is zone distortion (see § 7.5.1.1). Degradation of the samples is unlikely to be a serious issue. Nucleases of course separate from the nucleic acid once the electrophoresis is under way.

8.4.2.1. Use of basic Akroyd-type apparatus

The following is based on a convenient modification by De Wachter and Fiers (1971) of the apparatus and method originally due to Akroyd (1968).

Apparatus The gel is cast between two glass plates, $40 \times 20 \times 0.4$ cm. The space between the plates may be 2, 3 or 4 mm and is determined by the thickness of two Perspex strips, 1.5×40 cm, which close the cell at the sides, and are greased to provide a leak-proof joint with the glass. Spring clips (e.g. foldback paper clips) keep the plates firmly together. The lower side of the cell is closed by mounting in a plasticine block while the acrylamide solution is poured into it and allowed to polymerise (Fig. 8.6a). Slots for sample application are formed in the gel by inserting a Perspex slot former, 15×10 cm, and of the same thickness as the strips, into the liquid before polymerisation occurs. The number and width of the slots determines the number of samples that can be applied, a space of 1 cm being left between the slots.

For electrophoresis (Fig. 8.6b) the cell is stood in a $10 \times 10 \times 25$ cm glass tank, provided with a platinum wire or carbon rod electrode, which serves as lower buffer reservoir. Alternatively a plastic box of similar dimensions may be used for the reservoir. The gel is covered with a layer of buffer and electrical contact with a similar upper reservoir is established by a wick of Whatman 3 MM paper soaked with buffer. The wick is 16 cm wide, and one layer of paper is used per millimeter gel thickness. The distance between the cell and

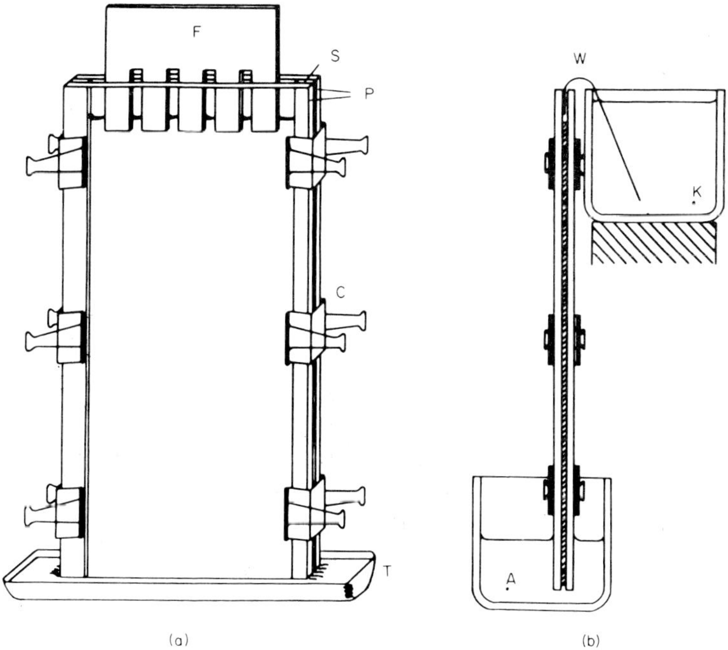

Fig. 8.6. Apparatus for gel slab electrophoresis. a) Assembly of the cell. Two glass plates (P), 400 × 200 × 4 mm are kept at a suitable distance by two Perspex strips (S), 400 × 15 × 2 or 3 or 4 mm. The assembly is made leakproof with grease and kept together with 6 steel clips (C). It is pushed vertically into a trough (T) filled with plasticine, to close the lower end. It is filled with acrylamide solution to 3 cm from the top and a Perspex slot former (F) is introduced to 1 cm below the liquid level. b) Electrophoresis (transverse section). The lower end of the gel slab is in direct contact with the buffer of the lower reservoir, which contains the anode (A), a platinum wire about 20 cm long. The top of the gel is covered by about 2 cm of buffer, and forms electrical contact with the upper reservoir containing the cathode (K) through a paper wick (W) soaked with buffer.

the buffer reservoir is kept as small as possible to minimise the electrical resistance of the wick. When a urea-containing buffer is used, the wick is covered with flexible polyethylene sheet to prevent crystallisation.

Composition of gels De Wachter and Fiers used this apparatus for the fractionation of fragments of RNA for sequencing, and have adapted it for a highly effective two-dimensional technique to give improved resolution. We give here their conditions for dealing with complex systems in different molecular weight ranges. Four types of gel are used. Their compositions are shown in Table 8.2, and they are made up by dilution from the stock solutions given below: 1) for gels of type 1: acrylamide, 190 g/l; bisacrylamide, 10 g/l; 2) for gels of types 2, 3 or 4: acrylamide, 400 g/l; bisacrylamide, 13 g/l; 3) Tris acetate buffer, 1 M, *p*H 8; 4) citric acid, 1 M; 5) urea, 9 M.

TABLE 8.2

Composition of gels used in vertical slab gel electrophoresis (De Wachter and Fiers 1971).

Gel type	Concentration of gelling agent (g/l)			Buffer
	Acryl-amide	Bis	Agarose	
1	19	1	5	Tris-acetate, 40 mM, *p*H 8
2	120	3.9	—	Tris-acetate, 40 mM, *p*H 8
3	200	6.5	—	Tris-acetate, 40 mM, *p*H 8
4	100	3.25	—	Citric acid, 25 mM, 6 M urea

De Wachter and Fiers also favour the inclusion of 1 g/l SDS and 10^{-5} M EDTA in the acrylamide solutions and bringing them to 100°C in a boiling water bath to denature traces of nucleases. Appropriate volumes of these solutions are mixed and diluted with distilled water to a total volume of 150, 200, or 250 ml for preparing slabs of 2, 3 or 4 mm thickness, respectively. The agarose used for type 1 gels is dissolved (§ 8.4.2.2) in water at 10 g/l immediately before use and diluted to half this concentration with appropriate amounts of hot stock solutions and water.

Catalyst is added to the mixtures immediately before they are poured into the cell. This comprises: 6) TEMED, 40 μl; ammonium persulfate, 100 g/l; 0.4 ml of this solution is added per 100 ml of acrylamide dilution to provoke polymerisation; 7) for acid gels (type 4), one adds to the acrylamide solution 0.4 ml of ferrous sulfate, $FeSO_4 \cdot 7 H_2O$, 2.5 g/l; 0.4 ml ascorbic acid, 100 g/l; and 0.4 ml hydrogen peroxide, 300 g/l.

The choice of gel concentration should be dictated by the size of the species to be separated, using Table 8.1 as an approximate guide. Acidic gels containing 6 M urea often resolve fragments which have the same mobility on neutral gels. De Wachter and Fiers found that bands obtained by fractionation of partial digests of bacteriophage RNA on neutral 12% gels could often be split into as many as ten components on this type of gel.

Preparation of gel slabs The glass plates are cleaned in hot detergent. Only plates that wet uniformly after this treatment are used. They are placed upright and allowed to dry. The surfaces should not be touched with the fingers.

A continuous thin line of grease, not wider than 1 mm, is applied 5 mm from the long edge of the plate. De Wachter and Fiers dispense vacuum silicone grease from a 5 ml hypodermic syringe, without a needle. The Perspex strips are then pressed against the greased edge until the grease forms an uninterrupted transparent band, showing that a leakproof joint is formed. The grease band should remain narrower than the Perspex strip and should not spread to the inside of the glass plate. Next, grease is applied to the tops of the strips and the second glass plate is put on top, with the same precautions. Finally 6 or 8 steel clips are put on the edges to keep the parts in place. The assembled cell is put upright and pushed firmly to a depth of about 8 mm into a bed of plasticine contained in a trough. This provides a leak-proof bottom which can withstand a hydrostatic pressure of 40 cm.

Catalyst is added to the solution of gelling agents and buffer and the mixture is poured into the cell, using a small funnel inserted into a length of flexible tubing projecting between the plates. The cell is filled to about 3 cm from the top. The slot former is then inserted to a depth of 4 cm from the top. After 0.5 hr, the top of the gel is covered with buffer and the slot former is carefully with-

Subject index p. 487

drawn. For preparation of type 1 gels, the freshly prepared hot agarose solution is cooled to 50°C by mixing with buffer, monomer solution and water, and the mixture with the added catalyst poured immediately into the cell.

The buffer reservoirs (Fig. 8.6b) are filled with the same buffer as that used in making the gel. The cell is put in the lower buffer compartment, resting on two glass rods lying on the bottom of the tank. Air bubbles trapped under the gel slab are removed with a bent Pasteur pipette. The paper wick is put in place and in De Wachter and Fiers' procedure the gel is subjected to one hour's pre-electrophoresis before the samples are applied. The run is performed in the cold.

Applying the sample The sample with added sucrose and bromophenol blue as before (§ 8.3.1.1), or xylene cyanol FF for acid electrophoresis, is carefully pipetted onto the surface of the gel in the slot. The volume should be such that the depth of the layer is no more than about 1 mm. The maximum volume thus ranges from 20 μl for a 1 cm slot on a 2 mm gel to 500 μl for a 13 cm slot on a 4 mm gel. Up to 10 μg of RNA per μl sample volume or per square mm of gel surface can be loaded on the gels. On the acid gels, De Wachter and Fiers state that carrier yeast RNA (BDH) should be added to the samples to give this total concentration. This evidently reduces spreading of labelled RNA behind and in front of the strongest zones which is otherwise observed in the acidic system.

Electrophoresis As soon as all the samples are loaded on the gel, the wick is replaced, the edge resting on the ridges that separate the slots. Electrophoresis can be carried out overnight in the cold at 250–600 V depending on the gel concentration. The voltage, current, and electrophoresis time, as well as migration distances found for RNA molecules of known molecular weight and for the dye markers, are summarised in Table 8.1. Finally, the apparatus is dismantled, the top plate is prised away with a fine spatula, so that the bottom plate, bearing the gel can be directly immersed in the staining bath. The

Perspex strips are first however removed, and the grease is wiped off with cotton wool wetted with acetone.

Staining The staining mixtures described under cylindrical gels (§ 8.3.1.3) are satisfactory, though De Wachter and Fiers give the following variant: 2 g of methylene blue are dissolved in one litre of 0.2 M acetic acid and 0.2 M Na acetate. The gel is immersed in this solution for 1 hr, and is then cleared by rinsing with running tap water overnight. For the indexing of zones to be detected by autoradiography, molecular weight markers in the form of ribosomal and tRNA in one channel of the gel are used. This is cut away and stained. Making correction for swelling, it is then possible to relate the positions of zones in the autoradiogram to the stained markers.

Autoradiography After dismantling the apparatus, the gel slab on its glass base is covered with a 50×30 cm sheet of thin plastic film (Gladwrap, Union Carbide Co. or Saran wrap, Dow Chemical Co.), which is folded back over the edges of the glass plate. This prevents the gel from drying out, but absorbs practically no radiation. Small labels marked with a radioactive ink are stuck on the plastic film on two opposite corners of the gel slab. The gel slab is then covered in the dark room with a 40×20 cm sheet of Kodak Royal Blue medical X-ray film or equivalent product. Good contact with the gel surface is obtained by putting a heavy glass plate or lead sheet on top. The exposure time depends on the activity in the sample, the number of bands in which it is distributed, and the thickness of the slab. In practice the time can vary between a few minutes and 24 hr. Longer times are not out of the question but diffusion of the RNA band then becomes appreciable. Dye bands diffuse faster.

8.4.2.2. Vertical acrylamide/agarose composite gels

The use of mixed acrylamide-agarose gels is described for those who prefer these to either low-concentration acrylamide gels or agarose alone, for any of the reasons given already. In the method of Peacock and Dingman (1967), the E-C apparatus is used. Agarose at 0.5% provides a satisfactory degree of mechanical rigidity, and the acrylamide concentration can then be varied to give molecular sieving in the desired molecular weight range.

Preparation of gels A warm solution of agarose which also contains all the reagents required for an acrylamide gel (acrylamide cross-linking reagent, accelerator, and catalyst) may be handled in either of two ways: 1) it may be kept above 40°C to prevent the agarose from gelling until acrylamide polymerises, and then subsequently cooled (method of Uriel and Berger, 1966); or 2) the solution may be cooled to 20°C to permit the agarose to gel and the acrylamide then allowed to polymerise. At acrylamide concentrations above 3.0% where the acrylamide alone forms a moderately firm gel, either method can be used. At lower acrylamide concentrations, however, where the polymerised acrylamide product was still fluid, the prior gelation of the agarose is necessary.

In the routine of Peacock and Dingman (1967) four solutions are used in the preparation of the gels: 1) 20% acrylamide monomer, 19 g of acrylamide and 1 g of *bis*acrylamide in 100 ml of water; 2) DMAEC, 6.4% in water (or, TEMED); 3) ammonium persulfate, 1.6% in water; 4) a buffer consisting of Tris (108 g), Na_2EDTA (9.3 g) and boric acid (55 g), in 1 l (*p*H 8.3).

To prepare 160 ml gel, water is added to 0.8 g of agarose in an amount depending on the required final concentration of acrylamide. Thus, for 2.0% final acrylamide, 0.8 g of agarose is suspended in 113 ml of water at room temperature in a 'Quickfit' flask. This is vigorously stirred magnetically, connected to a condenser, and refluxed at 100°C for 15 min. Alternatively it may simply be boiled over a naked flame with swirling until the agarose is dissolved, or left in a boiling water bath, and volume made up (e.g. by weight) to compensate for evaporation. The agarose solution is cooled under the tap to about 40°C. Meanwhile, buffer (16 ml), DMAEC (10 ml) and acrylamide solutions are mixed, the temperature is adjusted to about 35°C and 5 ml of 1.6% ammonium persulfate added with rapid mixing. This solution is at once poured into an electrophoretic cell. The slot former (precooled in ice water) is put in place and a chilled glass rod is placed in the front part of the cell to provide further cooling in this area. The agarose gels rapidly, and after 1 hr, the acrylamide has polymerised and the excess gel is removed from the cell.

Electrophoresis and evaluation The cell is set vertically, buffer (diluted 10-fold from stock) is added to the reservoirs, and the slot former is removed. In Peacock and Dingman's method the temperature of the circulating water is then reduced gradually over the next 0.75 hr to approximately 5°C. During this time, 200 V is applied at the electrodes by way of pre-electrophoresis. Samples are applied at the end of this time, and the electrophoresis is begun at 200 V. The time of the run, depending on requirements, is in general 1.5–2 hr for the 2% gels and up to 4 hr for the 10% gels. The same method may be used in uncooled apparatuses, but it is then advisable to decrease the applied voltage and extend the length of the run instead. Staining follows as before. Peacock and Dingman aver that the best of the common stains is methylene blue, which they use as a 0.2% solution.

For radioactivity measurements, in the range 3–5% acrylamide with 0.5% agarose, the gels are most easily sectioned by slicing segments with a microtome. The sections are then transferred one at a time from the cutting device to vials for liquid scintillation counting.

8.5. *Two-dimensional electrophoresis*

Two-dimensional electrophoresis has been used extensively to increase the resolution of protein mixtures. The discovery of the applicability of agarose and acrylamide gel electrophoresis to RNA has led to increasing demands on the resolving power of the technique (ch. 7), and it is not surprising therefore that two-dimensional techniques have been evolved to satisfy this demand.

The rationale of two-dimensional gel electrophoresis is that two species which co-migrate in the first dimension in one set of conditions may be separated in a second dimension if the buffer conditions are changed. The resulting separation may be due to one or a combination of reasons. Thus, 1) conditions may not be optimal to resolve all species in a mixture at once, e.g. high-molecular weight species may be resolved first in a gel of low acrylamide concentration, and smaller molecules unresolved in this medium may be separated in a gel of higher acrylamide concentration; 2) a combination of two types of electrophoretic separations, in particular a charge-based and a size-based separation, may lead to resolution of closely similar species (in acid solution for example the charge of a nucleic acid will become less negative to an extent depending on the base composition); 3) nucleic acid chains containing covalent breaks can be made to dissociate into their constituent fragments under denaturing conditions; 4) also nucleic acid-protein complexes such as viruses and ribosomes (ch. 9) may be dissociated into their constituents in the conditions used for the second dimensional run.

In general, it is found that better results are obtained if the conditions for two-dimensional gel electrophoresis are chosen so that the molecules migrate more slowly in the second dimension than in the first. This causes sharpening of the zone first generated, when it encounters the conditions of the second dimension. Thus, for (1) above, fractionation in the more dilute gel should precede the separation in the more concentrated gel. In separating nucleic acids at acid and neutral *p*H (De Wachter and Fiers 1972) the acid gel is chosen for the first dimension since in these conditions the RNAs, being less negatively charged and conformationally more expanded, travel slower than they do at neutral *p*H. It is usually advantageous in any case to use a gel of somewhat higher acrylamide concentration in the second dimension.

The arrangement used for two-dimensional gel electrophoresis may comprise various combinations of apparatus used for one-dimensional gel electrophoresis already described. Cylindrical gels used for the first dimension may be conveniently adapted to Akroyd type gels (§ 8.4.2.1) (Martini and Gould 1971). Alternatively, strips of Akroyd slab gels used in the first dimension may be applied to another gel slab of the same kind (Ehresman et al. 1972; De Wachter and Fiers 1972, and see below); gels of the type cast in the E-C Apparatus Co. equipment may be similarly used as described in § 8.5.2 (Peacock and Dingman 1967; Ikemura and Dahlberg 1973). Vigne and Jordan (1971) used this apparatus for the first dimension and the Akroyd-type slab for the second. Advantages of using the commercial device lie in the ease of assembly and cooling. The Akroyd-type apparatus also offers several advantages, notably that the gel dimension can be varied at will, and that several slabs can be run simultaneously (Figs. 7.10 and 7.11). The width of the gel may determine how many samples can be run in parallel in the first dimension, and the length determines the distance that they may be run so as not to outstrip the gel when applied at right angles. This possibility of increasing the dimensions may be critical in obtaining the desired resolution. For RNA sequence work 40 cm long slabs are frequently used (Adams et al. 1969).

8.5.1. Different pH in the two dimensions (De Wachter and Fiers 1972)

In this method, separations are carried out at *p*H 3.5 and *p*H 8. The electrophoresis cell is that designed by Akroyd (1968) with altered dimensions. The two glass plates are for this purpose separated by 2 mm thick Perspex side walls (Fig. 8.6). The dimensions of the gels are 40 × 20 cm for the separation in the first dimension and 30 × 25 cm for the second dimension.

Composition of the gels Since the net charge of an RNA molecule is appreciably lower at *p*H 3.5 than at *p*H 8 the acrylamide concentration of the acid gel must be lower than that for the neutral gel if the sample is to have comparable mobility in both dimensions. The acid gel is used as the first dimension; at the start of the second separation the RNA moves from a more dilute into a more concentrated gel, which results in a drop in mobility at the interface with concomitant zone sharpening. Because its charge in the second dimension is higher, the effect of the greater gel concentration once the sample has entered the second gel, will be offset by the accelerating effect of the higher *p*H. In this system the sample is first exposed to denaturing conditions so that species containing breaks in the chain, which are prevented by the secondary structure from becoming

TABLE 8.3

Composition of gels in two-dimensional gel slab electrophoresis (De Wachter and Fiers 1972).

Stock solution	Volume (ml) required for 150 ml gel			
	1st dimension, *p*H 3.5		2nd dimension, *p*H 8	
Final acrylamide concn. (%)	8	10	16	20
Monomer/buffer mixture (Acrylamide 400 g/l) (Bisacrylamide 13 g/l)	30	37.5	60	75
9 M urea	100	100	—	—
1 M citric acid	3.75	3.75	—	—
1 M Tris adjusted to *p*H 8 with citric acid	—	—	6	6
Catalyst:				
$FeSO_4 \cdot 7\ H_2O$, 2.5 g/l	0.6	0.6	—	—
Ascorbic acid	0.6	0.6	—	—
H_2O_2, 300 g/l	0.06	0.06	—	—
TEMED	—	—	0.06	0.06
Persulfate	—	—	0.6	0.6

manifest, will dissociate into their constituent fragments. In the second dimension these will then be separated on the basis primarily of their size.

The acrylamide concentration is chosen for the first dimension (acid gel), and may be 10% for fractionation of RNA mixtures containing maximum chain lengths of about 80 nucleotides (as applied by De Wachter and Fiers to a typical viral RNA partial digest), and is then made twice as high in the second (neutral) gel. The concentration of cross-linker (Bis) is 1/30 that of acrylamide. The buffer in reservoir and gel is 0.025 M citric acid, 6 M urea for the first dimension, and 0.04 M Tris–citric acid, *p*H 8, for the second dimension. Table 8.3 summarises the concentrations and amounts of stock solutions conveniently used for the preparation of each gel, as well as the catalyst, which is added immediately before the gel is poured.

Separation in the first dimension Cleaning of the glass plates, assembly of the cell, pouring of the slabs, loading of the sample and autoradiography are performed as described (§ 8.4.2.1). The slabs are subjected to a pre-run of about 1 hr before application of samples. The ethanol-precipitated, dried RNA is dissolved in 6 μl 6 M urea solution. The density is increased by addition of 3 μl of an aqueous solution containing per ml 500 mg sucrose or 300 g urea, and if required the dye markers, 5 μg trypan red. 2 μg xylene cyanol FF, and 2 μg bromophenol blue/ml of solution. The sample forms a layer of approximately 1 mm in the 5 mm-wide loading slot. The separations are carried out in the cold room at 4°C in the conditions described.

The run is stopped when the fastest marker, trypan red, reaches the end of the slab. An autoradiograph can be prepared at this point if needed. A rectangular strip of gel 1 cm wide and up to 20 cm long, is carefully cut out as shown in Fig. 8.7a using a scalpel or razor blade with a ruler as guide. The edge must be straight for good contact with the second gel.

Separation in the second dimension The strip is transferred with two pairs of forceps onto a glass plate, 25 × 30 cm, which will form the

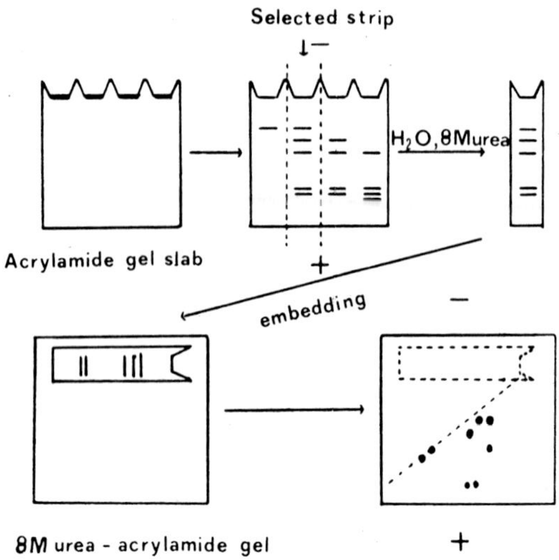

Fig. 8.7. Routine for two-dimensional acrylamide electrophoresis, from Vigne and Jordan (1971) (for explanation see text). Other workers prefer to embed the gel strip after the first separation at the bottom of the slab, for the samples to migrate upwards (as in Fig. 7.14).

TABLE 8.4

Conditions for two-dimensional gel electrophoresis and distance migrated by dyes.

	First dimension at *p*H 3.5		Second dimension at *p*H 8	
	8% acryl-amide	10% acryl-amide	16% acryl-amide	20% acryl-amide
Conditions				
Voltage (V)	900	900	350	350
Current (mA)	57	51	50	43
Time (hr)	4	6	15	15
Distance (cm)				
Xylene cyanol FF	16	17	10.5	7
Bromophenol blue	19	20	20	13.5
Trypan red	35	35	—	—

back wall of the electrophoresis cell in the second dimension. As illustrated in Fig. 8.7b, the strip is set 4 cm from the bottom edge of the plate, and parallel to it. The cell is then assembled, put upright into a trough in plasticine, and filled with the new acrylamide solution (Table 8.3) to 3 cm from the upper edge. Before polymerisation, some urea will have diffused out of the gel strip into the solution. This results in density gradients at the bottom and therefore a rather non-uniform gel below the strip. Since the RNA migrates from the bottom upwards in the second electrophoresis, this does not affect the quality of the separation.

Electrophoresis is carried out overnight under the conditions given in Table 8.4. At an early stage the colour of the bromophenol blue in the strip changes reflecting the equilibration of the sample to the new *p*H. After electrophoresis the cell is dismantled, and the gel is stained or subjected to autoradiography as described (§ 8.4.2.1.). The dye spots act as markers for locating particular zones of RNA when separations have to be reproduced.

8.5.2. Different gel concentrations in the two dimensions

In this procedure the only difference between the conditions in the two runs is the gel concentrations. This leads to somewhat improved separation by virtue of the different size-mobility law (§ 7.4.1) that applies under limiting conditions (away from the linear part of the log(molecular weight)-mobility plot).

Electrophoresis on polyacrylamide gel slabs (17 cm long × 13 cm wide) can be conveniently done in the vertical cell E-C 470 (Fig. 7.12) according to the procedure of Dahlberg and Ikemura (1973), which is given here with a few modifications. The electrophoresis buffer consists of 10.8 g of Tris base, 9.3 g of Na_2EDTA and 5.5 g of boric acid/l, giving a final *p*H of 8.3. Buffer is circulated between the top and bottom buffer reservoirs during electrophoresis. The details given here are for 10% gels, for RNA in the 4–5 S size range. The 10% polyacrylamide gel is polymerised in buffer containing 9.5% acrylamide, 0.5% Bis, 0.4% DMAEC (or TEMED), and 0.1% ammonium persulfate, at room temperature. For 5% or 20% gels, the concentrations of acrylamide and Bis are half or double the above, respectively. Small slots are used at this stage (1.5 mm × 3.5 mm wide). The RNA is applied (100 μg samples in say 20 μl), enriched as before with sucrose and tracker dye. If cooling is available (Dahlberg and Ikemura circulate coolant at 15°C) a high applied voltage of some 250 V may be employed for a run of 3 hr. Otherwise a lower voltage must be used.

After the run, a gel slice containing the RNA region is cut out with a scalpel or razor blade. The gel slice is put into the electrophoresis cell perpendicularly to the long axis, and set into the cell in a manner similar to that described above. The new acrylamide solution (20%) is poured into the cell and allowed to polymerise around and below the 10% strip. Because the 20% gel adheres tenaciously to the Perspex apparatus, it was found necessary to coat with fluorocarbon both the slot former and a region of about 2 cm around the two sides and bottom of the coolant plates that are in direct contact with the gel. Unless the cell is treated in this way, it is very difficult to remove the slot former after polymerisation or to dismantle the apparatus after the run. While the 20% gel polymerises, coolant is circulated to prevent the accumulation of air bubbles between the gel and the plates. Electrophoresis in the second dimension is carried out as in the first, but over a period of 17 hr at the same voltage.

8.5.3. Denaturing conditions in one dimension

We give here one further variant of the two-dimensional technique, which has given good results. Here denaturing conditions are used in the second dimension. The conditions, as given, are for RNA in the low-molecular weight range of partial digests. The procedure is due to Vigne and Jordan (1971).

The gel slab (13 × 18 × 0.3 cm) is prepared in the E-C Apparatus Co. electrophoresis cell and contains 12% acrylamide, 0.4% bisacrylamide, 0.1% TEMED and 0.04% ammonium persulfate made up in 0.04 M Tris acetate buffer at *p*H 8.4. It is run for 3–4 hr at 300 V with cooling. After completion of the run, the gel slab is removed from the apparatus and an autoradiograph prepared if required.

A strip bearing one of the samples run in the first electrophoresis is cut out from the slab and agitated gently in distilled water for 4–6 hr, then in 8 M urea (containing a trace of bromophenol blue, for 1–2 hr). There is little nucleotide loss in this time, and the ionic strength is reduced to cause zone-sharpening in the second dimension.

A 25% acrylamide gel slab made up with 8 M urea, 0.04 M Tris acetate, *p*H 8.4, initiator and catalyst is cast between two glass plates (20 × 40 cm) separated by 4 mm spacers. The solution is poured to a level 3 cm below the top of the plates, layered with water and allowed to set. The water is poured off, and then 10 ml of the same acrylamide solution containing urea and gelling agents but no buffer is poured on the gel, and into this solution the prepared strip is placed. After the new acrylamide layer has set, and embedded the strip, the second dimension electrophoresis is run as described in § 8.5.2. The bromophenol blue in the strip marks the progress of the run and reflects the zone-sharpening process. When the run has been completed staining and/or autoradiography is carried out by the procedures already described.

Practice of preparative gel electrophoresis of nucleic acids

Because of the low adsorptive capacity of polyacrylamide, the extraction of nucleic acids from gels is in principle not too difficult. We shall discuss in turn the extraction of zones cut from the gel, and the direct continuous electrophoretic elution of RNA from the end of the gel. The first method offers the better resolution if the nucleic acid concentration is kept within the range customarily employed in analytical work. It can sometimes be applied even to stained gels, and is the usual approach in sequencing work if the nucleic acid is strongly labeled, so that minute amounts will suffice for nucleotide mapping. The second approach is less arduous once it has been set up, and although comparable resolution is probably impossible, it can be scaled up. Again, however, a deterioration in resolution seems inevitable in practice. Because, as noted earlier, it is open to question whether gel electrophoresis is better than other (in particular chromatographic) methods for large-scale fractionation of nucleic acids, we shall concentrate primarily on methods involving the extraction of RNA from zones in the concentration range commonly occurring in analytical gels.

9.1. Extraction of RNA from gel slices

9.1.1. Detection of zones

The first problem in all methods of preparative electrophoresis is the location of the zones. A sure but tedious method is to slice the gel into segments of equal thickness (say 1 mm thick) with an apparatus such as that shown in Fig. 8.3, extract all of them individually, and thus determine the profile of RNA distribution throughout the gel. Another method is to stain either an identical gel (if one can be certain that the highest reproducibility between gels in a single run has been achieved), or track from a flat gel. The staining process of course is slow, and the likelihood of diffusion in the gel to be extracted considerable. It can be stored frozen, however, by immersion in liquid nitrogen, while the staining of the reference gel is effected. Another method is to 'pre-stain' the sample by addition of a small amount of a metachromatic dye such as acridine orange (McPhie et al. 1966), which is sensitively detected by its fluorescence under ultraviolet light (Woods glass filter lamp). If the sample is labeled with ^{32}P at high activity the zones can be detected by autoradiography in a short time. If the gel is sliced into equal segments, each segment may, as Watanabe et al. (1967) have shown, be simply introduced, together with some SDS to inhibit nuclease activity, into scintillation fluid (8:1 toluene:methanol) in a scintillation vial, counted directly and then extracted. ^{32}P can also be counted with a sacrifice of efficiency without scintillation fluid by Cerenkov radiation. A method for detecting ^{3}H- or ^{14}C-labeled zones is to cut a narrow strip of the gel longitudinally, use the slices from this for counting, and extract the RNA from the appropriate slices of the remainder. A simple method for cutting such a strip from cylindrical gels has been described by Tiollais et al. (1972), and consists in introducing a nylon thread to lie along the wall of the tube at the beginning of the experiment, and drawing it across the gel to produce a narrow sliver. Optical density amounts of closely migrating zones can be separated in the following way (Hamlyn and Martini, personal communication): The gel cylinder or strip is placed in a quartz cuvette and scanned in the ultraviolet, locating the zones approximately. A platinum wire is then introduced vertically into the cuvette between the estimated positions of the zones. The wire causes a sharp, vertical excursion of the pen on the gel scan and can be moved by successive approximation to a position equidistant between the peaks corresponding to the RNA zones. Finally the wire is used to section the gel between the two zones. We now consider how to recover the RNA from the fragment of gel containing (it is presumed) a single component from the initial mixture.

9.1.2. Extraction by diffusion

This is the simplest method, and works best with gels of low acrylamide concentration. Immersion of the slice in 0.5 ml of diluted EDTA (5 mM, as used by Bishop et al. 1967), overnight at 4°C with agitation extracts most of the RNA. Two such extractions with 0.5 ml each time led to recovery of 85–90% of the radioactivity of the slice of a 2.4% gel. The extraction process can be hastened, though at some risk of damage to the RNA, by heating. Thus Kourilsky et al. (1970) heated the slices for 1 hr at 100°C in 1 ml standard saline-citrate buffer per slice, and this appears to work also for more concentrated gels (Adesnik, 1970). The inclusion of denaturing agents (dimethylsulfoxide or urea) appears also to assist extraction.

9.1.3. Extraction by homogenisation

Efficient recovery can be achieved by homogenisation of the excised zone. A small Potter homogeniser works well: the gel slices are simply ground up with about 1 ml of buffer containing a denaturant (6 M urea for preference), and the resulting paste is vigorously centrifuged. This may be followed by a second extraction. A refinement of this primitive procedure is described by De Wachter and Fiers (1972), whose particular concern was extraction of RNA from zones in flat two-dimensional gels. Discs cut from cylindrical gels can be treated in the same way. A disc of filter paper (Whatman 52) is accurately cut (e.g. with a cork borer) to fit into the bottom of a plastic 2 ml disposable syringe barrel. The gel fragment is placed on top of the filter paper, and squashed by working the plunger with a rotary motion (De Wachter and Fiers suggest by pushing the end against a rubber-covered disc fitted onto the shaft of a slowly rotating electric motor). The plunger is then withdrawn cautiously so as to leave the paper and macerated gel in the barrel, and 0.5 ml 1 M NaCl solution is added. The syringe is then gently agitated on a vortex mixer so as to bring the gel into suspension, without disturbing the filter paper. The supernatant then percolates slowly through the filter paper and is collected, finally with pressure from the plunger.

The same authors (De Wachter and Fiers, 1972) have also made use of the strategy of Sanger and Brownlee, whereby the RNA is adsorbed and thus concentrated onto a disc of DEAE-cellulose paper. After homogenisation of the gel slice in 10 ml 0.2 M NaCl solution, the suspension is transferred to a Millipore funnel containing a disc (25 mm) of Whatman DE 81 paper. The suspension is allowed to settle for some minutes to prevent clogging of the paper by fines in the homogenate, and the supernatant is brought through by suction. De Wachter and Fiers observe that for the same reason the homogenisation should not be carried too far. The paper disc containing the RNA is then freed of gel by rinsing with water, and dried in a desiccator on a piece of filter paper. The RNA is recovered from the ion-exchange paper by folding this and introducing it into a conical micro-centrifuge tube, resting this in the top of another centrifuge tube, adding a buffer of high ionic strength (2 M triethylammonium bicarbonate, *p*H 10, is suggested), and centrifuging it through the paper into the receiver. Three successive extractions of 0.1, 0.075 and 0.05 ml are advocated. To the eluate, 0.05 ml acetic acid is added to bring the *p*H to about 5, and the RNA is precipitated with ethanol. The total recovery from the gel is about 75%.

Another way of dealing with an excised zone is described by Adesnik (1970), and has been adapted to strips of gel cut from broad slabs on which are run as much as 5 mg of RNA (Adams et al. 1969). The gel slice is coarsely chopped up and placed into a cylindrical tube 10 × 1 cm, one end of which is covered with DEAE paper, and over this a layer of cellophane attached to the tube with a rubber band. The tube is filled with buffer (0.04 M Tris acetate, *p*H 8.3) and placed in a disc electrophoresis apparatus. After electrophoresis the RNA is found trapped in the ion-exchange paper, from which it is eluted as before.

An even simpler method of elution from the paper is to trap it

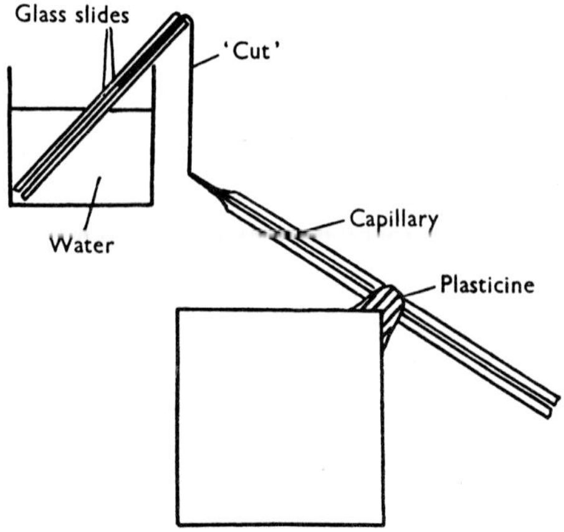

Fig. 9.1. Arrangement for elution of RNA from filter paper or ion-exchange paper. (In the latter case a high ionic-strength eluant would be used instead of water) (from Sanger and Tuppy, 1951.)

between two slides, one end protruding, and allow the eluant to be drawn through the paper and into a capillary pipette by capillarity (Fig. 9.1) (Sanger and Tuppy 1951).

9.2. Electroelution techniques

9.2.1. Small-scale methods

Ribonucleic acid can be eluted electrophoretically directly from the gel without the intervening process of searching for zones. For cylindrical gels, the simplest method is to cover the end of the tube with dialysis tubing, so as to leave a dead space, from which RNA can be recovered with a hypodermic syringe. This is, however, too primitive for most purposes, for one can only select one's fractions by guesswork.

Other contrivances involve flushing the RNA away by a continuous flow of buffer as it emerges from the gel, and collecting fractions. The most successful fractionations are obtained when the scale is small, and the many problems of heating, overlap and mixing of fractions, that beset attempts to scale up the basic analytical gel techniques, do not seriously obtrude. A simple adaptation of the cylindrical analytical gel system has been described by Mann and Huang (1969), who cast the gel in two tubes instead of one and join them by means of a sleeve equipped with an inlet and outlet tube. A 2-mm gap is left between the surfaces of the upper and lower gel segments in the sleeve and buffer is swept continuously through it with a pump (Fig. 9.2). An even simpler procedure is to attach an adaptor to the end of the tube containing an acrylamide gel of normal analytical dimensions. A very effective and simple design is that of Popescu et al. (1971) and the optimisation of the experimental variables is discussed by the same authors (Popescu et al. 1972).

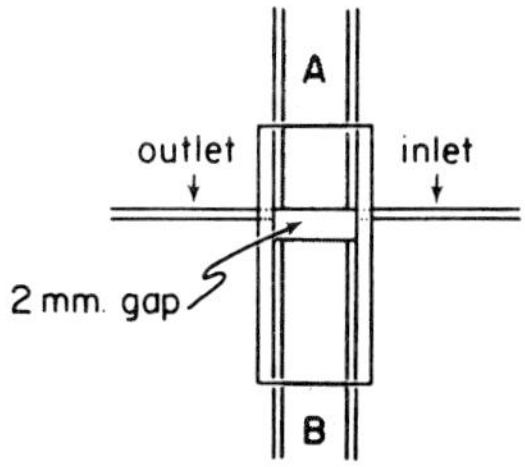

Fig. 9.2. Small-scale preparative electrophoresis device. Buffer is swept through the gap between the upper (A) and lower (B) parts of the cylindrical gel, and then to a fraction collector (Mann and Huang 1969).

An apparatus (Fig. 9.3) closely based on that of Popescu et al. has been used in the laboratory of one of the authors, and has given very satisfactory results. It requires no special machinery and can be rapidly set up. The adaptor consists of the sawn-off end of a 5 ml disposable plastic hypodermic syringe barrel. The glass tube containing the gel fits comfortably into the plastic cylinder, if slots are cut into this as shown. The plastic tubing is fitted, after softening over a Bunsen flame, over the syringe nozzle, and buffer is drawn through the compartment between the end of the gel and the conical end of the syringe barrel by a peristaltic pump working on the tubing. The eluate is monitored in the ultraviolet in a micro-flow cell (0.2 ml volume

Subject index p. 487

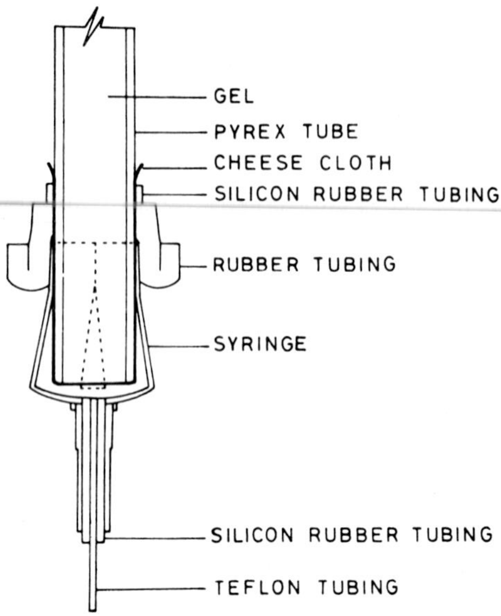

Fig. 9.3. Small-scale preparative electrophoresis apparatus by Popescu et al. (1971). The glass tube containing the gel (0.8 cm o.d.) fits into the sawn-off barrel of a 2 ml disposable plastic syringe, in which have been cut 2 mm wide slots. A peristaltic pump, working on the outlet tube causes buffer to be drawn through the compartment made up by the syringe bottom.

from Beckman RIIC) in a monitor or spectrophotometer (e.g. Beckman DB, at 260 or 280 nm, according to the concentration of the RNA), and thence to a fraction collector. For a typical fractionation, such as that of 16 S from 23 S RNA of *E. coli*, the following conditions are used: 2.4% acrylamide gel is set in the usual way in Tris acetate buffer (0.04 M Tris, 0.02 M Na acetate, *p*H 7.5), in a glass tube such as used in the analytical apparatus described above. Rather surprisingly a gel column of only 2 cm can afford very satisfactory separation. The quantity of RNA applied naturally limits the resolution, but 0.2 mg can be processed with little deterioration in the separation. Electrophoresis is allowed to proceed at 6 mA, through a single gel of the dimensions given. The pumping rate is 3 ml/hr, and separation requires about 3 hr.

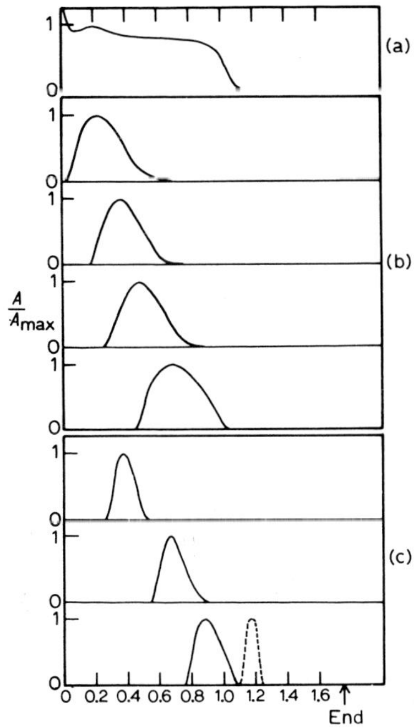

Fig. 9.4. Densitometer traces of stained poly(rA) zones after electrophoresis in 2.4% gels. a) Typical unfractionated sample. b) Fractions prepared by salt precipitation. c) Fractions made by preparative electrophoresis. The broken line is the profile of tRNA. Intensities are normalised at the peak. Mobilities are relative to bromophenol blue. The arrow indicates the end of the gel (from Pinder and Gratzer 1974).

Fractions of 0.5 ml are collected and the RNA is recovered by precipitation with ethanol and centrifugation. The use of this method for preparing narrow molecular-weight cuts from very polydisperse samples of polyadenylic acid is described by Pinder and Gratzer (1974) (see Fig. 9.4, in which the resolution is demonstrated by re-electrophoresis, in which the fractions run true). No doubt greater resolution could be achieved with longer gels, though at the cost of more diffusion, and probably therefore little resultant gain.

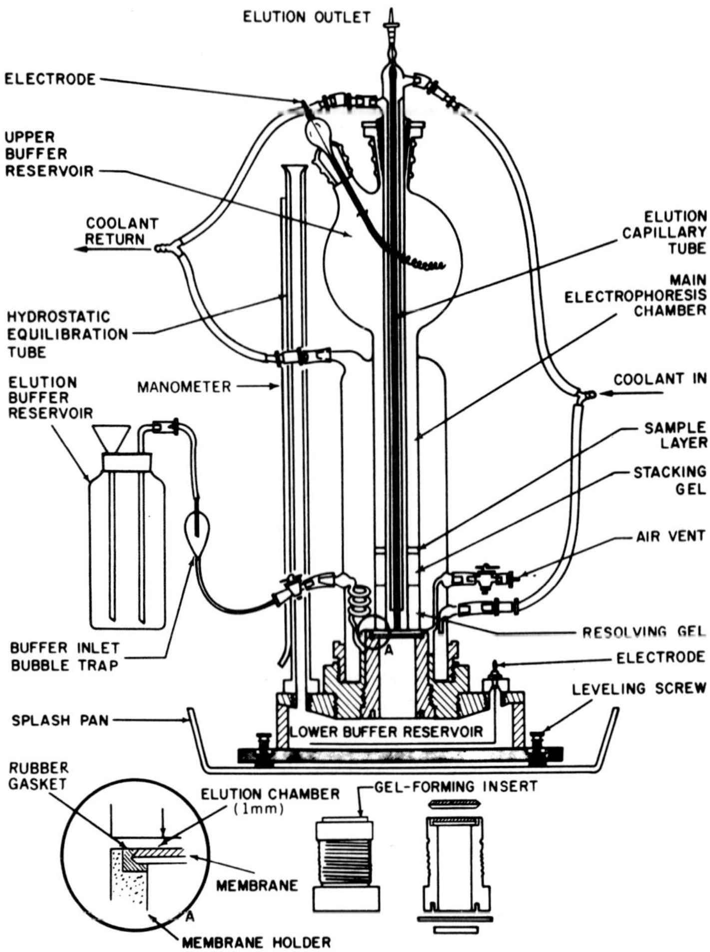

Fig. 9.5. Large-scale commercial preparative electrophoresis apparatus, based on the design of Jovin et al. (1964) (by courtesy of Buchler Instrument Co.).

9.2.2. *Large-scale electroelution*

As we have noted, preparative electrophoresis on a large scale presents considerable new problems, which do not appear to have been by any means completely overcome. Nevertheless, many apparatuses have been described, and several commercial designs are available, which with patience can be made to give quite good results if the highest degree of resolution is not demanded. A very successful application is that of Elson and Jovin (1969), using the apparatus (Fig. 9.5) sold by Buchler Instruments and devised by Jovin et al. (1964). The column is cooled by inner and outer circulating jackets. The gel is set within the annulus, closed by parafilm, and after setting, is mounted so that the bottom is above a porous glass membrane through which ionic contact is made to the lower buffer reservoir. The material which has migrated through the lower surface of the gel is swept into a capillary in the central cold finger and thence into collection vessels by a continuous buffer flow through the gap that forms the elution chamber. This apparatus has been used with gels at the extremes of concentration. Thus Morrison et al. (1970) have prepared haemoglobin messenger RNA by electrophoresis in 2.4% polyacrylamide, and 20% polyacrylamide has been used by Elson and Jovin (1969) for $(dAT)_n$ oligomers.

In the case of the dilute gels the major problem is that the gel tends to slip down the annulus in consequence of the hydrostatic pressure from the elution buffer. This was overcome (Lanyon et al. 1968) by maintaining a constant head of elution buffer only slightly higher than the level of buffer in the upper (inner) reservoir. The concentration of cross-links was also increased to 11% of the total monomer concentration to stiffen the gel. It has been found advantageous to place a circle of porous plastic (Vyon) underneath the column before sealing with parafilm. This may be left in place during the run and likewise prevents the gel from slipping and blocking the flow of elution buffer. Morrison et al. (1970) separated 5 mg haemoglobin messenger RNA on a 5 cm long gel at 700 mA constant current at 130 V across the gel. Fractions were eluted at the rate of 1 ml/min and samples collected every 5 min.

In the case of very concentrated gels the problems encountered by Elson and Jovin (1969) were that the gel tended to swell and thus block the elution chamber, and that the concentrated acrylamide solutions were difficult to layer sufficiently well in the normal way with buffer. The first obstacle was overcome by increasing the cross-linker concentration from 1 to 3% of the total monomer, the second by the use of *iso*butanol for layering. It was found that the current densities normally used for analytical scale electrophoresis

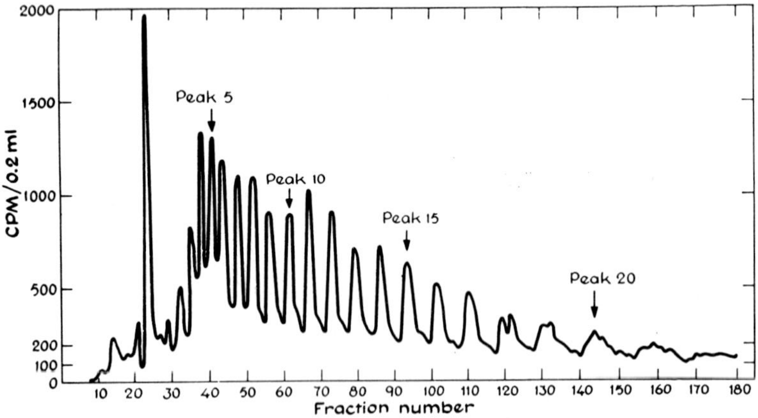

Fig. 9.6. Fractionation of oligonucleotides composed of alternating residues of adenylic and thymidylic acid d(AT) by preparative electrophoresis using the apparatus shown in Fig. 9.5 (Elson and Jovin 1969).

were too high for the thicker preparative gels. The current was therefore reduced to 2 mA/cm^2. Using a stacking gel of 2 cm, and a separating gel of 10–15 cm, a total volt drop of 200 V, and cooling at 15°C, oligomers of $(dAT)_n$ were separated over a period of 3–5 days. The upper and lower buffer reservoirs were changed every 24 hr. The resulting separations were comparable in resolution to those obtained on the analytical scale (Fig. 9.6).

Applications of gel electrophoresis

Since the introduction of gel electrophoresis as a means of studying nucleic acids some ten years ago, the increasing volume of the literature on its various ramifications reflects the power and versatility of the method. There is little doubt that gel electrophoresis is better than sedimentation analysis on almost all counts, and will come increasingly to replace it. A comprehensive account of all applications to date would be impossible, and we shall attempt here only to define the scope of the method, illustrating it with a few of the most successful or elegant examples.

10.1. Determination of molecular weight

The limitations of gel electrophoresis in aqueous solution for molecular-weight determination have been discussed (§ 7.6.1). Nevertheless useful estimates of molecular weights have often been obtained, on viral and ribosomal RNA species especially, and on the fragments generated by mild nuclease digestion. Where the molecular weight pertains to a species of defined conformation for which a homologous set of standards is available, the results are of course far less equivocal. One example of such a situation occurs for oligonucleotide fragments so small as to preclude any significant perturbation of the structure by base-pairing. Philippsen and Zachau (1972a, b) have shown how in this range precise determination of degree of polymerisation (DP) is possible. Superb resolution of

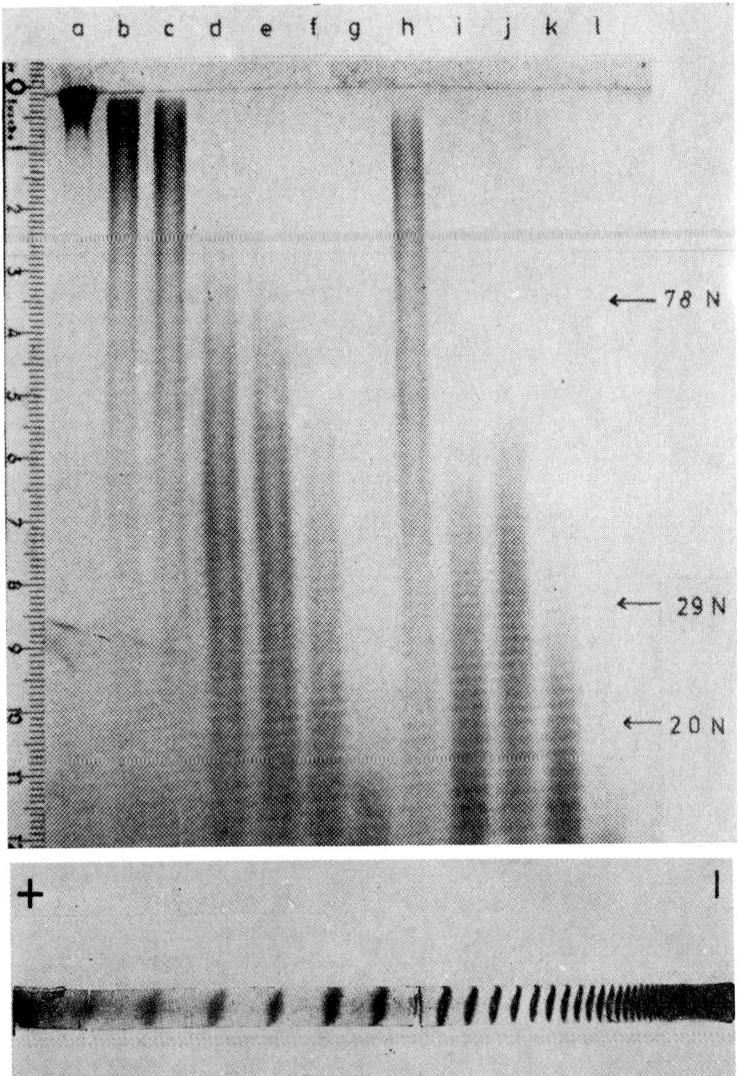

Fig. 10.1. Resolution of the low-molecular weight polynucleotide homologues by polyacrylamide gel electrophoresis: a) polyriboadenylic acid after degradation with kidney exonuclease. Samples, run on a 12% gel correspond to incubation with the enzyme under various conditions and for differing times (Philippsen and Zachau 1972a); b) pancreatic deoxyribonuclease partial digest of poly (dAT), alternating double helical polymer, run in 22% cylindrical gel (Elson and Jovin 1969).

oligoriboadenylic acids with separation of all successive homologues between 13 and 42 residues and the resulting calibration for chain length are shown in Figs. 10.1 and 10.2. Calibrations obtained by the same workers (Philippsen and Zachau 1972a) for tRNAs and their fragments are given in Fig. 10.3. Another case of an effectively homologous series arises in DNA, and in the low molecular weight range Elson and Jovin (1969) have separated a series of

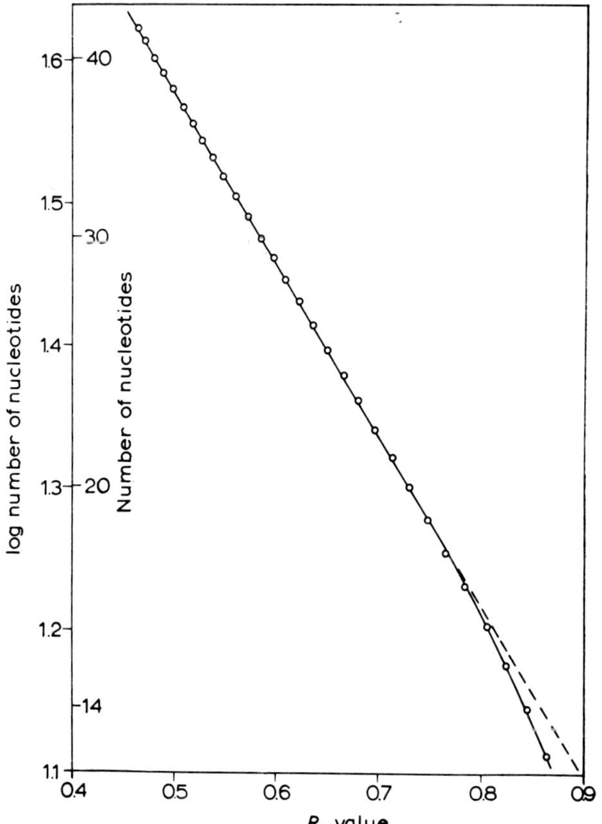

Fig. 10.2. Chain length-relative mobility relation for riboadenylic acid oligomers corresponding to the data shown in Fig. 10.1a (Philippsen and Zachau 1972b).

Subject index p. 487

alternating dAT oligomers with a resolution of one base-pair. The homology effect has proved valuable especially in the study of double-stranded viral DNAs, which have been mapped in terms of nucleotide fragments generated by highly selective nucleases, such as restriction enzymes (Danna and Nathans 1971; Danna et al. 1973; Pettersson et al. 1973).

A means of escaping from the uncertainty in the absolute molecular weights of external standards was found by Danna et al. (1973), who have taken advantage of the relatively small number of two-strand breaks introduced by the restriction enzyme, which ensure the recovery of all the DNA in large fragments; this makes it possible to express the size of fragments as a percentage of the total genome, which is sufficient for the purpose of the investigation. The precision is excellent, and the question of absolute accuracy does not arise (Figs. 10.4 and 10.5). An interesting finding, based on gel electrophoretic separation (Hewish and Burgoyne 1973) was that in nucleohistone the nuclease-labile regions, which are presumably determined by the protection of the remaining bulk of the DNA by histones, are regularly spaced along the sequence and these generate a regular progression of fragments, which are revealed as such by the resulting gel patterns. A different way with DNA, and one which is necessary for higher molecular weight species, because of their anomalous mobility-molecular weight relation (see above), is to examine the samples after irreversible alkaline denaturation; this evidently also produces a set of effective conformational homologues (Fig. 10.6).

This method is not effective for typical, partially base-paired RNA species, for internal complementarity of short regions ensures that denaturation is reversible. The most successful method of rendering all such species conformationally comparable, is, as has been noted, the use of formamide in the gels, and this technique has been fairly widely and successfully employed on such materials as viral RNA and its fragments (Duesberg and Vogt 1973), RNA formed in transcription of chromatin (Fig. 10.7), repressor binding sites on DNA (Maniatis and Ptashne 1973), nuclease fragments for sequencing (Brownlee et al. 1973), nuclear heterogeneous mRNA precursors and

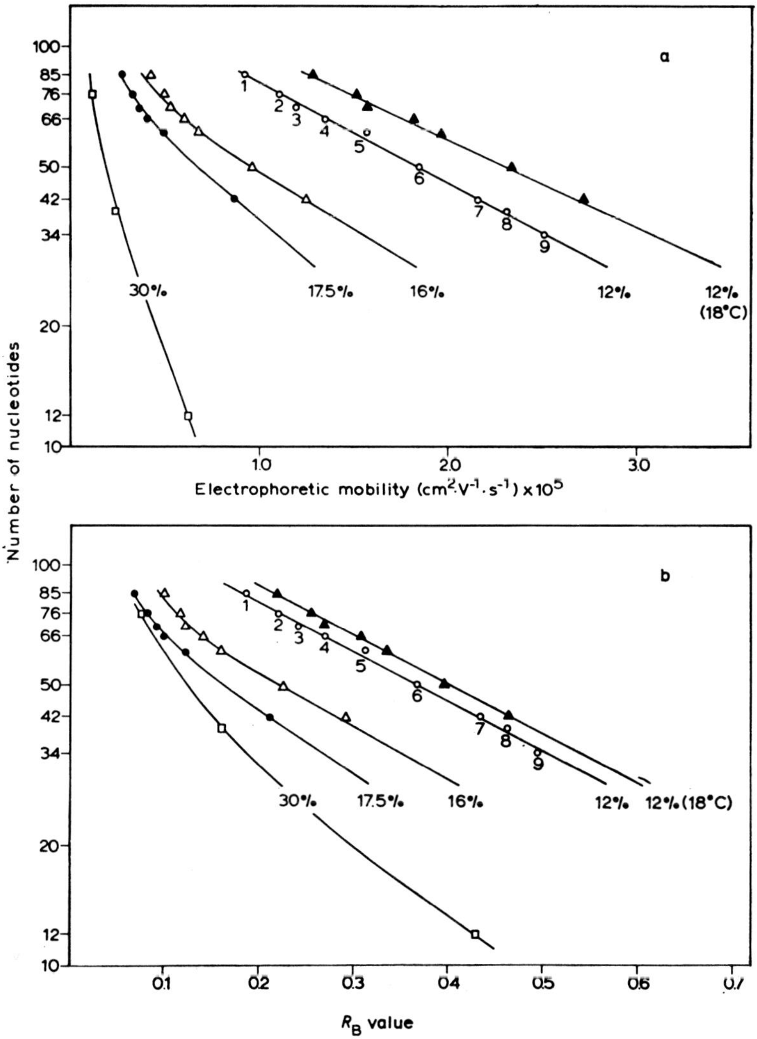

Fig. 10.3. Chain length-electrophoretic-mobility calibration for tRNA and known fragments of tRNAs at the different gel concentrations indicated. Mobilities on an absolute basis (a), and relative to dye marker (b). (Philippsen and Zachau 1972a).

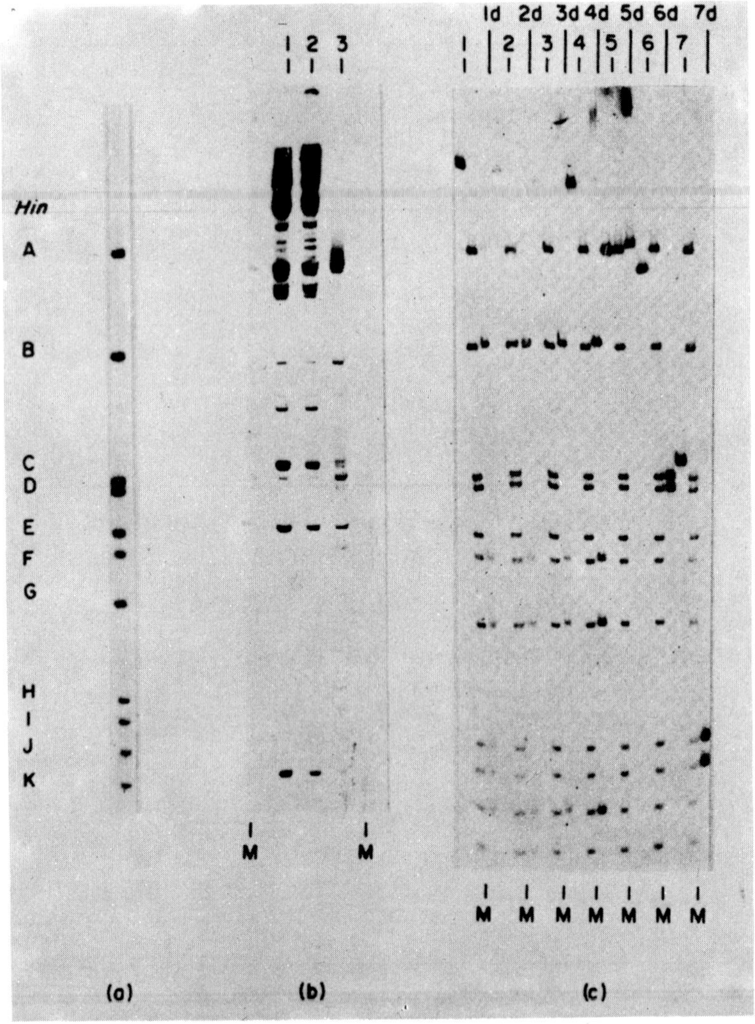

Fig. 10.4. Examples of partial and complete digests of ^{32}P-labeled SV40 DNA with restriction endonuclease from *Haemophilus influenzae*. Each plate is a radioautogram of a single gel slab following electrophoresis. The origin is at the top. a) A complete digest of SV40 DNA. b) Partial digest of SV40 DNA. 25 μg of ^{32}P-labeled SV40 DNA I (10^5 cpm/μg) were incubated in a vol of 0.1 ml with 0.016 of a unit of enzyme under standard conditions. Samples were removed after 20 min digestion (sample 2) and after 30 min digestion (sample 1). For sample 3, 23 μg of ^{32}P-labeled SV40 DNA

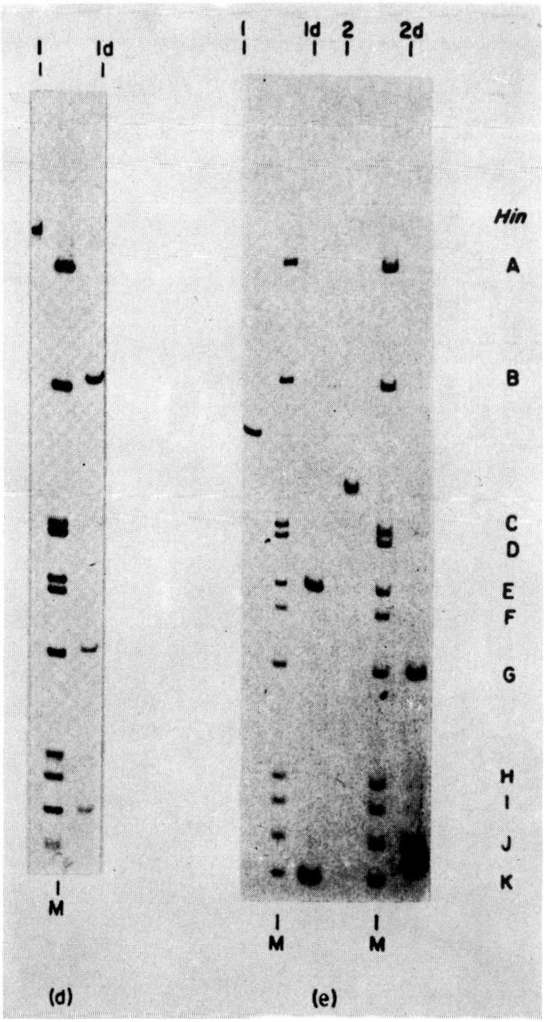

1(4.5×10^4 cpm/g) were incubated for 1 hr with 0.055 of a unit of enzyme in a vol of 0.32 ml. Samples of the partial digests (1.2 and 3) and of a complete digest marker (M) were electrophoresed. c), d) and e) Redigestion of partial digest products eluted from electrophoresis gels. For each sample the partial product (1, 2 etc) and the redigested partial products (1d, 2d etc.) were electrophoresed in the sample gel slab with a complete digest of SV40 DNA as marker (M).

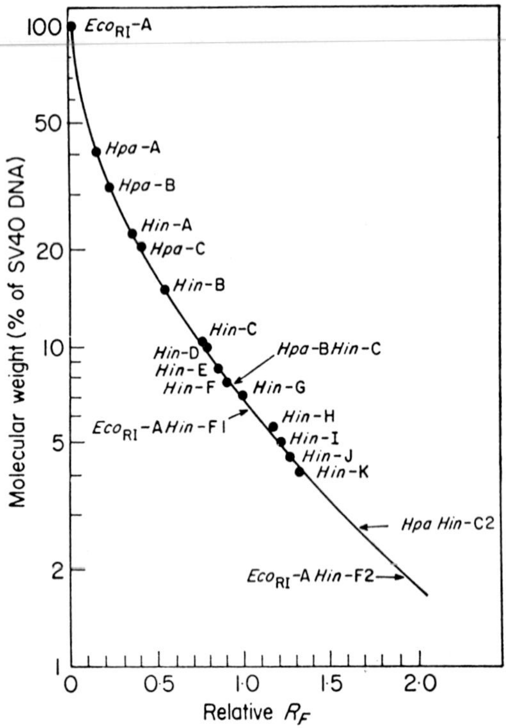

Fig. 10.5. Electrophoretic mobility-chain length calibration (4% acylamide gel) for double-stranded DNA, derived from fragments shown in Fig. 10.4. The relative mobility refers to one of the fragments (*Hin*-G) as the standard. Note that here the chain lengths are not expressed in absolute terms, but rather as a percentage of the total viral genome (Danna et al. 1973).

the messengers for α- and β-globin which separate only in formamide gels and are revealed thereby as having perceptibly different chain lengths (Gould and Hamlyn 1973, and Fig. 10.8).

Another set of natural homologues, as noted, are such homopolynucleotides as polyriboadenylic acid, which is of particular interest in that it occurs at the ends of many messenger RNAs. Pinder and Gratzer (1974) have shown that polyriboadenylic acids (in a higher molecular weight range than the oligomers of Philippsen and Zachau 1972a, depicted in Fig. 10.1) when run in acrylamide gels in aqueous solution fall on a single smooth calibration, which encompasses also the less structured (unstacked) series of polyribouridylic acids; single-stranded stacking, within the limits found in polyadenylic acid at room temperature, thus evidently has little effect on the electrophoretic mobility. These results are also of interest in providing a demonstration of the efficacy of the gel technique in dealing with polydisperse (as against paucidisperse) materials. Here again the technique proves itself greatly superior to sedimentation or other types of hydrodynamic analysis, for it gives a complete molecular weight distribution, which especially for a non-ideal, highly-charged species, such as a polynucleotide, is well-nigh impossible by conventional methods. Also, narrow molecular weight cuts can be prepared on a small scale by electrophoretic elution from the gels.

10.2. Conformational and related effects

The secondary, though important, effect of conformation on the electrophoretic mobility of RNA in gels has been discussed (§ 7.6). RNA species differing in conformation as mitochondrial and cytoplasmic ribosomal RNAs evidently do (Grivell et al. 1971; Dawid and Chase 1972) respond differently to changes in conditions, such as temperature or salt concentration, and these effects can be put to good use in improving fractionations: either one may simply adjust the available variables until good results are obtained, or one may use two-dimensional methods, varying the conditions between the two runs. A more general way of inducing a differential change in

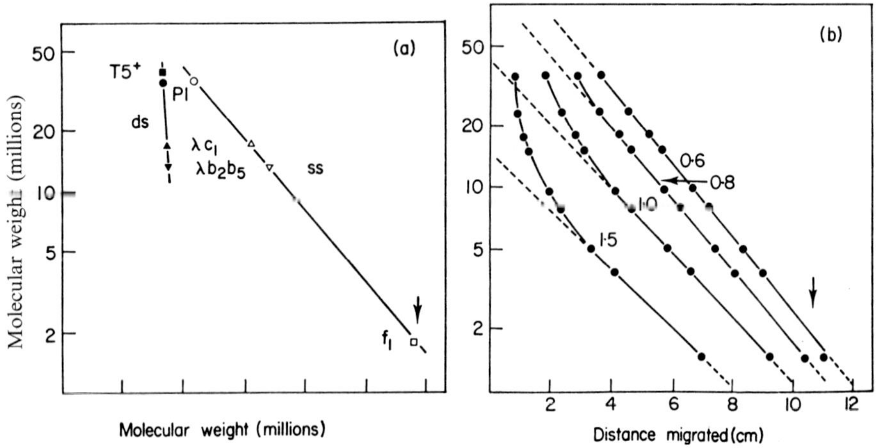

Fig. 10.6. Relation between molecular weight and electrophoretic mobility of DNA in agarose gels. A) comparison of double-stranded and single-stranded DNA. Electrophoresis of a series of reference ^{32}P-labeled DNA molecules was performed in 0.6% agarose gels. Distance migrated from the origin for each band in the autoradiograph is plotted against log molecular weight. For comparison, double-stranded forms of DNA are plotted at half-molecular weight positions. The vertical arrow shows the position of the tracking dye. Double-stranded DNA (ds) (filled symbols) were from bacteriophage T5 (■), P1 vir phage (●), λb2b5 phage (▼) and λc1 phage (▲). Single-stranded DNA (open symbols) were from P1 phage (○) λc1 phage (△) λb2b5 phage (▽) and f1 phage (□). B) Effect of gel concentration on the electrophoretic mobility of single-stranded DNA. Denaturated ^{32}P-labeled T5st (○) DNA was electrophoresed in agarose gels of indicated concentrations in Tris-acetate buffer. The mol.wt. of the T5 fragments determined in 0.6% agarose were used to calibrate the log mol.wt. against mobility relationship for the more concentrated gels. The curves are shown as solid lines with the linear regions extrapolated (broken line) to the theoretical exclusion limit for each gel. C) Estimation of T5 fragment molecular weights in the range 1.5 to 40 million by electrophoretic separation in 0.6% agarose gels, using single-stranded P1, λc1, λb2b5 and f1 as reference DNAs (○). Major T5 fragments (■); minor T5 fragments (●). D) Estimation of T5 fragment molecular weights in the range 0.1 to 5 million by electrophoretic separation in mixed 0.7% agarose-2.2% polyacrylamide gels and Tris-phosphate SDS buffer. Some of the larger T5 fragments with mol.wt. as determined in Fig. 10.6c were used as reference molecules. The mol.wt. values used for the RNA species (*E. coli* 16 S and 23 S rRNA, L-cell 18 S and 28 S rRNA) were those given by Loening (1969). The line connecting the

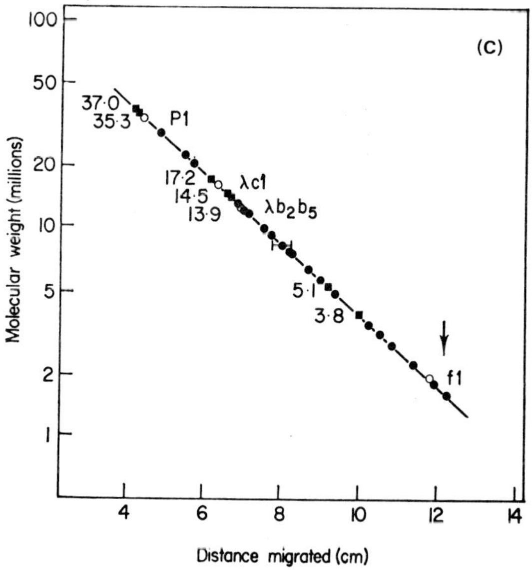

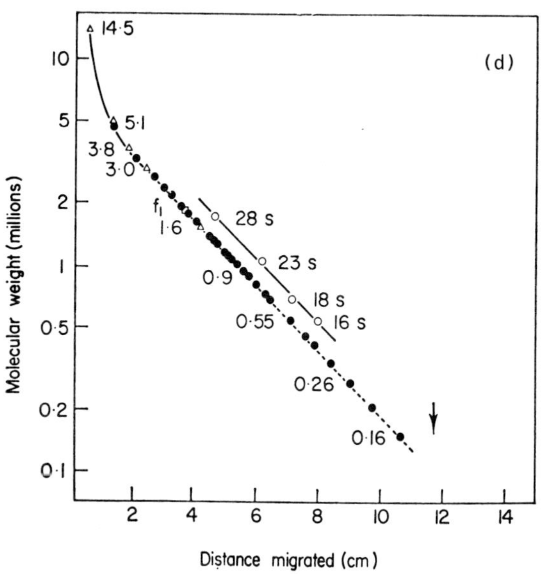

reference DNA points was extrapolated (broken line) for determining the mol.wt. of the small T5 fragments. Reference rRNA (○); reference f1 DNA (□); reference T5 DNA fragments (△); unknown minor fragments (●) (Hayward and Smith 1972).

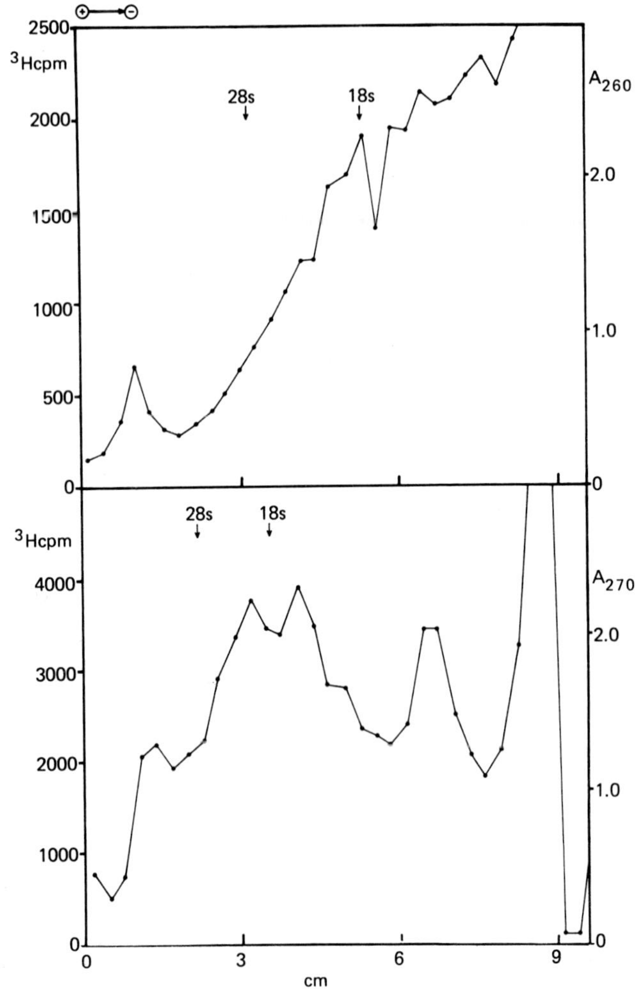

Fig. 10.7. RNA transcripts prepared on reconstituted reticulocyte chromation (i.e. chromatin prepared by mixing chicken erythrocyte DNA, chicken erythrocyte histone and chicken reticulocyte non-histone protein in high salt, urea and dialysing out the salt and urea). The upper panel shows the radioactivity distribution of the ^{3}H RNA synthesized in this system separated on 2.4% aqueous gels (cf. Loening 1967). The lower panel shows the same product run on 3% formamide gels. Sharper zones are obtained using the latter technique. The comparison also indicates the absence of hidden breaks in the bulk of the transcript (T. Barrett, personal communication).

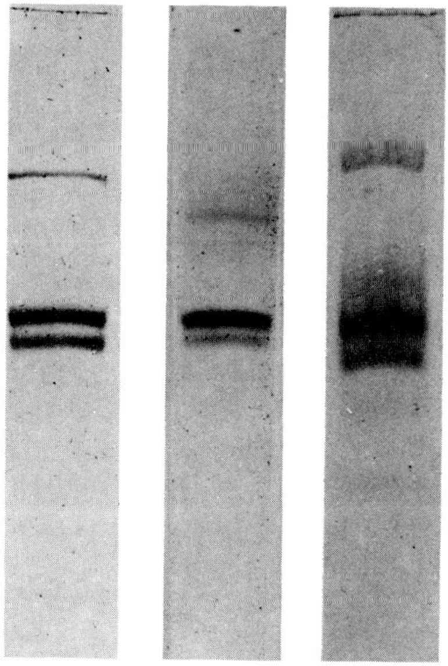

Fig. 10.8. Rabbit globin messenger RNA separated in formamide gels. The same preparation was run on (left) cylindrical gels in the apparatus shown in Fig. 7.7; (middle) vertical flat-bed gels of the Akroyd type (cf. Fig. 7.10); and (right) horizontal flat-bed gels in the apparatus described in Fig. 7.9. Despite the alleged disadvantages of the horizontal arrangement the α- and β-messengers are separated almost as well as in either vertical (cylindrical or flat-bed) arrangement, and the operations involved in setting up the apparatus are quickest with the apparatus shown in Fig. 7.9 (Hamlyn, personal communication).

mobility characteristics in a mixture of RNAs is to induce a partial denaturation in the second dimension, with a reagent such as urea, as has been done by De Wachter and Fiers (1972) or acid (see e.g. Reddy et al. 1974), with highly satisfactory results in terms of resolution. The most extreme conformational difference of course is that between a typical, partly base-paired, RNA, and a rod-like two-stranded species. These are readily resolved from one another and can be differentiated in terms of different mobility-gel concentration relationships (Harley et al. 1973; see Figs. 7.20 and 7.21), or even by different colours generated on staining (Dingman et al. 1970; Bevan et al. 1973).

The ability of gel electrophoresis to discriminate between conformational states that may differ in only minor degree in Stokes radius can be put to a number of good uses, for example in measuring the equilibria between the conformers of tRNA. Richards et al. (1973), working with 5 S RNA, have used gel electrophoresis to study the kinetics of interconversion between the 'native' state (defined by its ability to recombine with the 50 S ribosome) and the denatured. Although these forms are practically identical in the extent of base-pairing, they separate readily in gel electrophoresis, and their relative proportions can be measured by densitometry of the stained

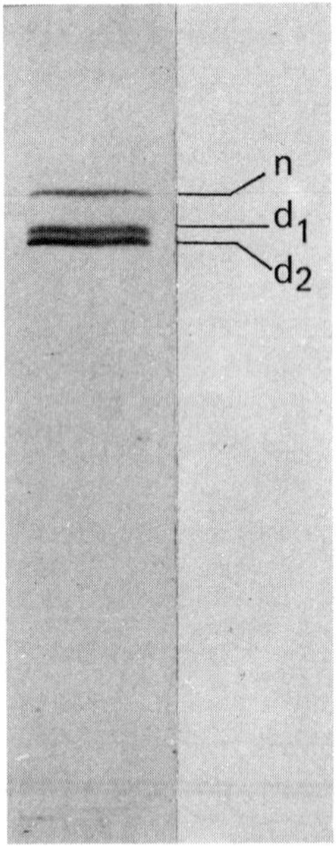

Fig. 10.9. Conformation-dependent separation in acrylamide gel: native and denatured 5 S RNA, and minor species (thought to be conformers) separated on 16% gels. The overall degree of base-pairing in the native and denatured forms is practically identical. The relative intensities have been measured and used to follow the kinetics of the conformation isomerisation process (Richards et al. 1972).

gels. Since under the conditions of the electrophoresis the rate of conversion is slow – many hours at room temperature – such a separation does not perturb the reaction, and accurately reflects the state of the equilibrium. The kinetics of the interconversion are observed at a higher temperature, and before electrophoretic analysis the aliquots of the reaction mixture, sampled at various times, are quenched by rapid cooling. Richards et al. obtained first-order rate constants for the reaction with excellent precision, as well as activation data obtained from a set of rate measurements at different temperatures. Gel electrophoresis has revealed (Richards et al. 1973) and is indeed probably the only method at present capable of revealing, that 5 S RNA appears able to enter more than these two conformational states (Fig. 10.9), and that a number of folding schemes may be energetically acceptable. It is possible that some the minor components seen in tRNA preparations may also have a similar origin.

Sensitivity of gel electrophoresis to the variants of conformation of DNA – linear, circular, nicked circular, supercoiled and single-stranded circular – has been mentioned (§ 7.6.3). So far there have been few applications of these promising findings, but there seems little reason to doubt that gel electrophoresis may come ultimately to replace isopycnic equilibrium sedimentation as a means of following conformational phemomena in DNA, such as the effects of various agencies including intercalating drugs on the degree of supercoiling.

10.3. Interacting systems

An interesting application of gel electrophoresis concerns associating systems. The analysis of boundary profiles in transport processes by analytical sedimentation and elution from gel filtration columns, has been developed to a high degree of sophistication, and is of great importance in the study of proteins. For zone transport phenomena studies have been less complete.

Eisinger (1971) and Eisinger and Blumberg (1972) have developed the theory of gel zone electrophoresis of species in rapid association-dissociation equilibrium. It is clear that in a monomer-dimer self-association two zones can never be generated, for as the monomer separates from the dimer, the disturbance of the equilibrium will cause the former to dimerise and the latter to dissociate. The result is a single skewed zone of mobility intermediate between those of monomer and dimer. The full theory, taking account of diffusion and zone profiles is complex, but experiment shows that its application gives the same result as the simplest intuitive treatment, i.e. for an equilibrium $2X \rightleftharpoons X_2$ with association constant K, the electrophoretic mobility u is given by

$$u = \alpha u_{X_2} + (1-\alpha) u_X \qquad (10.1)$$

where the suffixes refer to the mobilities of the pure dimer and monomer species and α the fraction of the monomers entering the associated state, i.e.

$$\alpha = (u - u_X)/(u_{X_2} - u_X) \qquad (10.2)$$

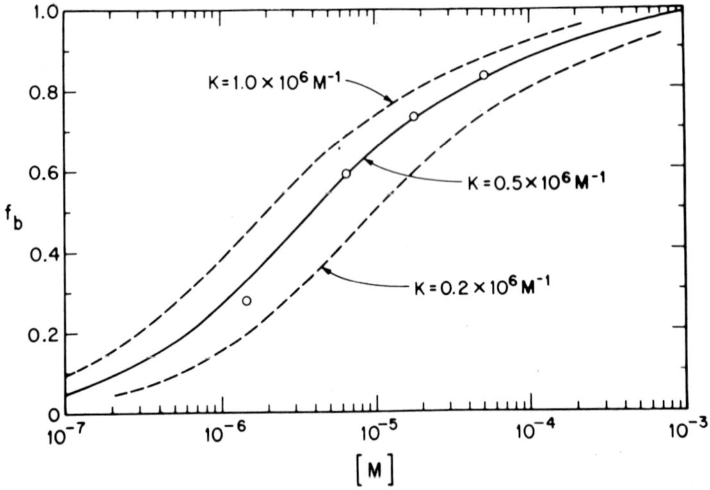

Fig. 10.10. Measurement of association constant for a system in rapid association equilibrium. The ordinate represents the extent of association of two tRNA species with mutually complementary anticodons, and is calculated at each total molar concentration M from the electrophoretic mobility of the single zone (see text). The curves are calculated for given values of the association constants (Eisinger 1971). For full details the original paper should be consulted.

Then if the total concentration (in monomer units) in the mixture is c

$$K = \alpha/(1-\alpha)^2 c \tag{10.3}$$

Thus α and hence K can be evaluated if u_X and u_{X_2} are known or inferrable. In fact it is easy to obtain at least u_X from limiting conditions (e.g. the mobility in circumstances that lead to no association); u_{X_2} can be obtained from the mobility-molecular weight relationship for the gel or can be treated as an independent variable, since a series of data can and should be obtained by varying c. Moreover, if quartz electrophoresis tubes are used, mobilities can be obtained directly with good precision to yield an association constant for two tRNA species that possess mutually complementary anticodons, and so bind strongly to each other. The results are shown in Fig. 10.10; the paper should be consulted for further details.

It is possible that similar situations involving rapid association-dissociation equilibria have been encountered in ribosomes, which under appropriate conditions exist in a reversible equilibrium 70 S $\rightleftharpoons$ 50 S + 30 S.

10.4. Enzymic degradation

Perhaps the most important application of gel electrophoresis of RNA is that of sequence determination. The work done by Sanger and his colleagues, by Fiers and his group, and by others on the sequences of high molecular weight RNA species, which are amongst the major achievements of modern molecular biology, depended on the production and isolation of suitable fragments. *A priori* it would have been expected that with only four types of residues in the RNA chain, and only a rather low nearest-neighbour preference by the known endonucleases, the chances of generating such fragments would be low. Only with the advent of gel electrophoresis was it discovered that both pancreatic and T_1 nucleases at low levels of digestion in fact produced a wide spectrum of essentially (or wholly) monodisperse fragments from ribosomal RNA (McPhie et al. 1966;

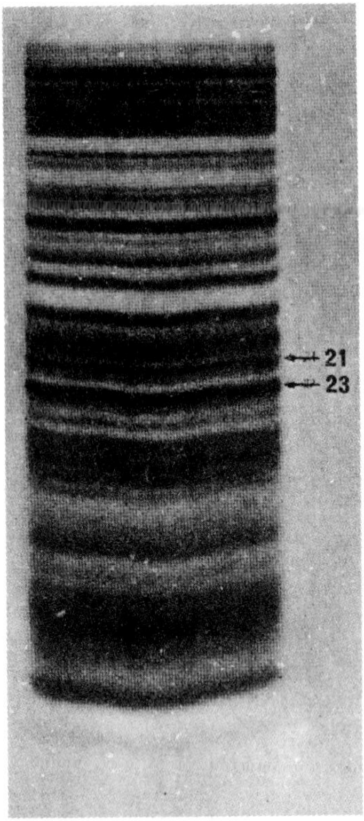

Fig. 10.11. Autoradiograph of partial T1-ribonuclease digest of ^{32}P-labeled R17 virus RNA. The bands indicated were cut out and used for sequence determination (Adams et al. 1969).

Gould, 1966). It was soon established that viral species like R17 RNA were similarly specifically cleaved (see e.g. Adams et al. 1969), and with highly labelled material the RNA extracted from a single zone in an analytical gel (see e.g. Fig. 10.11) was sufficient for fingerprinting and sequencing.

The digestion patterns are often highly reproducible and can be used as a kind of 'fingerprint', dependent only on structural features of the RNA, and offer possibilities of taxonomic applications (Gould et al. 1966; Gould 1968). Thus not only can evolutionary changes be observed over a wide variety of species, but the method can be used to establish identity, or at least close similarity, between for example two species of bacteria (Pinder et al. 1969). A quantitative criterion for describing the degree of congruence of two digestion patterns has been developed (Pinder and Gratzer 1972).

Digestion patterns have also been put to use in conformational studies. Both tRNA and 5 S ribosomal RNA can exist, as noted (§ 10.2), in two or more stable conformationally distinct forms. These show different and characteristic susceptibilities to nucleases, and the cleavage points when identified have led to partial characterisation of the conformational differences between the two forms (Jordan 1971; Streeck and Zachau 1971). Examination of fragments generated by digestion of ribosomes with nucleases, and comparison with the patterns derived from the free RNA, or from ribosomes in different states of digestion or unfolding, can in principle give information on the accessibility and conformation of the RNA in the ribosome. An analysis along these lines has been described by Pinder and Gratzer (1972). Similarly the formation of a regular set of products apparently successive multiples of a molecular weight unit by mild digestion of chromatin has, as mentioned (§ 10.1), been used to argue for a regularity in the structure of the chromatin complex (Hewish and Burgoyne 1973).

A further application is in enzymology, namely the study of nuclease specificity. The differences in the fragments generated by T_1 and pancreatic ribonucleases has been noted (Gould et al. 1966). Pinder and Gratzer (1970) examined T_1 ribonuclease digests of formaldehyde-treated essentially structureless RNA, and obtained the same digestion pattern as from the native material despite a very much higher lability. The results seem to exclude any explanation of the specific fragmentation in terms solely of conformation, instead they suggest that sequences were recognised by subsites on the enzyme, in the way already observed in proteases and amylases. The corollary is that different enzymes with the same primary specificity may differ in the fragmentation patterns produced on mild digestion; this appears indeed to be the case. The preferred cleavage modes of mammalian

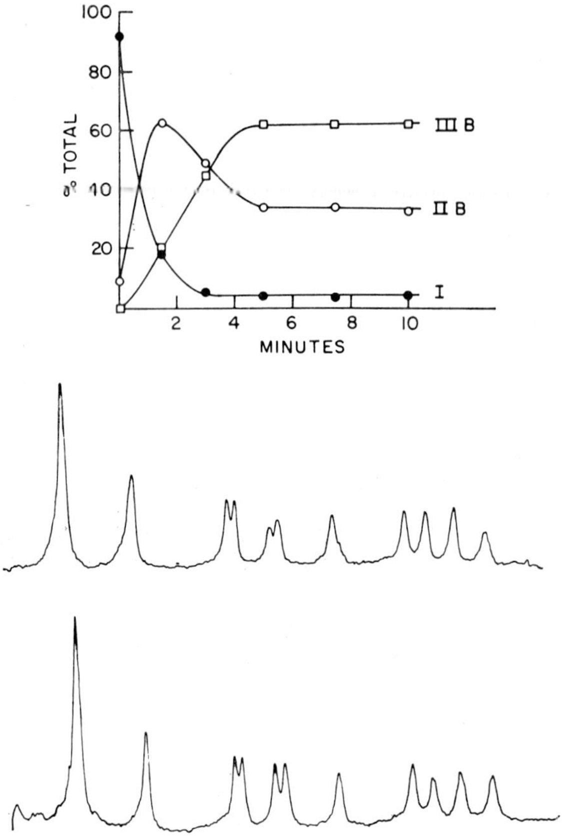

Fig. 10.12. a) Kinetics of cleavage of SV40 DNA by an *E. coli* B restriction enzyme as measured by gel electrophoresis of substrate (I) and products (IIB and IIIB). b) Use of gel electrophoresis as a 'fingerprint' to identify the products of cleavage of the parent SV40 DNA (top) and of the fragment IIIB (bottom), by *H. influenzae* restriction nuclease (Adler and Nathans 1973). Patterns represent densitometer tracing of autoradiograms.

tissue nucleases have been studied by separation and identification of cleavage products from tRNA and 5 S RNA molecules of known sequence by Philippsen and Zachau (1972a, b).

One of the most elegant applications has been in the study of restriction enzymes. The distinction between different restriction enzymes and the recognition of the sequence specificity of a given enzyme, and of the state of the DNA on which it acts, have been uniquely accomplished by examination of gel patterns. The attack of restriction enzymes from *E. coli* B strains and from *Haemophilus influenza* on SV40 DNA, in respect both of kinetics and identification of products, has been studied by Adler and Nathans (1973 and Fig. 10.12).

10.5. Nucleoprotein particles

Since this does not altogether fall within the province of the present account, only a brief survey will be given. It has long been known (e.g. Dessev et al. 1969) that whole ribosomes will migrate in agar or acrylamide gels and that 30, 50 and 70 S (or 40, 60 and 80 S) particles can be readily separated. Careful surveys of the resulting patterns turned up a number of interesting features, not apparent in sedimentation profiles. Kokileva et al. (1971) for instance found some very considerable and unexpected differences between migration rates of the 60 S subunits from the livers of eight species of vertebrates. These differences were precisely mirrored in differences in the extracted 28 S RNA, which thus evidently determines the size, or at any rate the mobility characteristics, of the nucleoprotein particle. Neither the 40 S particles nor their extracted RNA showed any differences whatever, which leads to the conclusion that evolutionary changes in eukaryotic ribosomes manifest themselves most significantly in the large subunit.

Examination of the corresponding patterns from the molecular biologist's favourite organism *E. coli* also reveals a dramatic effect. Dahlberg et al. (1969) first noted an unexpected heterogeneity in the subunits, and later Bosch and his colleagues (Talens et al. 1973) resolved both 70 S and 50 S ribosomes into four or even more components, and the 30 S into three. These workers took great pains to show that the effects did not result from an electrophoretic artefact, and it must be supposed at this stage that they represent a biological

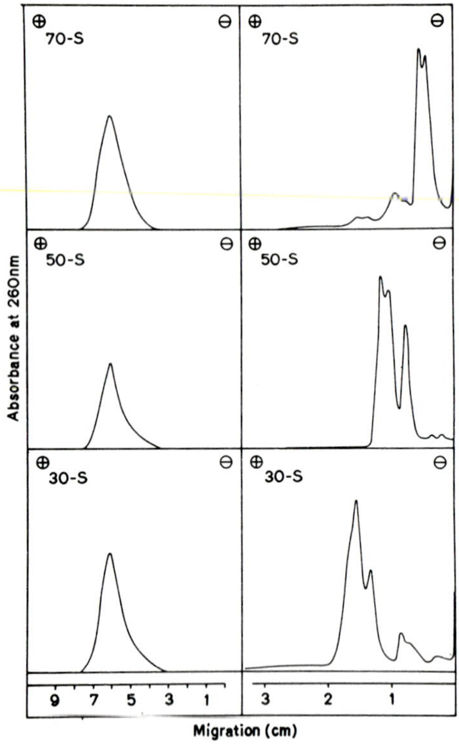

Fig. 10.13. Heterogeneity of 70 S *E. coli* ribosomes and of their subunits as revealed by electrophoresis in 4% polyacrylamide gels (right-hand panels). As the left-hand panels show, the heterogeneity is not apparent from sucrose density gradient sedimentation profiles (Talens et al. 1973).

heterogeneity (Fig. 10.13). Analysis of the proteins extracted from the various fractions may perhaps reveal the origins of the differences between the components. Most importantly, it also appears as though gel electrophoresis may be able to distinguish between some at least of the functional states of ribosomes as they pass through the protein synthesis cycle. This is one area not yet fully explored and confused by misinterpretation of sedimentation data. However, there seems no

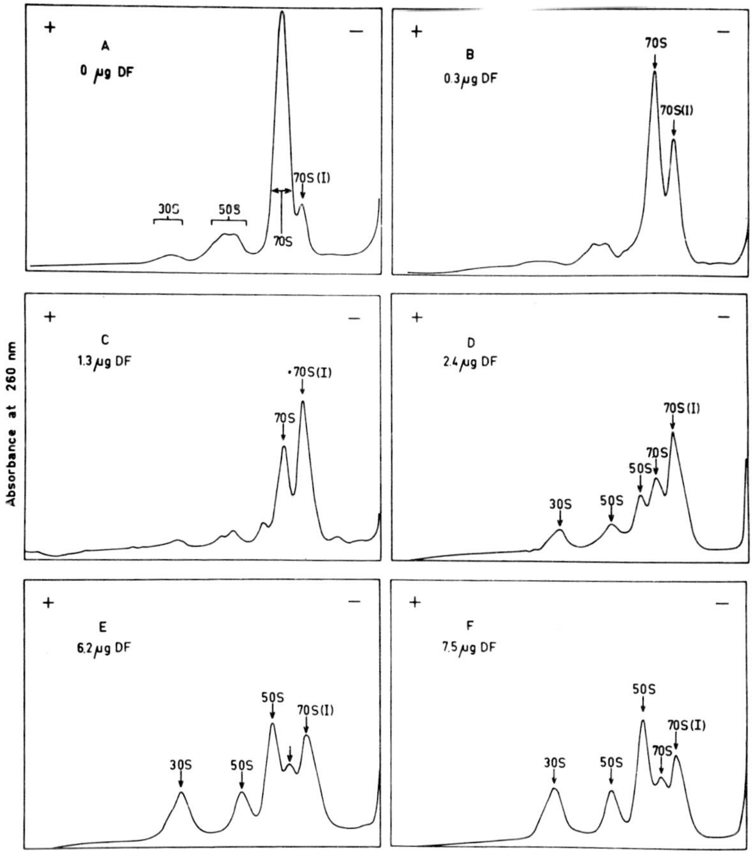

Fig. 10.14. The use of polyacrylamide gel electrophoresis to follow dissociation of *E. coli* ribosomes by increasing concentrations (as indicated) of dissociation factor (Talens et al. 1970).

doubt that a genuine intermediate of distinct conformational character appears transiently in the dissociation of the 70 S ribosome by a dissociation factor (Talens et al. 1970; Fig. 10.14). The first effect of introducing this factor into the system is the appearance of a new component which migrates more slowly than the 70 S particle. This may be an expanded state of the ribosome. When more of the dissociation factor is added both the pristine and modified 70 S particles progressively disappear to give place to the 30 and 50 S subunits.

In weak composite acrylamide-agarose gels Dahlberg et al. (1969) reported that not only ribosomes but polysomes could be made to migrate, and this provides indeed an elegant and convenient procedure for the analysis of polysome populations (Fig. 10.15). Addition of the antibiotic streptomycin which is known to bind to ribosomes, causes

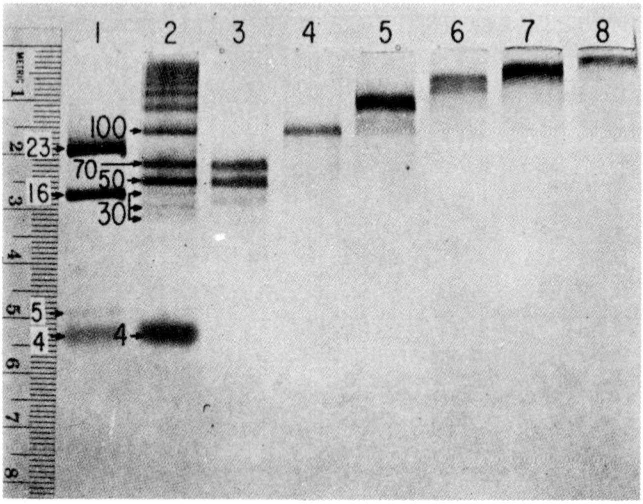

Fig. 10.15. Observations of *E. coli* polysome patterns in 2.25–0.5% polyacrylamide agarose composite gels. The samples are: (1) ribosomal RNA marker, (2) total polysomes, and (3)–(8) successive cuts of the sucrose density gradient sedimentation profile of the polysomes, from the 70 S (3) to the 28 S (8) region of the gradient (Dahlberg et al. 1969).

an unequivocal change in the mobilities of all components in the system, with no accompanying dissociation. The streptomycin may therefore exert its effect, which involves misreading of the messenger, not merely by binding to a functionally implicated ribosomal protein, but at a remove, by provoking a fairly extensive disturbance of the structure as a whole, great enough to change the hydrodynamic characteristics appreciably).

At the other end of the molecular-weight range, gel electrophoresis has been used to separate nucleolytic fragments of ribosomes in studies aimed at determining the protein contacts in the particle (Brimacombe et al. 1971; Allet and Spahr 1971). Smaller fragments of RNA carrying one or a few ribosomal proteins have also been detected by gel electrophoresis (see e.g. Garrett et al. 1971, and Fig. 10.16), taking advantage of the ability of small nucleoprotein fragments to stain both for RNA and for protein, with standard protein dyes such as Coomassie Blue or Amidoblack. The fragments have been isolated, and the RNA extracted and subjected to fingerprint

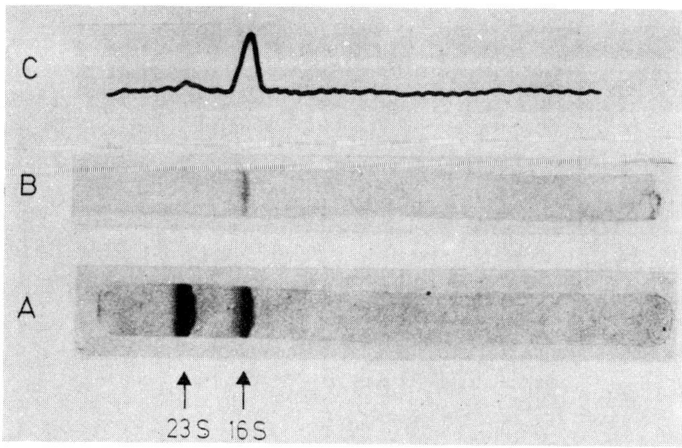

Fig. 10.16. Detection of binding of a ribosomal protein to 16 S ribosomal RNA. The presence of protein S 4 in the 16 S zone, shown in electrophoresis result (A), causes it to give a positive response to the stain Coomassie Brilliant Blue represented photographically in B and densitometrically in C (Garret et al. 1971).

analysis, so as to determine the sequences associated with the particular ribosomal proteins.

There have been a number of applications of gel electrophoresis in the virus field. We mention only a typical example: this is the analysis by Bozarth et al. (1971), of one of the polyhedral viruses found in *Penicillium* species. The RNA by gel electrophoresis is heterogeneous, with several two-stranded and single-stranded species. Two separate

Subject index p. 487

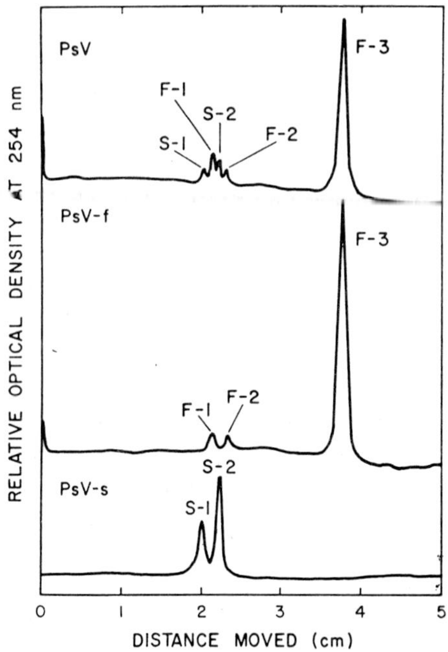

Fig. 10.17. Polyacrylamide gel electrophoresis of total RNA from different serotypes of *Penicillium stoloniferum.* F3 is a single-stranded RNA, the remainder are double-stranded (Bozarth et al. 1971).

serotypes of the virus could be isolated, and possessed different gel electrophoretic mobilities. When the RNAs were extracted from the two types they were found to be different, the one type giving rise to three double-stranded and one single-stranded component, the other to two double-stranded species, different in molecular weight from any found in the other serotype (Fig. 10.17). A similar serotype-dependent heterogeneity in double-stranded reovirus RNA is shown in Fig. 10.18 from the work of Shatkin et al. 1968).

Many new applications of gel electrophoresis will undoubtedly be devised, and the method should prove itself as generally versatile and advantageous in the study of viruses, nucleohistones, nucleo-

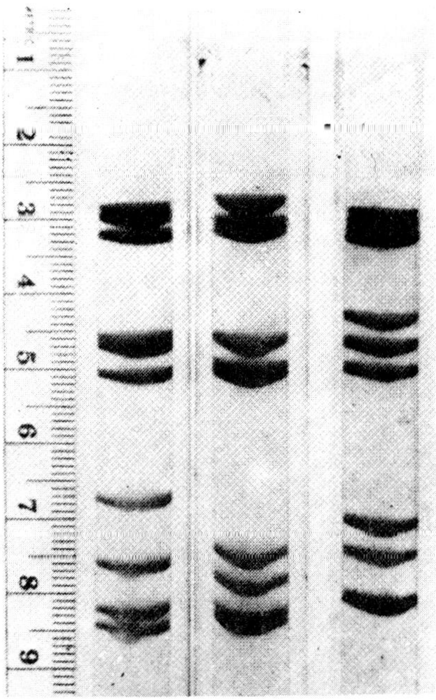

Fig. 10.18. Gel electrophoretic analysis in 2.5% acrylamide of the double-stranded RNA species present in three different reovirus serotypes. The molecular weights lie between 0.8 and 7.5 million (Shatkin et al. 1968).

protamines and ribosomes as it already has in nucleic acid chemistry and biochemistry.

10.6. Metabolic studies

Work on the metabolism of the nucleic acids has been of central interest in many areas of molecular biology, and the diversity of the applications of gel electrophoresis in this sphere no doubt reflects the very wide interest that attaches to it, as well as the advantages inherent in the method. Essentially the desired attributes of a fractionation method in such work are high resolution, rapidity, economy in terms of material and easy detection and quantitation of radioactive labels in the components. We shall give here some prominent if arbitrarily chosen examples of work of this nature, which best illustrate the extent to which these requirements are met.

Among the most successful uses of analytical gels has been the detection of precursor molecules, from which the mature species is derived by degradation. The precursor may differ little in molecular weight from its product and the resolving power of the gel method

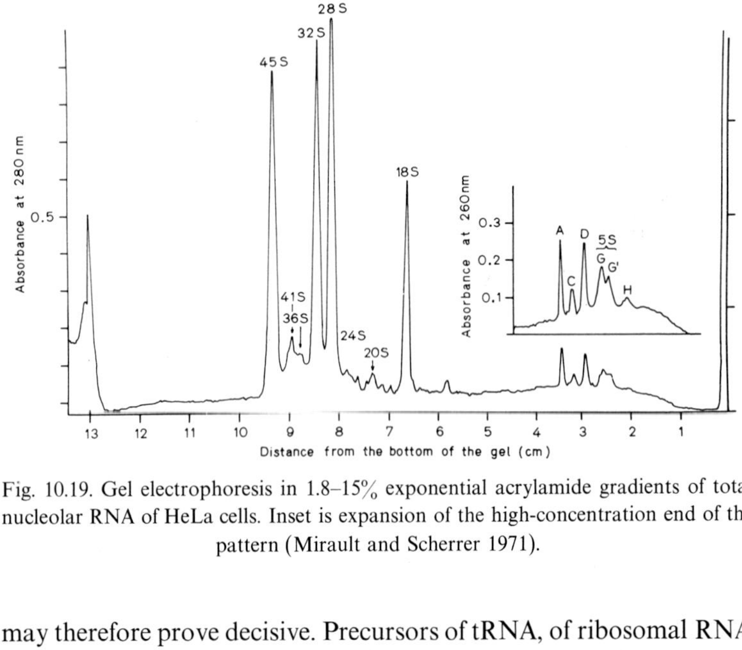

Fig. 10.19. Gel electrophoresis in 1.8–15% exponential acrylamide gradients of total nucleolar RNA of HeLa cells. Inset is expansion of the high-concentration end of the pattern (Mirault and Scherrer 1971).

may therefore prove decisive. Precursors of tRNA, of ribosomal RNA and of messenger have all been observed in this way. We show here however the observation of ribosome precursors isolated from the nucleolus of HeLa cells (Mirault and Scherrer 1971). Fig. 10.19 shows gel electrophoresis (on an acrylamide gradient which allows good resolution throughout the range) of the total nucleolar RNA extract. Fig. 10.20 demonstrates the identity of the precursors, which are rapidly labeled with tritium, relating them to the ultraviolet-

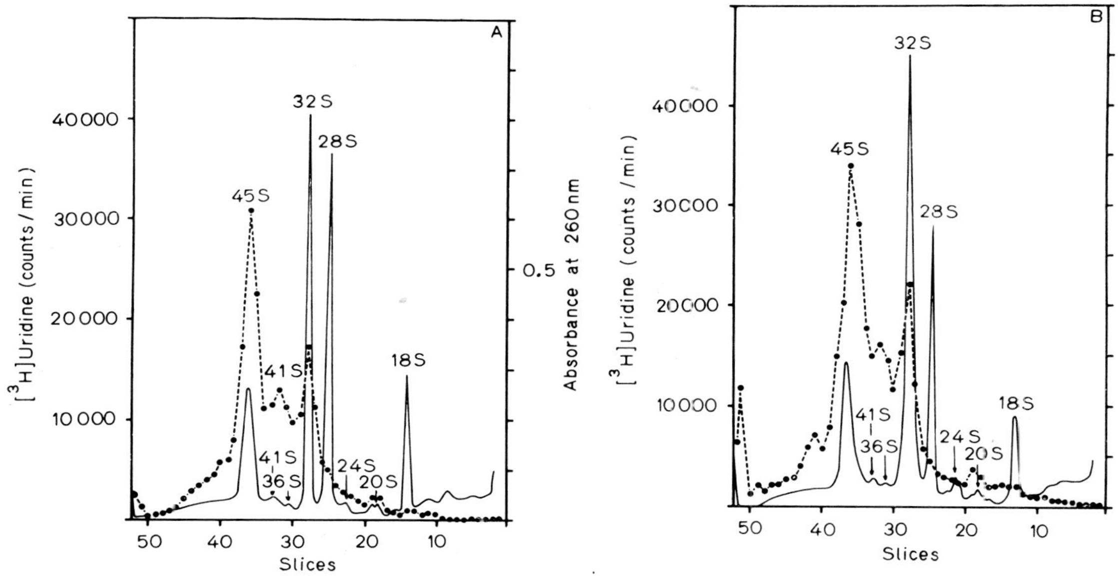

Fig. 10.20. RNA from nucleoli and from isolated preribosomes. HeLa cells were labeled for 30 min with (^{3}H)uridine (1 μCi/ml, 2 μM uridine, 2×10^6 cells/ml) and fractionated to obtain nucleoli. A) shows the pattern of the nucleolar RNA; B) pattern of the RNA released from the isolated preribosomes. Electrophoresis on 2–6% polyacrylamide exponential gel gradients (15 hr at 10 V/cm). ——, absorbance at 260 nm; - - - -, ^{3}H-radioactivity (Mirault and Scherrer, 1971).

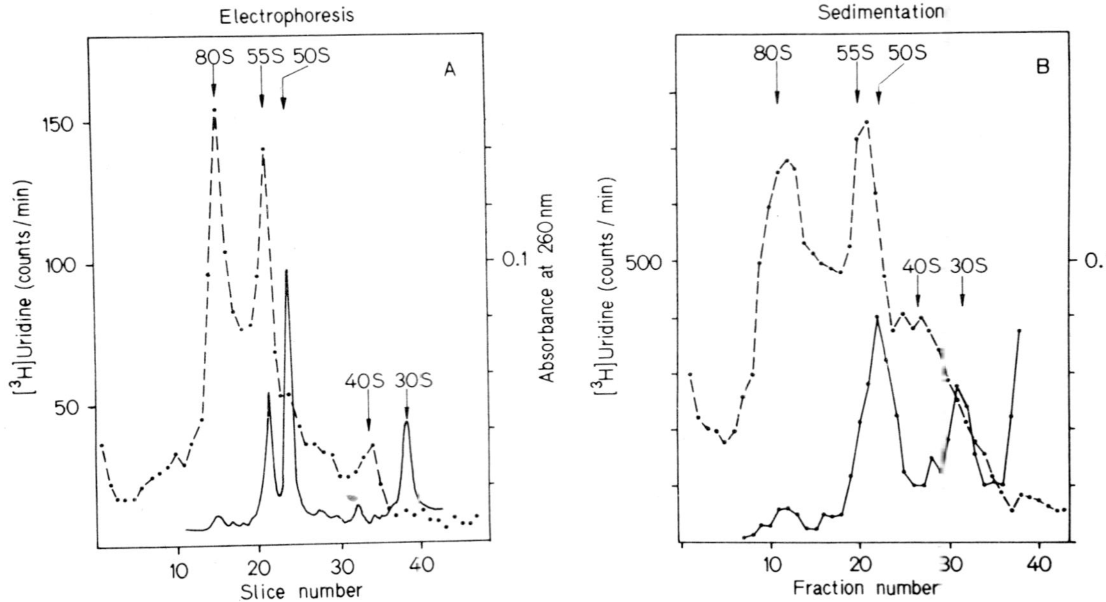

Fig. 10.21. Comparative analysis of nucleolar preribosomes by electrophoresis and sedimentation. Cells were labeled for 30 min with (^{3}H)uridine (0.3 μCi/ml, 1.2 μM uridine, 4×10^5 cells/ml) and nucleoli prepared from which the preribosomes were extracted. A) one part of these preribosomes with some cytoplasmic ribosomes as markers were analysed by electrophoresis on a 2.2% uniform polyacrylamide gel; B) Another part was analysed by sedimentation on a 5–20% sucrose gradient in EDTA-buffer (40000 rev/min 2.5 hr, 4°C, Spinco, SW40) ——, absorbance at 260 nm; ----, ^{3}H-radioactivity. This profile shows that the 55 S precursor resolves readily from the 50 S subunit of the matured ribosomes, from which it is indistinguishable in density gradient centrifugation (Mirault and Scherrer, 1971).

absorbing zones. The label is found in the 80 S, 55 S and 40 S particles, and it is to be noted how well the 55 S zone separates from the 50 S, from which it is unresolved in density gradient sedimentation. Examination of the RNA reveals that the 80 S particle contains 45 S precursor RNA, the 55 S particle 32 S RNA and the 40 S particle 20 S RNA. The fractionation of the extracted RNA, identifying the above species as precursors is shown in Fig. 10.21. In these experiments acrylamide gradients of 2–6% were used, and to obviate the difficulties of handling such gels the scans were performed directly in the quartz tubes in which the gels were set and run.

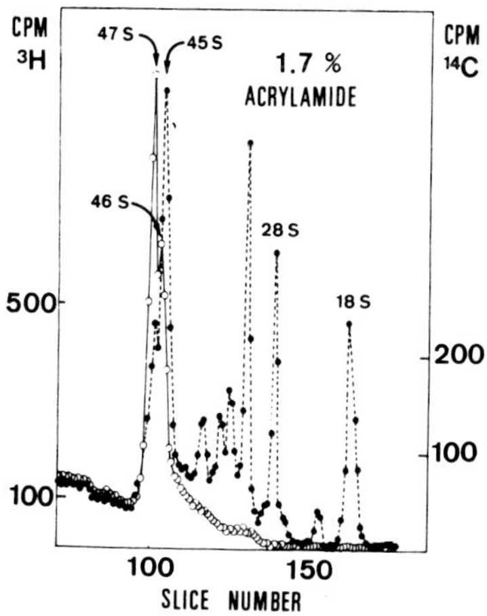

Fig. 10.22. Demonstration by gel electrophoresis of heterogeneity in the 45 S ribosomal precursor RNA from mammalian cells. Three species, nominally 45, 46 and 47 S are resolved. The visualisation of the different peaks is enhanced by labelling at different times with ^{3}H (○) and ^{14}C (●) (Tiollais et al. 1971).

An example of a result wholly dependent on the superlative resolution of acrylamide gels is shown in Fig. 10.22 (Tiollais et al. 1971). This shows that on closer examination the 45 S precursor is not homogeneous, but contains three resolvable populations, revealed by labelling for different times with the labels, ^{3}H and ^{14}C. The peaks correspond to a nominal 45, 46 and 47 S.

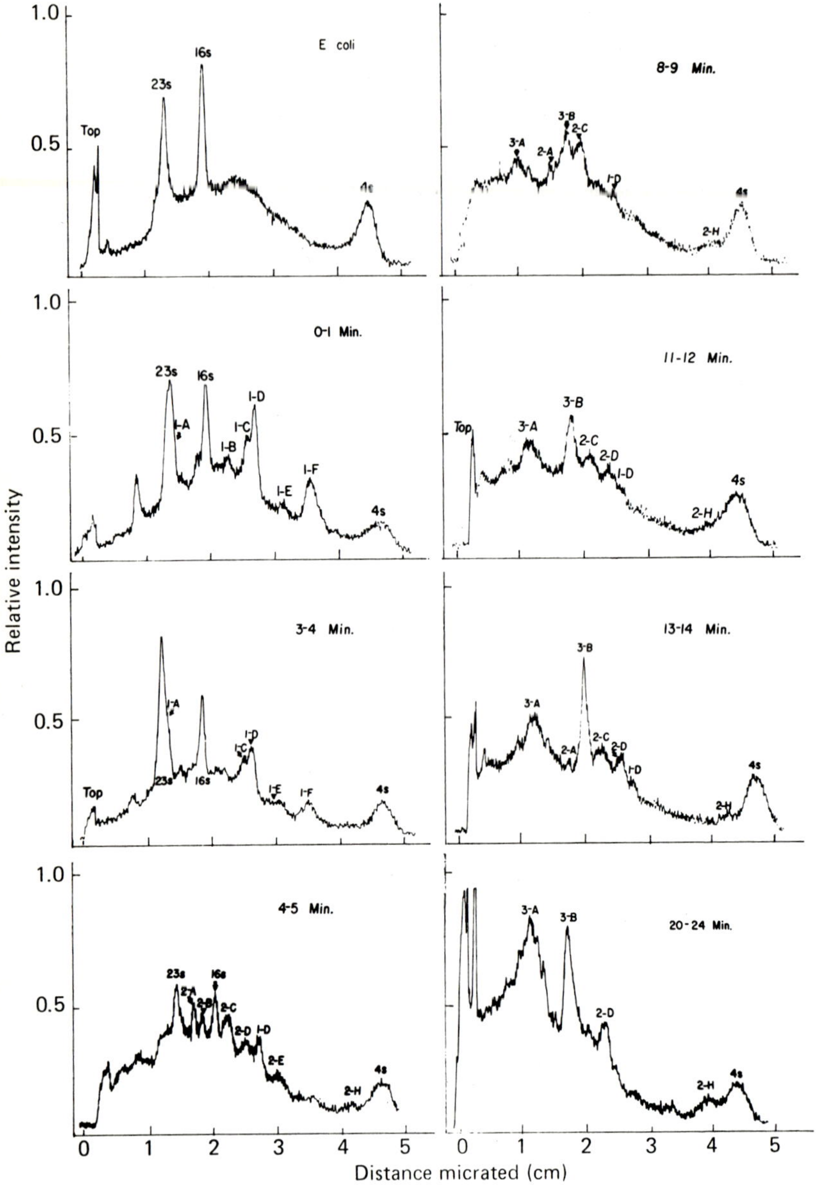
E coli
Top
23s
16s
4s
0-1 Min.
1-A
1-B
1-C
1-D
1-E
1-F
3-4 Min.
4-5 Min.
2-A
2-B
2-C
2-D
2-E
2-H
8-9 Min.
3-A
3-B
11-12 Min.
13-14 Min.
20-24 Min.
Relative intensity
Distance micrated (cm)

Another important application of gel electrophoresis has been to the events of viral infection in both bacterial and mammalian cells. Among many beautiful examples one may pick out the work of Sirbasku and Buchanan (1970), who have followed by autoradiography in acrylamide gels the events following the entry of T5 bacteriophage into *E. coli* cells (Fig. 10.23). A detailed kinetic description emerges. After transfer of the phage genome, three phage-specific types of RNA are induced, the synthesis of the first beginning immediately and continuing some 4 min. The second form begins to appear at 3–5 min and continues for perhaps 36 min. The third type puts in an appearance at 9 min and persists 45–60 min. If only a small fraction of the T5 DNA is allowed to enter, the first RNA alone subsequently appears. The manufacture of corresponding protein is needed for the cessation of RNA synthesis thereafter. The RNA in question is a product of T5 transcription, as demonstrated by hybridisation. The induced RNA types appear in phase with protein synthesis and turn up in polysomes, and are therefore presumably messengers.

Finally we give an instance of the numerous applications of gel electrophoresis to turnover studies in cellular events. Fig. 10.24 shows the labeling changes that characterise the behaviour of RNA in mitochondria. Penman et al. (1970) indicate that at least 3 different RNA polymerase systems operate in mammalian cells. By the use of specific inhibitors, such as cordycepin, it is possible to discriminate between the modes of behaviour of these systems, and in an interesting feature of the mitochondrial RNA species is that after shut-off of RNA synthesis, all the high molecular-weight species seem to decay (half life about 3 hr) in much the same manner as cytoplasmic messenger. The tRNA from the mitochondria on the other hand appears not to be subject to this degradation process, and persists for long

Fig. 10.23. Gel electrophoretic analysis of RNA synthesis in T5-bacteriophage infected *E. coli* cells. After pulse-labeling with ^3H for one minute the RNA was analysed electrophoretically at the times indicated. The profiles are densitometry traces of autoradiographs of the gels. These are used for the metabolic identification of the different classes of RNA synthesised (Sirbasku and Buchanan, 1970).

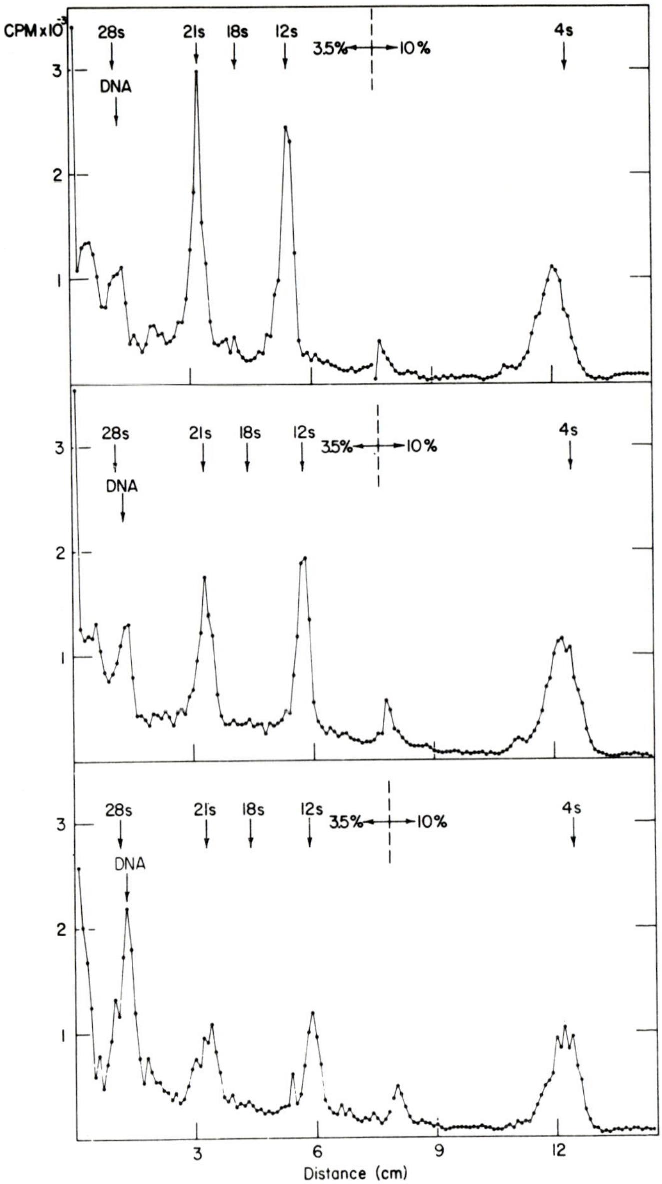
CPM x 10⁻³
28s
21s
18s
12s
3.5% ← → 10%
4s
DNA
3
2
1
3
6
9
12
Distance (cm)

periods. The labeling kinetics of the various species can, as Fig. 10.24 indicates, be readily studied individually by electrophoretic analysis.

In the same general category of applications one may include the search for new species of RNA. A number of these have come to light, and because of their low proportions to the major recognised types of RNA, and often the small extent in which they differ from some of the latter in molecular weight, could only have been detected by gel electrophoresis. Indeed the first examination by this method of a tRNA preparation revealed the presence of a number of minor components, one of them 5 S ribosomal RNA, the others of unknown character. Further evidence of such heterogeneity was adduced by Hindley (1967), and one of the unknown species, a 6 S RNA, was extracted in highly labeled form from the electrophoretic gels and its sequence determined (Brownlee 1971). Its function and origin are still unknown. At higher resolution and especially in a two-dimensional system (Ikemura and Dahlberg 1973) *E. coli* yields no less than 20 or so electrophoretic species in the 70–400 nucleotide size range, and their appearance in the cell may be followed separately by pulse labeling experiments (c.f. also the observations of Reddy et al. 1974, on the RNA of mammalian cells). Similar heterogeneity, involving a number of well-defined minor components, has been reported in *E. coli* ribosomal RNA (Shaup et al. 1969). This has been interpreted as representing a true biological heterogeneity, rather than merely adventitious degradation of the 23 S ribosomal RNA. As noted above, many examples have also been found of molecular weight heterogeneity of viral nucleic acids as extracted from the native particles. Clearly in regard to the detection of microheterogeneity the gel electrophoresis method is by far the best now available.

Fig. 10.24. Gel electrophoresis in discontinuous polyacrylamide gel (3.5 and 10% gels set in tandem, with the concentration discontinuity at the point indicated) of mitochondrial RNA after exposure to the inhibitor cordycepin (cytoplasmic RNA synthesis previously stopped with actinomycin D). From top to bottom, analyses of (^{3}H)-uridine-labeled RNA, 30, 90 and 180 min after addition of cordycepin (Penman et al. 1970).

Other techniques

11.1. Gel filtration

This technique has already been discussed fully in this series (Fischer 1969) and its application to small oligonucleotides has been mentioned (§ 1.1). Different gel types separate different useful molecular weight ranges up to about 10^8 dalton. For good resolution the sample volume must be small compared with the column volume and the viscosity must be low. So, large columns are required for preparative work. These are available commercially (e.g. Pharmacia Fine Chemicals AB).

The behaviour of nucleic acids on agarose gels has been described by Oberg and Phillipson (1967). They succeeded in partially separating, in one run, on a 2.1×60 cm column of agarose gel equivalent to Sepharose 2B, 1 mg of high molecular weight DNA, poliovirus RNA (molecular weight $= 2 \times 10^6$ daltons), ribosomal RNA and transfer RNA. The elution positions of ribosomal RNA and transfer RNA changed when the flow rate was increased from 2 to 8 ml cm^{-2} hr^{-1}. The two ribosomal RNAs were not resolved at all.

In general, the resolution is inferior to acrylamide gel electrophoresis and zone centrifugation but in situations where high resolution is not required gel filtration is a useful, reliable and predictable preparative technique.

The experimental procedure is outlined above (§ 6.6; Fischer 1969).

11.2. Sedimentation

The speed dx/dt, with which a molecule moves under the action of a centrifugal force, $\omega^2 x$, is given by $dx/dt = S\ \omega^2 x$ where S is the sedimentation coefficient for the molecule under these conditions. If the experiment is performed in water at 20°C and extrapolated to zero concentration the usually quoted sedimentation coefficient, $S_{20,w}$ is obtained. (In the ultracentrifuge x is the distance of the molecule from the centre of rotation and ω is the angular velocity in radians per second.)

The sedimentation coefficient depends on the mass of the molecule and its frictional properties, mainly surface area. For example, for single-stranded DNA in alkaline solutions $S^0_{20,w} = 0.0528\ M^{0.400}$ where M is the molecular weight; for neutral denatured DNA $S^0_{20,w} = 0.0882\ M^{0.346}$ (Studier 1965). Some fractionation of nucleic acids on the basis of sedimentation coefficient differences can be achieved in the preparative ultracentrifuge using swinging bucket rotors or, on a large scale, zonal rotors.

The details of these methods are not covered in this manual but a further introduction can be found in, for example, 'An Introduction to Ultracentrifugation' by Bowen (1970) and a great deal of detailed theory in Schachman (1959). Experimental techniques using zonal rotors are reviewed in a monograph edited by Anderson (1966) and some more recent developments are in 'Methodological Developments in Biochemical Separations' and 'Methodological Developments with Zonal Rotors' both edited by Reid (1972).

11.3. Isopycnic centrifugation

The sedimentation velocity of a molecule becomes zero when the density of the molecule equals the density of its solvent. This condition is readily obtained with DNA molecules in concentrated caesium chloride solutions. If such a solution is spun in an ultracentrifuge at speeds between 25,000 and 50,000 rev/min, the caesium chloride forms a density gradient in the rotor and the DNA molecules move to the region where their density equals that of the solvent. Apparent densities of DNA molecules (around 1.7 g ml^{-1} in CsCl) can be measured to an accuracy of ± 0.0002 g ml^{-1} and preparative fractionation of molecules differing in density by as little as 0.01 g ml^{-1} can be achieved. Such an experiment takes at last 18 hr or as much as 6 days in the centrifuge (Vinograd 1963). Preforming the gradient makes only a small saving in time.

The width of the band formed by a homogeneous macromolecule depends on the gravitational field, $\omega^2 x$, the density gradient, $d\rho/dx$, and the molecular weight of the macromolecule, M;

$$\sigma^2 = \frac{RT}{M\bar{v}} \frac{dx}{d\rho} \frac{1}{\omega^2 x} \tag{11.1}$$

where σ is the width at half height of the Gaussian band, R is the universal gas constant, T is the temperature in K, and $\bar{v}$ is the partial specific volume of the macromolecule. In practice this limits the molecular weight range of the method to DNA having $M > 10^5$ dalton approximately. RNA will not band in CsCl but can be banded in Cs_2SO_4; RNA-DNA hybrids and denatured DNA will band in CsCl at higher densities than the corresponding native double-stranded DNA.

The density, ρ, of a double stranded DNA molecule, and hence its position in the gradient, depends primarily on its nucleotide composition (eq. 2.2 gives $\rho = 1.660 + 0.098$ (GC)). The relation does not hold for DNAs containing glucosylated, methylated or other modified residues, nor for DNAs of very simple sequence such as synthetic polynucleotides, crab poly dAT (Wells et al. 1970) and 'centromeric' DNA. Single stranded DNA is denser than double stranded DNA and isopycnic centrifugation can be used to separate them.

11.3.1. Preparing the gradient

The following conditions are routinely used for isopycnic banding of sonicated DNA, molecular weight around 5×10^5 dalton. The preferred rotor for preparative runs is an angle rotor such as the 8×35 ml angle rotor for MSE preparative ultracentrifuge. This type of rotor gives better resolution than swing-out or angle rotors with the tubes less nearly vertical (Flamm et al. 1969). Each 35 ml tube contains 20.0 g water or dilute buffer, 25.4 g CsCl (AnalaR grade from B.D.H. is satisfactory for routine preparative work) and 1 mg solid DNA. Larger loads reduce resolution, partly because the high viscosity in the band makes collection difficult. This gives a CsCl solution of density 1.70 g ml^{-1} which is suitable for DNA with a G+C content of 42%. The density can be checked by measuring the refractive index with an Abbe refractometer and using the equation:

$$\rho = (10.8601 \times \mu_D) - 13.4974 \tag{11.2}$$

where ρ is density in g/cm^3 and μ_D is the refractive index at 25°C at the wavelength of the sodium D line (Ifft et al. 1961; Brunier and Vinograd 1965). The volume of the gradient is (20.0+25.4)/1.70= 26.7 ml. Data for other densities and volumes are given in Table 11.1. When sharp, well characterised, bands are being centrifuged smaller volumes of CsCl are quite adequate.

The tube is then filled with liquid paraffin, to stabilise the gradient and reduce tube collapse. The small vacuum seal Allen Screw is

TABLE 11.1

Making up CsCl solutions.

Density 25°C g ml^{-1}	CsCl concentrations % w/w	Mass of water*	Mass of CsCl*	μ_D
1.66	54.2	7.6	9.0	1.3957
1.67	55.1	7.5	9.2	1.3966
1.68	55.4	7.5	9.3	1.3975
1.69	55.9	7.45	9.45	1.3985
1.70	56.2	7.45	9.55	1.3994
1.71	56.7	7.4	9.7	1.4003
1.72	57.0	7.4	9.8	1.4012
1.73	57.2	7.4	9.9	1.4021
1.74	58.0	7.3	10.1	1.4031
1.75	58.3	7.35	10.15	1.4040
1.76	58.6	7.4	10.2	1.4049

* For 10 ml final volume.

removed from a stainless steel cap (CsCl attacks aluminium) and the cap is fitted to the tube and tightened. The screw is then replaced and the tube wiped free from liquid paraffin. The tubes are loaded into the rotor and spun, usually at 20°C or 25°C. Nuclease activity is strongly inhibited in concentrated CsCl solution so degradation of the DNA is not usually a problem.

TABLE 11.2

Conditions for isopycnic equilibrium in CsCl solutions at 25°C. DNA molecular weight $> 10^7$ dalton. For smaller DNAs use longer gradients and spinning times. These conditions are not exclusive; many variations are useful.

Rotor	Gradient volume ml	Gradient length cm	Speed rev·min^{-1} $\times 10^{-3}$	Time of run hr
MSE 10 × 10 ml	4.5	1.8	35	60
MSE 10 × 10 ml	4.5	1.8	42	22
MSE 8 × 50 ml	10	1.9	30	70
MSE analytical	0.65	1.2	45	20
Beckman 40	4.5	1.6	33	60
Beckman SW 39	3.0	2.8	33	60
Beckman 30	10	1.9	25	90

The speed of the centrifuge is limited because stainless steel caps reduce the top rotor speed by 25% and the mean density of the gradient and paraffin in the tube may be more than 1.2 g ml^{-1}. Low speeds give shallower gradients and better separation of bands although the band width also increases. The time required to reach equilibrium is greater at lower speeds. For an overnight run, 18 hr, a speed of 40,000 rpm is recommended. For maximum resolution a speed of 28,000 rpm for 6 days has been used. Conditions for other rotors are given in Table 11.2.

11.3.2. Collecting the gradient

DNA is not normally visible in solution, although it can be stained

(§ 11.3.3), so the band(s) must be located by ultraviolet absorption or other means. In general, the gradient must be collected either in fractions or through a continuous flow monitor. Complete semi-automatic systems for this process are available commercially (e.g. Isco; International Equipment Co.).

If these systems are not used the gradient can be collected from the top or bottom of the tube. Fig. 11.1 shows an arrangement for collecting from the top. The tube cap is removed and the liquid paraffin taken off the top of the gradient, together with any pellicle

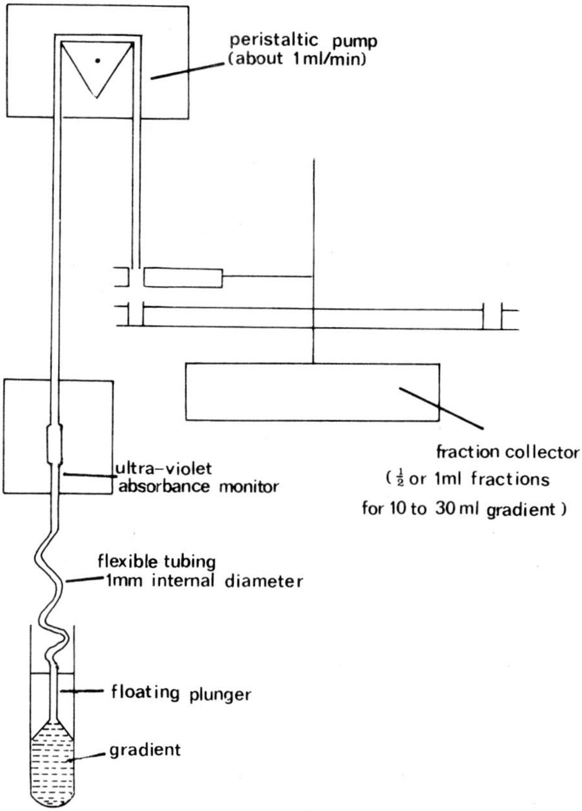

Fig. 11.1. Fractionating a density gradient from the top.

(the skin formed by proteins and other less dense materials). A plunger, machined from PTFE (polytetrafluoroethylene) to be a sliding fit in the centrifuge tube, is placed on the gradient which is then sucked out, the plunger floating down as the gradient is removed. The diagram shows an ultraviolet absorbance monitor and a fraction collector but these are not essential. Other methods for collection from the top use dense CsCl or mineral oil to displace the gradient from the bottom. The dense liquid is introduced through a hole punched in the bottom or the side of the tube or through a hollow needle carefully lowered into the gradient from the top.

The gradient can be collected from the bottom of the tube by punching a hole in the bottom and allowing the gradient to drip out. Dripping by gravity is not very reliable and so the gradient is forced out by liquid paraffin introduced through the top, Fig. 11.2. This requires an airtight seal at the top which is most easily obtained by drilling a 1-mm diameter hole through one of the Allen screws that provides the vacuum seal in the centrifuge tube cap and then fitting a stainless steel or PTFE tube on the top. After centrifuging with a normal Allen screw the centrifuge tube cap is left fitted to the centrifuge tube and the Allen screw is simply removed and replaced with the modified one. The top of the tube is then clamped off (leave open during fitting to centrifuge tube to prevent pressure building up inside the tube). The hole in the bottom is made with a large dissecting needle or hand drill. Under the conditions described no air bubble will be sucked in at the bottom and only a very little of the gradient will leak out when the needle is removed from the hole. If the gradient is to be passed through a monitor an open, dry hollow needle (syringe needle) is used and left in the centrifuge tube so that the gradient will pass out through it.

If a monitor is not used the gradient may be forced out with a pump or a syringe. In the syringe method a fixed volume, for example, 0.5 or 1 ml for a 10 to 25 ml gradient, of liquid paraffin is forced in at the top and an equal volume of gradient is collected from the bottom of the centrifuge tube. This is repeated until the whole gradient is collected (Fig. 11.2a). If a continuous flow monitor

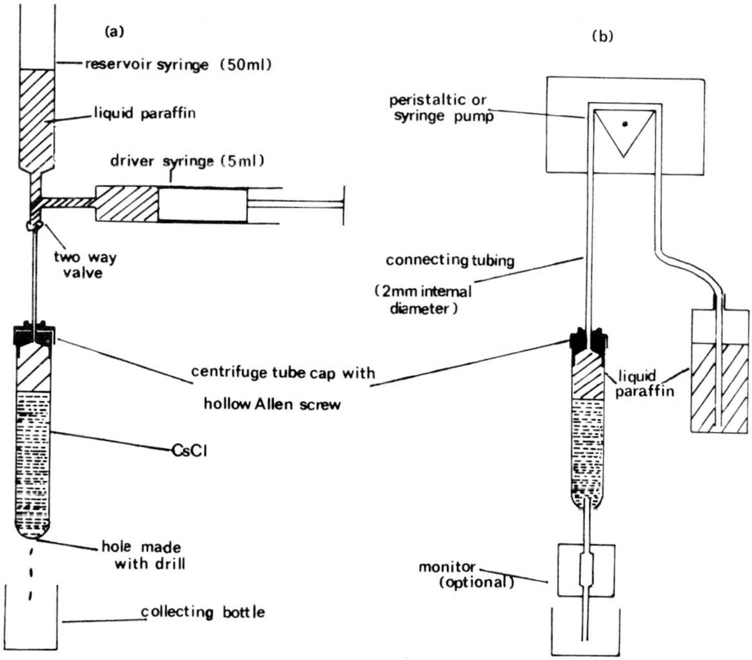

Fig. 11.2. Fractionating a density gradient from the bottom. a) manual syringe method; b) pump method.

is used the pump method is essential and the gradient is pumped out continuously using the monitor indication, drop counting, weighing or timing to collect fractions (Fig. 11.2b). A syringe pump is particularly suitable for this application because of its smooth action and limited volume required. The density of the gradient can be continuously monitored using a refractive index monitor, a vibrating tube monitor (Stanton Redcroft Ltd), or a β-particle absorption monitor (Atherton et al. 1972; Cope and Matthews 1972). Otherwise the density of individual fractions can be calculated from their refractive indices.

The density gradient fractionator marketed by MSE provides a useful stand for these methods. The hollow Allen screw adaptor can be fitted to the top mount and the bottom mount can be used as supplied for the hollow needle methods. It is essential that the bottom assembly is completely dry when it is used to pierce the tube. If it is wet, air bubbles can be introduced at the bottom and wreck the gradient as they float up to the top.

11.3.3. Some general hints

i) The presence of liquid paraffin around the tube vacuum seal seems to help to keep it air-tight during fractionation of the gradient; ii) connecting tubing and flow cell(s) carrying the gradient should be

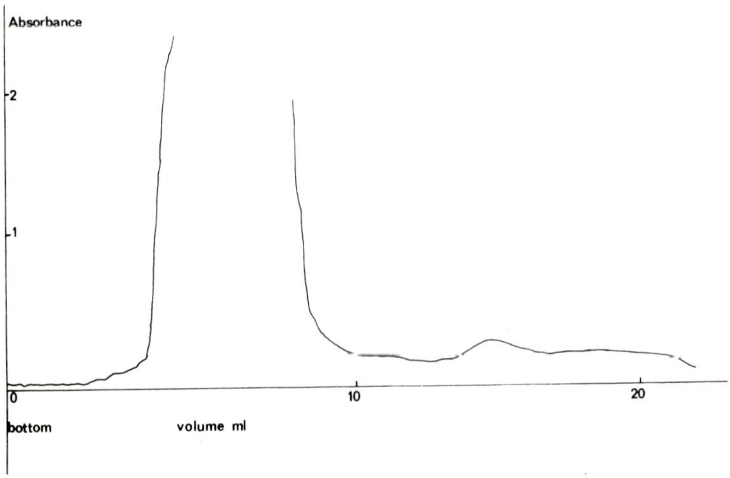

Fig. 11.3. Record obtained from monitoring a preparative CsCl gradient containing 1 mg DNA using the arrangement of Fig. 11.2b.

arranged vertically if possible so that the gradient stabilises the flow as in Figs. 11.1 and 11.2; iii) don't mistake a glycogen (or other polysaccharide) band sensitive to α-amylase but not ribonuclease or deoxyribonuclease, for a DNA satellite (Brunk and Hanawalt 1966).

The result of passing a preparative gradient of sonicated *Physarum polycephalum* DNA in CsCl through an ultraviolet absorbance monitor is shown in Fig. 11.3. The ultraviolet absorbing region can be collected by watching the monitor output. Alternatively, 1 ml fractions can be measured after fractionation (Fig. 11.4). These results were obtained by the pump and hollow needle method of collecting from the bottom (Fig. 11.2b).

The DNA can be seen directly in the CsCl gradient by reversibly staining with ethidium bromide (Firtel and Bonner 1971). Solid CsCl is added to the DNA solution to make the density up to about 1.55 g ml^{-1} (0.97 g CsCl to each 1 ml original DNA solution) followed by 1/20 volume of ethidium bromide solution (10 mg/ml in water). Spinning time is 48 hr at 40,000 rev/min. RNA and

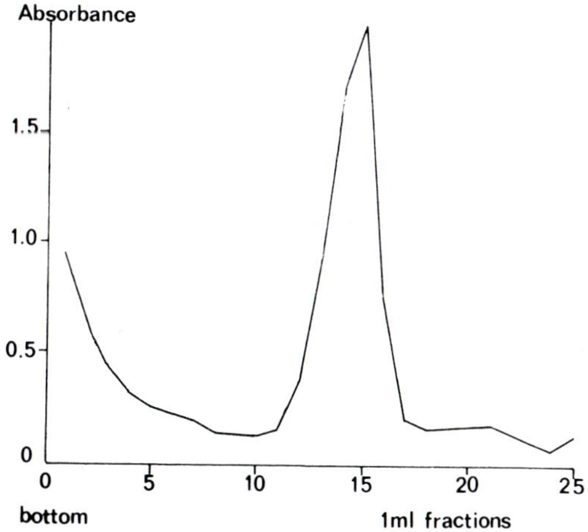

Fig. 11.4. Ultraviolet absorbance measurements on individual fractions from a CsCl gradient. The centre peak is DNA. The absorbance at the bottom of the gradient is probably due to RNA.

protein are stained red and appear banded, at the bottom and at the top respectively. The DNA density is reduced by the ethidium bromide so it bands well above any polysaccharide. The stained DNA can be seen readily using fluorescence in near ultraviolet light. The ethidium bromide is removed by diluting the DNA band with 3 vol of water and extracting twice with an equal volume of *iso*pentyl alcohol. The DNA can then be precipitated with two volumes of 2-ethoxyethanol.

11.3.4. Analytical isopycnic centrifugation

Standard conditions are 20 hr at 45,000 rev/min using 1 to 5 μg DNA. Densities are normally calculated with reference to a DNA of known density which is present in the centrifuge cell with the DNA to be analysed. Usually a standard DNA density 10 or 20 mg/ml above or below the sample DNA can be used (e.g. *Micrococcus lysodeiktius*, $\rho = 1.731$ g/ml; *Escherichia coli* or T7 phage, $\rho = 1.710$ g/ml; Sober 1968). The density is given by

$$\rho = \rho_0 + 4.2\,\omega^2 (r^2 - r_0^2)\,10^{-10}\ \text{g cm}^{-3} \tag{11.3}$$

where ρ is the density of a band distance r from the centre of rotation, ρ_0 is the density of the reference band at r_0 and ω is the angular velocity in radians s^{-1} (Vinograd 1963). The reference DNA and the density assumed for it must always be clearly stated.

In the special case of a homogeneous DNA the width of the band can be used to determine the molecular weight (Vinograd 1963, eq. 10.1).

Glycogen can be recognised in the analytical ultracentrifuge by its high index of refraction and low ultraviolet absorbance if Schlieren and absorbance traces of the same run are compared (Brunck and Hanawalt 1966).

11.3.5. Silver and mercury complexes in Cs_2SO_4 gradients

Silver and mercury ions bind to the bases in a DNA molecule with a preference for G-C base pairs. The complex appears denser in Cs_2SO_4 solutions and so the resolution of two DNA species, differing in G+C content, by density gradient centrifugation can be increased by a partial binding of silver or mercury to the component which is already the denser (Nandi, Wang and Davidson 1965; Jensen and Davidson 1966). The binding is reversible.

The method given by Jensen and Davidson (1966) is as follows:

add a small volume of purified concentrated DNA solution in 0.01 M Na_2SO_4 to a stock solution of Cs_2SO_4 in 0.1 M cacodylate buffer *p*H 8.0. Add a small volume of concentrated $Ag(NO_3)_2$ solution and stir gently. Spin the solution to equilibrium. By adding successive aliquots of silver nitrate the conditions for the resolution can be found.

The density of DNA in Cs_2SO_4 is much less than in CsCl because of different hydration. In the absence of added ions *E. coli* DNA, for example, bands near $\rho = 1.43$ g cm^{-3}. Added silver ions raise the density in proportion to added silver up to $\rho = 1.58$ g cm^{-3} at a molar ratio of silver added to DNA phosphate of about 0.55. The density at 25°C, ρ, of Cs_2SO_4 solutions is given by

$$\rho = 13.6986 n_{\mathrm{D}}^{25} - 17.3233 \tag{11.4}$$

where n_{D}^{25} is the refractive index at 25°C of the sodium D line (Vinograd and Hearst 1962) but the constant changes slightly to 17.3108 in the presence of 0.1 M cacodylate buffer *p*H 8.0 (Jensen and Davidson 1966).

The solutions must be free from silver complexing agents like chloride, EDTA or Tris buffer.

11.3.6. Applications

Preparative gradients have been widely used for preparing ‘satellite’ DNAs such as the highly repetitous mouse satellite, the DNA sequences coding for ribosomal RNA and mitochondrial DNA (e.g. Flamm et al. 1969). They can be used for separating RNA-DNA hybrids from native and denatured DNA for preparative and analytical purposes (e.g. Birnstiel et al. 1968). DNA can be density-labelled with deuterium, ^{15}N and bromo-deoxyuridine and normal and heavy DNA separated (e.g. Meselson, Stahl and Vinograd 1957; Braun and Wili 1969).

11.4. Hydroxyapatite (HAP)

Hydroxyapatite is an insoluble form of calcium phosphate. The mechanism of DNA binding to hydroxyapatite (HAP) is not understood, but it is well established that native and denatured DNA can be quantitatively separated using the property that although both types of DNA bind in low concentrations of phosphate buffer (equal volumes of 0.03 M KH_2PO_4 and K_2HPO_4 or the respective sodium phosphates), denatured DNA is selectively released by 0.12 M phosphate buffer and native DNA can then be recovered using 0.3 M phosphate buffer (Bernardi 1969). The presence of other salts does not seem to be important but urea and/or a detergent such as sodium dodecyl sulphate (SDS) are used to improve recovery of high molecular weight DNA and calcium complexing agents like citrate and ethylenediamintetraacetic acid (EDTA) must be absent. Bernardi (1971) has recently described the use of HAP for nucleic acid fractionation.

11.4.1. Preparing HAP

Hydroxyapatite is available commercially (e.g. Bio-Rad Laboratories). The crystals should be treated carefully to avoid breaking them and fines should be decanted thoroughly before use.

It can also be made in the laboratory from cheaper chemicals by the following method (Tiselius et al. 1956). First, dissolve 2 g of $Ca(OH)_2$ in 1 l of distilled water in cold room and keep this as a saturated calcium hydroxide solution. Take a 1 l beaker containing 120 ml 0.5 M sodium phosphate *p*H 6.8 (equimolar amounts of Na_2HPO_4 and NaH_2PO_4) and stir very vigorously at room temperature; add 100 ml 0.5 M $CaCl_2$ drop-wise and continue stirring for 1 hr. Let the precipitate settle and pour off the supernatant. Wash the precipitate once with 600 ml distilled water. Add another 600 ml distilled water and transfer the slurry to a 5-l beaker. Add 750 ml saturated $Ca(OH)_2$, make the solution up to 4 l and boil for at least 30 min with stirring. Add more $Ca(OH)_2$ if the *p*H drops below 8.5 during the boiling. Decant the supernatant while hot to remove small crystals and then wash the precipitate 7 times with 600 ml 5 mM phosphate buffer *p*H 6.7. Treat the crystals gently as they are fragile and a large crystal size is required. Store the hydroxyapatite wet under 50 ml 5 mM phosphate buffer at *p*H 6.7.

An improvement in crystal size and reproducibility can be obtained by boiling the hydroxyapatite in 50 mM phosphate buffer 6.7 before use, whatever its source. Hydroxyapatite can in principle be regenerated by washing in 0.5 M or stronger phosphate buffer and then boiling in dilute buffer as above. Fresh hydroxyapatite is probably more popular.

11.4.2. Column method

Columns of hydroxyapatite are packed and operated in the same ways as other columns except that high operating pressures cannot be used. Stepwise and gradient elution are both used and high operating temperatures, up to 100°C, may be required. This can be achieved by circulating hot water through the column jacket. The temperature of the column is measured with a thermometer, preferably thermocouple or thermistor, in the eluting buffer just above the top of the bed of hydroxyapatite. The buffers must be thoroughly degassed and kept at the temperature the column is being operated at. This is simply arranged by using a water-bath with a circulating pump to heat both buffer solutions and the jacketed column. Suitable apparatus is manufactured by for example, Grant Instruments Ltd. (Water bath and circulating pump); Pharmacia Fine Chemicals AB (column); Comark Electronics Ltd. (thermo couple probe, and thermometer). For temperatures over 90°C glycerol can be added to the circulating water (Miyazawa and Thomas 1965).

11.4.3. Centrifuge method

Step-wise elution from a column can be replaced by centrifugation and washing. This is particularly advantageous where a simple absorption and/or elution procedure is carried out on a number of samples. The column and the centrifuge give identical results (Brenner, Fanning, Rake and Johnson 1969). A small bench centrifuge taking 10 ml glass tubes is normally used. For temperatures above 25°C the centrifuge is heated or placed in an oven. A suitable heated centrifuge is available from Laboratory Thermal Equipment Ltd. who use an MSE minor centrifuge and a heating jacket with thermostat control up to 80°C. The hydroxyapatite slurry and solution to be assayed or the elution buffer are gently mixed, incubated at the temperature required for 3 min then mixed again and spun just hard enough to sediment the hydroxyapatite (e.g. 500 rpm, for 1 min including acceleration and slowing down without braking in a small swing-out rotor). The supernatant can be poured or pipetted off and further elution steps carried out. Incubation can be carried out in the centrifuge but for higher temperatures, such as 60°C, a water bath is recommended because of the poor heat transfer in the centrifuge.

For both methods the capacity of hydroxyapatite to absorb DNA is very approximately 100 μg DNA per ml packed hydroxyapatite or 400 μg DNA per g dry hydroxyapatite.

11.4.4. Applications

The use of hydroxyapatite for DNA-fractionation exploits either the process of DNA denaturation or DNA reassociation. DNA denaturation is the separation of the two complementary strands of native DNA by heat or agents like formamide or other methods. Denaturation takes place more easily the higher the A+T content of the DNA. Reassociation is the forming of a complementary double helix from single strands of DNA. This depends mainly on the concentrations of the complementary strands and hence on the repetition frequency of the sequence involved (Britten and Kohne 1966, 1968).

11.4.4.1. DNA denaturation

The separation on hydroxyapatite of DNAs on the basis of their A+T content can utilise progressive DNA denaturation. The DNA is bound to hydroxyapatite in 0.12 M phosphate buffer at room temperature. The hydroxyapatite is washed with 0.12 M phosphate buffer at a temperature below that at which denaturation is expected, e.g. 75°C for a 60% A+T DNA (§ 2.4.2) and repeatedly washed with this buffer at suitable temperature increments, e.g. 2.5°C, until all the DNA is eluted. As the DNA denatures, due to temperature rise, it will be eluted from the hydroxyapatite in 0.12 M phosphate buffer as single-stranded DNA. If, at any point, the remaining double-stranded DNA is required it can be eluted with 0.3 M phosphate buffer. Although this method works (Miyazawa and Thomas 1965; McCallum and Walker 1967), it is not often used because isopycnic centrifugation in caesium chloride solutions (§ 11.3) has advantages in practice, provided an ultracentrifuge is available and the DNA is fully native (but see, for example, Saunders et al. 1972).

11.4.4.2. DNA reassociation

Hydroxyapatite is frequently used to assay DNA reassociation (Britten and Kohne 1968). The precision of reassociation depends critically on the conditions of incubation and a detailed discussion of these is beyond the scope of this manual (but see Britten and Kohne 1968; Church and McCarthy 1968; Wetmur and Davidson 1968; Seidler and Mandel 1971). For preparative purposes the method is largely used to prepare denatured DNA or reassociated DNA that is not usually perfectly matched.

The general principle is to prepare denatured DNA by heating native DNA dissolved in 0.12 M phosphate buffer at 100°C for 10 min and then incubating the solution at $(T_m - 25)$°C. T_m is the thermal denaturation temperature of the native DNA in 0.12 M phosphate buffer. If the initial absorbance of the DNA solution was A_{260} at a wavelength of 260 nm and 10 mm path length then the incubation time is characterised by the parameter C_0t where

$$C_0t = 0.500 \times A_{260} \times \text{incubation time in hr} \qquad (10.5)$$

C_0t has the units of moles of nucleotides × sec × litres^{-1}. The T_m and hence temperature of incubation can be reduced by lowering the ionic strength of the buffer or adding agents like formamide.

After this incubation the solution is added to hydroxyapatite (column or centrifuge tube) usually at $(T_m - 15)$°C and the unreassociated, single-stranded, DNA is eluted with 0.12 M phosphate buffer. Reassociated, double-stranded, DNA is eluted with 0.30 M phosphate buffer.

Subject index p. 487

The single-stranded DNA can be incubated further and fractionated again. The following scheme has been used by Britten and Smith (1970) and Saunders et al. (1972) for mammalian DNA. Denature DNA and incubate to $C_0t=10$. Separate single-stranded (S) and double-stranded (D) fractions. Incubate fraction S to a total $C_0t=50$ and separate single stranded (S,S) and double stranded (S,D) fractions. Denature and incubate fraction D to $C_0t=0.05$ and separate single stranded (D,S) and double stranded (D,D) fractions. Incubate fraction D,S to total $C_0t=1$ and separate single stranded (D,S,S) and double stranded (D,S,D) fractions. Denature and incubate fraction D,D to $C_0t=0.02$ and separate single stranded (D,D,S) and double stranded (D,D,D) fractions. Fraction S,S is called 'single copy' or 'unique' DNA; fractions S,D+D,S,S are called 'slowly reassociating' DNA; fractions D,S,D+D,D,S are called 'intermediate' DNA and fraction D,D,D is called 'fast' or 'rapidly reassociating' DNA. Different C_0t values are needed for organisms with different genome sizes.

A simpler separation into 'unique' and 'repeated' DNA can be achieved in one or two incubations designed with a C_0t large enough to reassociate the repeated DNA but not the 'unique' DNA. For example, a C_0t of 225 can be used to prepare 'unique' DNA from *Dictyostelium discoideum* (Firtel and Bonner 1971).

11.5. Affinity chromatography

Complementary base pairing between single-stranded nucleic acid chains can be used as a separation method if one strand is bound to an insoluble matrix. This approach has found widespread use in preparing messenger RNA (mRNA) molecules most of which are found to have poly (A) sequences at their 3′ ends. These poly (A) sequences will bind to poly (U) or poly (T) oligonucleotides in high salt at neutral *p*H and low temperature e.g. 0.12 M NaCl, 10 mM Tris *p*H 7.4, 1 m M EDTA at room temperature and will be freed by relaxing these conditions, e.g. 0.2% sodium dodecyl sulphate (SDS), 10 mM Tris, *p*H 7.4, 1 mM EDTA at 37°C. The use of temperatures above room temperature can be avoided by eluting in the presence of a denaturing agent such as 50% formamide (Jacobson et al. 1974; Ojala and Attardi 1974). The insoluble matrix can be cellulose powder or filters (Sheldon et al. 1972) or Sepharose (agarose gel beads) (Wagner et al. 1971). The absorbent can be obtained ready for use from Miles Laboratories Ltd. (poly (U) and poly (T) cellulose) and Pharmacia Fine Chemicals (poly (U) – Sepharose).

Appendix

Addresses of manufacturers and suppliers mentioned in the text

Amersham, The Radiochemical Centre, Amersham, Bucks, England.
Ashland Chemicals, Columbus, Ohio, U.S.A.
Baker, J. T., Chemical Co., Phillipsburg, N.J., U.S.A.
Balston, W. and R., Ltd., Springfield Mill, Maidstone, Kent, England.
Beckman Instruments, Glenrothes, Scotland, U.K.
BioRad Laboratories, 32nd Avenue, Richmond, Calif. 94804, U.S.A.
British Drug Houses (BDH) Ltd., Poole, Dorset, England.
Buchler Instruments Inc., 1327 16th Street, Fort Lee, N.J., U.S.A.
Camlab (Glass) Ltd., Cambridge, England.
Cargille Laboratories Inc., Cedar Grove, N.Y., U.S.A.
Chromatronix, 2743 Ninth Street, Berkeley, Calif. 94710, U.S.A.
Comark Electronics Ltd., Brookside Ave., Rustington, Sussex, England.
Dow Chemical Coy., Midland, Michigan, U.S.A.
Drummond Scientific Coy., Broomall, Penn., U.S.A.
Dupont de Nemours & Co. Inc., Instrument Products Division, Wilmington, D.E. 19898, U.S.A.
Eastman-Kodak, Liverpool, England.
E-C Apparatus Coy., 226 South 40th Street, University City, Philadelphia, Penn. 19104, U.S.A.
Fisons, Scientific Apparatus, Bishop Meadow Rd., Loughborough, Leicestershire, England.

Gilford Instruments Inc., 132 Artino Street, Oberlin, Ohio 44075, U.S.A.

Grant Instruments (Cambridge) Ltd., Barrington, Cambridge CB2 5QZ, England.

L'Industrie Biologique Française, 35 Quai de Moulin de Cage, Gennevilliers (Seine), France.

International Equipment Co., 300 2nd Avenue, Needham Heights, Mass., U.S.A.

International Specialities Co. (ISCO), 47000 Superior Street., Lincoln, Nebraska 68504, U.S.A.

Joyce-Lobel Ltd., Princes Way, Team Valley, Gateshead, England.

Laboratory Thermal Equipment Ltd., Greenfield, Nr. Oldham, Lancashire, England.

LKB Produkter AB, S-161 Bromma 1, Sweden.

Measuring and Scientific Equipment Ltd. (MSE), Manor Royal, Crawley, Sussex, England.

Marine Laboratories Ltd., P.O. Box 37, Stoke Court, Stoke Poges, Slough SL2 4LY, England.

Merck, E., 6100 Darmstadt, Germany.

Mickle Laboratories, Mill Works, Gomshall, Surrey, England.

Nuclear Chicago, 2000 Nuclear Drive, Des Plaines, Ill. 60018, U.S.A.

Packard Instrument Coy. Inc., 2220 Warrenville Road, Downers Grove, Ill. 60515, U.S.A.

Pharmacia Fine Chemicals AB, Uppsala, Sweden.

Porous Plastics Ltd., now Porvair Ltd., Kings Lynn, Norfolk, England.

Pye Unicam Ltd., York Street, Cambridge CB1 2PX, England.

Reeve Angel Scientific Ltd., 14 New Bridge Str., London EC4V 6AY, England.

Savant Instruments Inc., 221 Park Ave., Hicksville, N.Y. 11801, U.S.A.

Sephadex, Registered Trade Mark of Pharmacia Fine Chemicals AB.

Serva Feinbiochemica GmbH, D-6900 Heidelberg 1, Germany.

Shandon Southern Ltd., Camberley, Surrey, England.

Stanton-Redcroft Ltd., Copper Mill Lane, London SW17, England.

Ultraviolet Products, Santa Barbara, Calif., U.S.A.

Subject index p. 487

Varian Aerograph, 2700 Mitchell Drive, Walnut Creek, Calif. 94598, U.S.A.

Waters Associates Inc., 61 Fountain Street, Framingham, Mass. 01701, U.S.A.

Whatman, Registered Trade Mark of W. and R. Balston, Ltd.

Worthington Biochemical Corp., Freehold, N.J. 07728, U.S.A.

Zeiss Instruments, Oberkochen, West Germany.

References

AAIJ, C. and P. BORST (1972) Biochim. Biophys. Acta *269*, 192.

ABRAHAMS, R. (1951) Arch. Biochem. Biophys. *30*, 44.

ADAMS, J. M., P. G. N. JEPPESEN, F. SANGER and B. G. BARRELL (1969) Nature *223*, 1009.

ADESNIK, M. (1973) Methods in Enzymology, ed. Colowick and Kaplan, p. 125.

ADESNIK, M. and C. LEVINTHAL (1970) J. Mol. Biol. *48*, 187.

ADLER, S. P. and D. NATHANS (1973) Biochim. Biophys. Acta *299*, 177.

AKROYD, P. (1968) *In*: I. Smith, ed., Chromatographic and Electrophoretic Techniques, Vol. 2 (Heinemann, London) p. 458.

ALLET, B. and P. F. SPAHR (1971) Eur. J. Biochem. *19*, 250.

ANDERSON, N. G. (1966) Nat. Cancer Inst. Monograph, *21*.

ANDERSON, N. G., J. G. GREEN, M. L. BARBER SR. and F. C. LADD (1963) Anal. Biochem *6*, 153.

ANKER, H. S. (1970) FEBS Lett. *7*, 293.

APGAR, J., G. A. EVERETT and R. W. HOLLEY (1965) Proc. Nat. Acad. Sci. U.S. *53*, 546.

APGAR, J., G. A. EVERETT and R. W. HOLLEY (1966) J. Biol. Chem. *241*, 1206.

ARMSTRONG, A., H. HAGOPIAN, V. M. INGRAM, I. SJOQUIST and J. SJOQUIST (1964) Biochemistry *3*, 1194.

ATHERTON, R. S., I. S. BOYCE, C. G. CLAYTON and A. R. THOMSON (1972) E. Reid. ed. Methodological Developments of Zonal Rotors (Longmans).

BARTOS, E. M., G. W. RUSHIZKY and H. A. SOBER (1963) Biochemistry *2*, 1179.

BAYEV, A. A., T. V. VENKSTERN, A. D. MIRZABEKOV, A. I. KRUTILINA, L. LI and V. D. AXELROD (1965) Biochim. Biophys. Acta *108*, 162.

BAYEV, A. A., T. V. VENKSTERN, A. D. MIRZABEKOV, A. I. KRUTILINA, V. A. AXELROD, L. LI and V. A. ENGELHARDT (1967) D. Shugar, ed., Genetic Elements (Academic Press).

BELL, D., R. V. TOMLINSON and G. M. TENER (1964) Biochem. *3*, 317.

BENEY, L. and M. SZEKELY (1966) Biochem. J. *100*, 17c.

BEVAN, E. A., A. J. HERRING and D. J. MITCHELL (1973) Nature *245*, 81.

BERNARDI, G. (1966) Procedures in Nucleic Acid Research. G. L. Cantoni and D. R. Duvies, ed., Vol. 1, Harper.

BERNARDI, G. (1969) Biochim. Biophys. Acta *174*, 423, 425.

BERNARDI, G. (1971) *In*: L. Grossman and K. Moldave, eds., Methods in Enzymology *21* D p. 95.

BIRNSTIEL, M., J. SPEIRS, I. PURDOM, K. JONES and U. E. LOENING (1968) Nature *219*, 454.

BISHOP, D. H. L. and D. E. BRADLEY (1965) Biochem. J. *95*, 82.

BISHOP, D. H. L., J. R. CLAYBROOK and S. SPIEGELMAN (1967) J. Mol. Biol. *26*, 373.

BJORK, G. and I. SVENSSON (1967) Biochim. Biophys. Acta *138*, 430.

BLATTNER, F. R. and H. P. ERICKSON (1967) Anal. Biochem. *18*, 220.

BOEDTKER, H. (1960) J. Mol. Biol. *2*, 171.

BOEDTKER, H. (1971) Biochim. Biophys. Acta *240*, 448.

BOLLUM, F. J. (1962) J. Biol. Chem. *237*, 1945.

BOZARTH, R. F., H. A. WOOD and A. MANDELBROT (1971) Virology *45*, 516.

BRAM, S. (1971) Nature New Biol. *232*, 174.

BRAUN, R. (1967a) Biochim. Biophys. Acta *142*, 267.

BRAUN, R. (1967b) Biochim. Biophys. Acta *149*, 601.

BRAUN, R. and H. WILI (1969) Biochim. Biophys. Acta *174*, 246.

BRENNER, D. J., G. R. FANNING, A. V. RAKE and K. E. JOHNSON (1969) Anal. Biochem. *28*, 447.

BRIMACOMBE, R., J. M. MORGAN and R. A. COX (1971) Eur. J. Biochem. *23*, 52.

BRITTEN, R. J. and D. E. KOHNE (1966) Carnegie Inst. Year Book *65*, 78.

BRITTEN, R. J. and D. E. KOHNE (1968) Science *161*, 529.

BROOKES, P. and C. HEIDELBERGER (1969) Cancer Res. *29*, 157.

BROWNLEE, G. G. (1971) Nature New Biol. *229*, 147.

BROWNLEE, G. G. (1972) Determination of sequences in RNA, *In*: T. S. Work and E. Work, eds., Laboratory Techniques in Biochem. and Molecular Biology, Vol. 3, Part 1 (North Holland, Amsterdam).

BROWNLEE, G. G. and F. SANGER (1967) J. Mol. Biol. *23*, 337.

BROWNLEE, G. G., F. SANGER and B. BARREL (1967) Nature *215*, 735.

BROWNLEE, G. G., E. M. CARTWRIGHT, N. J. COWAN, J. M. JARVIS and C. MILSTEIN (1973) Nature New Biol. *244*, 236.

BRUNER, R. and J. VINOGRAD (1965) Biochim. Biophys. Acta, *108*, 18.

BRUNK, C. H. and P. C. HANAWALT (1966) Exp. Cell Res. *42*, 406.

BUDOWSKY, E. I. and V. P. DEMUSHKIN (1964) Biokhimiya *29*, 1063.

CANTOR, C. R. and I. TINOCO (1965) J. Mol. Biol. *13*, 65.

CARRARA, M. and G. BERNARDI (1968a) Biochim. Biophys. Acta *155*, 1.

CARRARA, M. and G. BERNARDI (1968b) Biochemistry *7*, 1121.

CATON, J. E. and G. GOLDSTEIN (1971) Anal. Biochem *42*, 14.

CHERSI, A., A. BERNARDI and G. BERNARDI (1966) Biochim. Biophys. Acta *129*, 12.

CHOULES, G. L. and B. H. ZIMM (1965) Anal. Biochem. *13*, 336.

CHRAMBACH, A. (1966) Anal. Biochem. *15*, 544.

CHURCH, R. B. and B. J. McCARTHY (1968) Biochem. Genet. *2*, 55.

CLARKE, J. T. (1964) Ann. N.Y. Acad. Sci. *121*, 428.

COHN, W. E. (1955) *In*: E. Chargaff and J. M. Davidson, eds., The Nucleic Acids *1*, (Academic Press, New York).

COHN, W. E. and D. G. DOHERTY (1956) J. Am. Chem. Soc. *78*, 2863.

CONN, H. J. (1946) Biological Stains, 5th Ed. Biotech. Publications, Geneva, N.Y.

COPE, J. R. and H. R. MATTHEWS (1972) *In*: E. Reid, ed., Methodological Developments with Zonal Rotors (Longmans).

CRANE, R. K. and F. LIPMANN (1953) J. Biol. Chem. *201*, 235.

DAHLBERG, A. E., C. W. DINGMAN and A. C. PEACOCK (1969) J. Mol. Biol. *41*, 139.

DANNA, K. and D. NATHANS (1971) Proc. Nat. Acad. Sci. *68*, 2913.

DANNA, K. J., G. H. SACK and D. NATHANS (1973) J. Mol. Biol. *78*, 363.

DAVIS, B. J. (1963) Enzyme Analysis 3b, Canalco Inst. Publications.

DAVIS, B. J. (1964) Ann. N.Y. Acad. Sci. *121*, 404.

DAWID, I. B. and J. W. CHASE (1972) J. Mol. Biol. *63*, 217.

DESSEV, G. N., C. D. VENKOV and R. G. TSANEV (1969) Eur. J. Biochem. *7*, 280.

DE WACHTER, R. and W. FIERS (1971) *In:* L. Grossman and K. Moldave, eds., Methods in Enzymology, Vol. 21 (Academic Press, N.Y.) p. 167.

DE WACHTER, R. and W. FIERS (1972) Anal. Biochem. *49*, 184.

DINGMAN, C. W., M. P. FISHER and T. KAKEFUDA (1972a) Biochemistry *11*, 1242.

DINGMAN, C. W., T. KAKEFUDA and A. ARONOW (1970) Biochim. Biophys. Acta *224*, 114.

DINGMAN, C. W., T. KAKEFUDA and M. P. FISHER (1972b) Anal. Biochem. *50*, 519.

DIRHEIMER, G. and J. P. EBEL (1967) Bull. Soc. Chim. Biol. *49*, 447.

DRYSDALE, J. W. and P. RIGHETTI (1972) Biochemistry *11*, 4044.

DUESBERG, P. H. and P. K. EBEL (1973) J. Virol. *12*, 594.

DUTTING, D., H. FELDMAN and H. G. ZACHAU (1966) Hoppe Seylers Z. Physiol. Chem. *347*, 249.

EGYHAZI, E., U. RINGBORG, B. DANEHOLT and B. LAMBERT (1968) Nature *220*, 1036.

EHRESMANN, C., P. STIEGLER, P. FELLNER and J.-P. EBEL (1973) Biochimie *54*, 901.

EHRLICH, S. D., J. THIERY and G. BERNARDI (1972) J. Mol. Biol. *65*, 207.

EISENBERG, H. and G. FELSENFELD (1967) J. Mol. Biol. *30*, 17.

EISINGER, J. (1971) Biochem. Biophys. Res. Commun. *44*, 1135.

EISINGER, J. and W. E. BLUMBERG (1973) Biochemistry *12*, 3648.

ELSON, E. and T. M. JOVIN (1969) Anal. Biochem. *27*, 193.

FAIRBANKS, G. JR., C. LEVINTHAL and R. H. REEDER (1965) Biochem. Biophys. Res. Commun. *20*, 393.

FAWCETT, J. S. and C. J. O. R. MORRIS (1966) Separation Sci. *1*, 9.

FIERS, W., R. DE WACHTER, L. LEPOUTRE and L. VANDENDRIESSCHE (1965b) J. Mol. Biol. *13*, 451.

FILIPSKI, J., J.-P. THIERY and G. BERNARDI (1973) J. Mol. Biol. *80*, 177.

FIRTEL, R. A. and J. BONNER (1971) Unpublished communication.

FISCHER, L. (1969). An introduction to gel chromatography, *In*: T. S. Work and E. Work, eds., Laboratory Techniques in Biochemistry and Molecular Biology, Vol. 1 Part II (North Holland, Amsterdam).

FISHER, M. P. and C. W. DINGMAN (1971) Biochemistry *10*, 1895.

FLAMM, W. G., M. L. BIRNSTIEL and P. M. B. WALKER (1969) *In*: G. D. Birnie and S. M. Fox, eds., Subcellular Components – Preparation and Fractionation (Butterworths, London).

FORGET, B. G. and S. M. WEISSMAN (1969) J. Biol. Chem. *244*, 3148.

FRESCO, J. R., L. C. KLOTZ and E. G. RICHARDS (1963). A New Spectroscopic Approach to the Determination of Helical Secondary Structure in Ribonucleic Acids. Cold Spr. Harb. Symp. Quant. Biol. *28*, 83.

GARRETT, R. A., K. H. RAK, L. DAYA and G. STOFFLER (1972) Mol. Gen. Genet. *114*, 112.

GASSEN, H. G. (1969) J. Chromatogr. *39*, 147.

GHYSEN, A. and J. E. CELIS (1974) J. Mol. Biol. *83*, 333.

GIDDINGS, J. C. (1961) *In*: E. Heftmann, ed., Chromatography (Rheinhold: N.Y.).

GOLDSTEIN, G. (1967) Anal. Biochem. *20*, 477.

GORDON, A. H. (1969) Electrophoresis of proteins in polyacrylamide and starch gels, *In*: T. S. Work and E. Work, eds., Laboratory Techniques in Biochemistry and Molecular Biology, Vol. 1, Part I (North-Holland, Amsterdam).

GOULD, H. J. (1966) Biochemistry *5*, 1103.

GOULD, H. J. (1968) *In*: J. G. Hawkes, ed., Chemotaxonomy and Serotaxonomy (Academic Press, N.Y.) p. 131.

GOULD, H. J. and P. H. HAMLYN (1973) FEBS Lett. *30*, 301.

GOULD, H. J., S. BONANOU and K. KANAGALINGHAM (1966) J. Mol. Biol. *22*, 397.

GOULD, H. J., J. C. PINDER, H. R. MATTHEWS and A. H. GORDON (1969) Anal. Biochem. *29*, 1.

GRIVELL, L. A., L. REIJNDERS and P. BORST (1971) Eur. J. Biochem. *19*, 64.

GROOT, P. H. E., C. AAIJ and P. BORST (1970) Biochem. Biophys. Res. Commun. *41*, 1321.

GROSS, D. (1961) J. Chromatogr. *5*, 194.

GROSSBACH, U. and I. B. WEINSTEIN (1968) Anal. Biochem. *22*, 311.

GURR, E. (1962) Staining Animal Tissues (Hill, London).

HACHMAN, J. and H. G. KHORANA (1969) J. Am. Chem. Soc. *91*, 2749.

HADDEN, N., F. BAUMANN, F. MACDONALD, M. MUNK, R. STEVENSON, D. GERE, F. ZAMARONI and R. MAJORS (1971) Basic liquid chromatography (Varian Aerograph, Walnut Creek, California U.S.A.).

HALL, R. H. (1963) Biochem. Biophys. Res. Commun. *12*, 429.

HALL, R. H. (1964) Biochemistry *3*, 769.

HALL, R. H. (1965) Biochemistry *4*, 661.

HALL, J. B. and R. L. SINSHEIMER (1963) J. Mol. Biol. *6*, 115.
HARLEY, E. H., J. S. WHITE and K. R. REES (1973) Biochim. Biophys. Acta *299*, 253.
HAYES, F. N., E. HANSBURY and V. E. MITCHELL (1964) J. Chromatogr. *16*, 410
HAYWARD, G. S. and M. G. SMITH (1972) J. Mol. Biol. *63*, 383.
HEPPEL, L. A., D. R. HARKNESS and R. J. HILMOE (1962) J. Biol. Chem. *237*, 841.
HEWISH, D. R. and L. A. BURGOYNE (1973) Biochem. Biophys. Res. Commun. *52*, 504.
HIMMELHOCH, S. R. and E. H. PETERSON (1966) Anal. Biochem. *17*, 383.
HINDLEY, J. (1967) J. Mol. Biol. *30*, 125.
HIRSCHMAN, S. Z. and G. FELSENFELD (1966) J. Mol. Biol. *16*, 347.
HJERTEN, S. (1970) D. Glick, ed., Methods of Biochemical Analysis *18* (Wiley, N.Y.) pp. 55.
HJERTEN, S., S. JERSTEDT and A. TISELIUS (1965) Anal. Biochem. *11*, 219.
HOHN, T. and W. POLLMANN (1963) Z. Naturforsch. *18b*, 919.
HOHN, T. and H. SCHALLER (1967) Biochim. Biophys. Acta *138*, 466.
HOLIDAY, E. R. (1937) J. Sci. Inst. *14*, 166.
HOLLEY, R. W. (1965) Science *150*, 921.
HOLTON, R. A., D. M. SPATZ, E. E. VAN TAMELEN and W. WIERENGA (1974) Biochem. Biophys. Res. Commun. *58*, 605.
HUNTER, A. R. and R. J. JACKSON (1971) Eur. J. Biochem. *19*, 316.
HURLBERT, R. B., H. SCHMITZ, A. F. BRUMM and V. R. POTTER (1954) J. Biol. Chem. *209*, 23.
IFFT, J. B., J. E. HEARST and J. VINOGRAD (1961a) Proc. Nat. Acad. Sci. *47*, 1015.
IFFT, J. B., D. H. VOET and J. VINOGRAD (1961b) J. Phys. Chem. *65*, 1138.
IKEMURA T. and J. E. DAHLBERG (1973) J. Biol. Chem. *248*, 5024.
JACOBSON, A., A. R. FIRTEL and H. F. LODISH (1974) J. Biol. *82*, 213.
JACOBSON, D. H. (1971) Ph.D. Thesis, Massachusetts Institute of Technology.
JENSEN, R. H. and N. DAVIDSON (1966) Biopolymers *4*, 17.
JOHNS, E. W. (1967) Biochem. J. *104*, 78.
JORDAN, B. R. (1971) J. Mol. Biol. *55*, 423.
JORDAN, E. M. and S. RAYMOND (1969) Anal. Biochem. *27*, 205.
JOVIN, T. M., A. CHRAMBACH and M. A. NAUGHTON (1964) Anal. Biochem. *9*, 351.
KAISER, I. J. (1969) Biochemistry *8*, 231.
KATZ, S. and D. J. COMB (1963) J. Biol. Chem. *238*, 3065.
KAWATA, I. and K. MIURA (1970) J. Mol. Biol. *51*, 247.
KELMERS, A. D. and D. E. HEATHERLY (1971) Anal. Biochem. *44*, 486.
KIDBY, D. K. (1970) Anal. Biochem. *34*, 478.
KIRK, J. T. O. (1963) Biochem. Biophys. Acta *76*, 417.
KIRK, J. T. O. (1967) Biochem. J. *105*, 673.
KOKILEVA, L., I. MLADENOVA and R. TSANEV (1971) FEBS Lett. *16*, 17.
KOURILSKY, P. H., S. MANTEUIL, M. H. ZAMENSKY and F. GROS (1970) Biochem. Biophys. Res. Commun. *41*, 1080.
LAGOKVIST, U. and P. BERG (1962) J. Mol. Biol. *5*, 139.

LANE, B. G. (1963) Biochim. Biophys. Acta *72*, 110.
LANYON, W. G., J. PAUL and R. WILLIAMSON (1972) Eur. J. Biochem. *31*, 38.
LASKOWSKI, M. (1966) *In*: G. L. Cantoni and D. R. Davies, eds., Procedures in Nucleic Acid Research (Harper, N.Y.).
LAURENT, T. C. and J. KILLANDER (1964) J. Chromatogr. *14*, 317.
LEBOY, P. S., E. C. COX and J. G. FLAKS (1964) Proc. Nat. Acad. Sci. *52*, 1367.
LEDER, P. and M. NIRENBERG (1964) Proc. Nat. Acad. Sci. *52*, 420.
LEWICKI, P. P. and A. J. SINSKEY (1970) Anal. Biochem. *33*, 273.
LISHANSKAYA, A. I. and M. I. MOSEVITSKY (1973) Biochem. Biophys. Res. Commun. *52*, 1213.
LLOYD, D. A. and S. MANDELES (1970) Biochemistry *9*, 932.
LOENING, U. E. (1967) Biochem. J. *102*, 251.
LOENING, U. E. (1968) J. Mol. Biol. *38*, 355.
LOENING, U. E. (1969) Biochem. J. *113*, 131.
MCCALLUM, M. and P. M. B. WALKER (1967) Biochem. J. *105*, 163.
MCPHIE, P., J. HOUNSELL and W. B. GRATZER (1966) Biochemistry *5*, 988.
MADEN, B. E. H., M. SALIM and D. F. SUMMERS (1972) Nature New Biol. *237*, 5.
MADISON, J. T. (1966) Cold Spring Harbour Symp. Quant. Biol. *31*.
MADISON, J. T., G. A. EVERETT and H. KUNG (1966) Science *153*, 531.
MAIZEL, J. V. (1966) Science *151*, 988.
MANDELES, S. and H. O. KAMMEN (1966) Anal. Biochem. *17*, 540.
MANIATIS, T. and M. PTASHNE (1973) Proc. Nat. Acad. Sci. *70*, 1531.
MARKHAM, R. and J. D. SMITH (1952) Biochem. J. *52*, 565.
MARMUR, J. and P. DOTY (1959) Nature *183*, 1427.
MARMUR, J. and P. DOTY (1962) J. Mol. Biol. *5*, 109.
MARSHAK, A. and H. J. VOGEL (1951) J. Biol. Chem. *189*, 597.
MARTIN, A. J. P. and R. L. M. SYNGE (1941) Biochem. J. *35*, 1358.
MARTINI, O. H. W. and H. J. GOULD (1973) Biochim. Biophys. Acta *295*, 621.
MATTHEWS, H. R. (1968a) Ph. D. Thesis, University of London.
MATTHEWS, H. R. (1968b) J. Chromatogr. *36*, 302.
MATTHEWS, H. R. (1968c) J. Gen. Virol. *3*, 403.
MATTHEWS, H. R. (1968d) Eur. J. Biochem. *7*, 96.
MATTHEWS, H. R., E. M. BRADBURY, R. J. INGLIS and N. SARNER (1971) Abstr. Commun. 7th FEBS Mtg. p. 182.
MESELSON, M., F. W. STAHL and J. VINOGRAD (1957) Proc. Nat. Acad. Sci. *43*, 581.
MEZZASOMA, I. and B. FARINA (1966) Bull. Soc. Ital. Biol. Sper. *42*, 1449.
MEZZASOMA, I. and B. FARINA (1966) Bull. Soc. Ital. Biol. Sper. *43*, 29.
MICHELSON, A. M. (1963) The Chemistry of Nucleosides and Nucleotides (Academic Press, London and N.Y.).
MICHL, H. (1958) J. Chromatogr. *1*, 93.
MILLAR, D. B. and R. W. BYRNE (1967) Arch. Biochem. Biophys. *119*, 398.

MIRAULT, M.-E. and K. SCHERRER (1971) Eur. J. Biochem. *23*, 372.

MIRZABEKOV, A. D., A. I. KRUTILINA and A. A. BAYEV (1966) Biochim. Biophys. Acta *129*, 429.

MIYAZAKI, M., M. KAWATA and S. TAKEMURA (1966a) J. Biochem. *60*, 519.

MIYAZAKI, M. and S. TAKEMURA (1966b) J. Biochem. *60*, 526.

MIYAZAKI, M., M. KAWATA, K. NAKAZAWA and S. TAKEMURA (1967) J. Biochem. *62*, 161.

MIYAZAWA, Y. and C. A. THOMAS (1965) J. Mol. Biol. *11*, 223.

MOLDAVE, K. and L. GROSSMAN (1971) Methods Enzymol. *20*, part C. pp. 3–83.

MORRIS, C. J. O. R. (1966) Protides Biol. Fluids *14*, 543.

MORRISON, M., R. WILLIAMSON, G. LANYON and J. PAUL (1970) Biochem. J. *119*, 59 p.

MUNDY, K. W. (1965) Technicon Fifth International Symposium: Automation in Analytical Chemistry, London.

NANDI, U. S., J. C. WANG and N. DAVIDSON (1965) Biochemistry, *4*, 1687.

NAUGHTON, M. A. and H. HAGOPIAN (1962) Anal. Biochem. *3*, 276.

NEUHOFF, V. (1973) Micromethods in Molecular Biology (Springer Verlag, Berlin).

NISHIMURA, S., F. HARADA, U. NARUSHIMA and T. SENO (1967) Biochim. Biophys. Acta *142*, 133.

OBERG, B. and L. PHILLIPSON (1967) Arch. Biochem. Biophys. *119*, 504.

OGSTON, A. G. (1958) Trans. Faraday Soc. *54*, 1754.

OGSTON, A. G. and C. F. PHELPS (1961) Biochem. J. *78*, 827.

OHSAKA, A., J. I. MUKAI and M. LASKOWSKI (1964) J. Biol. Chem. *239*, 3498.

OJALA, D. and G. ATTARDI (1974) J. Mol. Biol. *82*, 151.

OWEN, R. J., L. R. HILL and S. P. LAPAGE (1969) Biopolymers *7*, 503.

OLIVERA, B. M., P. BAINE and N. DAVIDSON (1964) Biopolymers *2*, 245.

ORNSTEIN, L. (1963) Enzyme Analysis (Canalco Inst. Publications).

ORNSTEIN, L. (1964) Ann. N.Y. Acad. Sci. *121*, 321.

PEACOCK, A. C. and C. W. DINGMAN (1967) Biochemistry *6*, 1818.

PEACOCK, A. C. and C. W. DINGMAN (1968) Biochemistry *7*, 668.

PEARSON, R. L., J. F. WEISS and A. D. KELMERS (1971) Biochim. Biophys. Acta *228*, 770.

PENMAN, S., H. FAN, S. PERLMAN, M. ROSBASH, R. WEINBERG and E. ZYLBER (1970) Cold Spring Harbor Symp. Quant. Biol. *35*, 561.

PENSWICK, J. R. and R. W. HOLLEY (1965) Proc. Nat. Acad. Sci. *53*, 543.

PETERSON, E. A. and H. A. SOBER (1959) Anal. Chem. *31*, 857.

PETERSON, E. A. and H. A. ROWLAND (1961) J. Chromatogr. *5*, 330.

PETERSON, E. A. (1971) Ion-exchange chromatography, *In:* T. S. Work and E. Work, eds., Laboratory Techniques in Biochemistry and Molecular Biology, Vol. 2, Part II (North-Holland, Amsterdam).

PETERSEN, G. B. and J. M. REEVES (1966) Biochim. Biophys. Acta *129*, 438.

PETTERSSON, U., C. MULDER, H. DELIUS and P. A. SHARP (1973) Proc. Nat. Acad. Sci. *70*, 200.

PHILIPPSEN, P. and H. G. ZACHAU (1972a) Biochim. Biophys. Acta *277*, 523.

PHILIPPSEN, P. and H. G. ZACHAU (1972b) Biochim. Biophys. Acta *277*, 539.

PINDER, J. C. and W. B. GRATZER (1970) Biochemistry *9*, 4519.
PINDER, J. C. and W. B. GRATZER (1972) Eur. J. Biochem. *26*, 73.
PINDER, J. C. and W. B. GRATZER (1974) Biochim. Biophys. Acta *349*, 47.
PINDER, J. C., H. J. GOULD and I. SMITH (1969) J. Mol. Biol. *40*, 289.
PINDER, J. C., D. Z. STAYNOV and W. B. GRATZER (1974a) Biochemistry *13*, 5367.
PINDER, J. C., D. Z. STAYNOV and W. B. GRATZER (1974b) Biochemistry *13*, 5373.
POPESCU, M., L. H. LAZARUS and N. GOLDBLUM (1971) Anal. Biochem. *40*, 247.
POPESCU, M., L. H. LAZARUS and N. GOLDBLUM (1972) Anal. Biochem. *45*, 35.
RAJBHANDARY, U. L. and H. P. GHOSH (1969) J. Biol. Chem. *244*, 1104.
RAJBHANDARY, U. L. and A. STUART (1966) Ann. Rev. Biochem. *35*, 759.
RAJBHANDARY, U. L., A. STUART, R. D. FAULKNER, S. H. CHANG and H. G. KHORANA (1966) Cold Spring Harbor Symp. Quant. Biol. *31*, 425.
RAJBHANDARY, U. L., S. H. CHANG, A. STUART, R. D. FAULKNER, R. N. HOSKINSON and H. G. KHORANA (1967) Proc. Nat. Acad. Sci. *57*, 751.
RANDERATH, E. and K. RANDERATH (1967a) J. Chromatogr. *31*, 485.
RANDERATH, K. and E. RANDERATH (1967b) J. Chromatogr. *31*, 500.
RAYMOND, S. (1962) Clin. Chem. *8*, 455.
RAYMOND, S. and L. WEINTRAUB (1959) Science *130*, 711.
REDDY, R., T. O. SITZ, T. S. RO-CHOI and H. BUSCH (1974) Biochem. Biophys. Res. Commun. *56*, 1017.
REID, E. (1972) Ed. Methodological Developments in Biochemical Separations *and* Methodological Developments with Zonal Rotors (Longmans, London) (in press).
REIJNDERS, L., P. SLOOF, J. SIVAL and P. BORST (1973) Biochim. Biophys. Acta *324*, 320.
REYNOLDS, J. A. and C. TANFORD (1970a) Proc. Nat. Acad. Sci. *66*, 1002.
REYNOLDS, J. A. and C. TANFORD (1970b) J. Biol. Chem. *245*, 5161.
RICHARDS, E. G. and R. LECANIDOU (1971) Anal. Biochem. *40*, 43.
RICHARDS, E. G. and W. B. GRATZER (1968) *In*: I. Smith, ed., Chromatographic and Electrophoretic Techniques, Vol. 2 (Heinemann, London) p. 419.
RICHARDS, E. G. and C. J. TEMPLE (1971) Nature Phys. Sci. *230*, 92.
RICHARDS, E. G., J. A. COLL and W. B. GRATZER (1965) Anal. Biochem. *12*, 452.
RICHARDS, E. G., R. LECANIDOU and M. E. GEROCH (1973) Eur. J. Biochem. *34*, 262.
RINGBORG, U., E. EGYHAZI, B. DANEHOLT and B. LAMBERT (1968) Nature *220*, 1037.
RODBARD, D. and A. CHRAMBACH (1970) Proc. Nat. Acad. Sci. *65*, 970.
RODBARD, D., A. CHRAMBACH and G. H. WEISS (1974) *In*: R. C. Allen and H. R. Maurer, eds., Electrophoresis and Isoelectric Focusing in Polyacrylamide Gel (de Gruyter, Berlin) p. 62.
ROLFE, R. and M. MESELSON (1959) Proc. Nat. Acad. Sci. *45*, 1039.
RUSHIZKY, G. W. and C. A. KNIGHT (1960) Virol. *11*, 236.
RUSHIZKY, G. W. and H. A. SOBER (1962) J. Biol. Chem. *237*, 834.
RUSHIZKY, G. W. and H. A. SOBER (1963) J. Biol. Chem. *238*, 371.
RUSHIZKY, G. W. and W. W. MILLER (1967) Anal. Biochem. *20*, 181.
RUSHIZKY, G. W. and H. A. SOBER (1962) J. Biol. Chem. *237*, 2883.

RUSHIZKY, G. W., E. N. BARTOS and H. A. SOBER (1964) Biochemistry *3*, 626.

RUSHIZKY, G. W., I. H. SKAVENSKI and H. A. SOBER (1965) J. Biol. Chem. *240*, 3984.

SANGER, F. and G. G. BROWNLEE (1967) *In*: D. Shugar, ed., Genetic Elements (Academic Press N.Y. and London) p. 303.

SANGER, F. and H. TUPPY (1951) Biochem. J. *49*, 463.

SANGER, F., G. G. BROWNLEE and B. G. BARRELL (1965) J. Mol. Biol. *13*, 373.

SAUNDERS, G. F., S. SHIRAKAWA, P. P. SAUNDERS, F. E. ARRIGHI and T. C. HSU (1972) J. Mol. Biol. *63*, 323.

SCHACHMAN, H. K. (1959) Ultracentrifugation in Biochemistry (Academic Press N.Y. London).

SCHAUP, H. W., J. B. BEST and A. B. GOODMAN (1968) Nature *221*, 864.

SCHILDKRAUT, C. L. and J. J. MAIO (1969) J. Mol. Biol. *46*, 305.

SCHILDKRAUT, C. L., J. MARMUR and P. DOTY (1962) J. Mol. Biol. *4*, 430.

SCHWARTZ, A. N. and B. A. ZABIN (1966) Anal. Biochem. *14*, 321.

SCHWARTZ, A. N., A. W. G. YEE and B. A. ZABIN (1965) J. Chromatogr. *20*, 154.

SEILDER, R. J. and M. MANDEL (1971) J. Bacteriol. *106*, 608.

SHAPIRO, H. S. and E. CHARGAFF (1963) Biochim. Biophys. Acta *76*, 1.

SHELDON, R., C. JURALE and J. KATES (1972) Proc. Nat. Acad. Sci. *69*, 417.

SINHA, N. K., R. K. FUJMURA and P. KAESBERG (1965) J. Mol. Biol. *11*, 84.

SINHA, N. K., M. D. ENGER and P. KAESBERG (1965) J. Mol. Biol. *12*, 299.

SIRBASKU, D. A. and J. M. BUCHANAN (1970) J. Biol. Chem. *245*, 2679.

SHACK, J. and B. S. BYNUM (1964) J. Biol. Chem. *239*, 2602.

SHATKIN, A. J., J. D. SIPE and P. LOH (1968) J. Virol. *2*, 986.

SMITH, A. E. and K. A. MARCKER (1970) Nature *226*, 607.

SMITH, I. (1968) *In*: I. Smith, ed., Chromatographic and Electrophoretic Techniques, Vol. 2 (Heinemann, London) p. 365.

SMITH, J. D. (1955) *In*: E. Chargaff and J. N. Davidson, eds., The Nucleic Acids (Academic Press N.Y.).

SMITH, J. D. and D. B. DUNN (1959) Biochim. Biophys. Acta *31*, 573.

SMITHIES, O. (1955) Biochem. J. *61*, 629.

SOBER, H. A. (1968) A Handbook of Biochemistry (The Chemical Rubber Company, Cleveland).

SPENCER, E. W., V. M. INGRAM and C. LEVINTHAL (1966) Science *152*, 1722.

SPENCER, E. W., V. M. INGRAM and C. LEVINTHAL (1967) Science *153*, 1336.

SPENCER, J. H. and E. CHARGAFF (1963a) Biochim. Biophys. Acta *68*, 9.

SPENCER, J. H. and E. CHARGAFF (1963b) Biochim. Biophys. Acta *68*, 18.

STAEHELIN, M. (1963) *In*: J. N. Davidson and W. E. Cohn, eds., Progress in Nucleic Acid Research (Academic Press N.Y. and London) *2*, 169.

STANTON, M. G. (1965) Anal. Biochem. *12*, 310.

STEINER, R. F. and R. F. BEERS (1961) Polynucleotides (Elsevier, Amsterdam) p. 301.

STAYNOV, D. (1972) Anal. Biochem. *47*, 13.

STAYNOV, D. and G. STAINOV (1969) J. Sci. Inst. *2*, 1114.

STAYNOV, D., J. C. PINDER and W. B. GRATZER (1972) Nature New Biol. *235*, 108.
STEINER, R. F. and R. F. BEERS (1961) Polynucleotides (Elsevier, Amsterdam) p. 301.
STOCKX, J. and L. VANDENDRIESSCHE (1963) Biochim. Biophys. Acta *72*, 137.
STREECK, R. E. and H. G. ZACHAU (1971) FEBS Lett. *13*, 329.
STUDIER, F. W. (1965) J. Mol. Biol. *11*, 373.
SUEOKA, N. (1959) Proc. Nat. Acad. Sci. *45*, 1480.
SUEOKA, N. (1961) J. Mol. Biol. *3*, 31.
SUGIYAMA, T. (1965) J. Mol. Biol. *11*, 856.
SUGIYAMA, T. and H. FRAENKAL-CONRAT (1961) Proc. Nat. Acad. Sci. *47*, 1393.
SULKOWSKI, E. and M. LASKOWSKI (1962) J. Biol. Chem. *237*, 262.
TAKEISHI, K., T. UKITA and S. NISHIMURA (1968) J. Biol. Chem. *243*, 5761.
TAKAHASHI, M., T. OGINO and K. BABA (1969) Biochim. Biophys. Acta *174*, 183.
TALENS, A., O. P. VAN DIGGELEN, M. BRONGERS, L. M. POPA and L. BOSCH (1973) Eur. J. Biochem. *37*, 121.
TALENS, J., F. KALOUSEK and L. BOSCH (1970) FEBS Lett. *12*, 4.
THACH, R. E. (1966) *In*: G. L. Cantoni and D. R. Davies, eds., Procedures in Nucleic Acid Research (Harper and Row, N.Y. and London).
THIRION, J.-P. and P. KAESBERG (1968) J. Mol. Biol. *33*, 379.
TIOLLAIS, P., F. GALIBERT and M. BOIRON (1971) Proc. Nat. Acad. Sci. *68*, 1117.
TIOLLAIS, P., F. GALIBERT, A. LEPETIT and M. A. AUGER (1972) Biochimie *54*, 339.
TISELIUS, A., S. HJERTEN and O. LEVIN (1956) Arch. Biochem. Biophys. *65*, 132.
TOMLINSON, R. V. and G. M. TENER (1962) J. Am. Chem. Soc. *84*, 2644.
TOMLINSON, R. V. and G. M. TENER (1963) Biochemistry *2*, 697.
TSANEV, R. and D. STAYNOV (1964) Biokhimyia *29*, 1126.
TSANEV, R., D. STAYNOV, L. KOKILEVA and I. MLADENOVA (1969) Anal. Biochem. *30*, 66.
TYNDALL, R. L., K. B. JACOBSON and E. TEETER (1964) Biochim. Biophys. Acta *87*, 335.
UCHIDA, T. and F. EGAMI (1966) *In*: G. L. Cantoni and D. R. DAVIES, eds., Procedures in Nucleic Acid Research (Harper and Row, N.Y. and London).
URIEL, J. and J. BERGER (1966) C. R. Acad. Sci. Paris *262*, 164.
UZIEL, M. and W. E. Cohn (1965) Biochim. Biophys. Acta *103*, 539.
UZIEL, M. and H. G. Gassen (1969) Biochemistry *8*, 1643.
VANDENBUSSCHE, P. and W. FIERS (1966) Biochim. Biophys. Acta *114*, 182.
VASU, S. S. (1969) St. Cerc. Biochim. *12*, 393.
VESTERGAARD, P., C. WITHERALL and T. PITI (1967) J. Chromatogr. *31*, 337.
VIGNE, R. and B. R. JORDAN (1971) Biochimie *53*, 981.
VINOGRAD, J. and J. E. HEARST (1962) *In*: Progress in Chemistry of Organic Natural Products (Springer Verlag, Berlin) *20*, 395.
VINOGRAD, J. (1963) Methods Enzymol. *6*, 854.
VISCHER, E. and E. CHARGAFF (1948) J. Biol. Chem. *176*, 715.
DE WACHTER, R. and W. FIERS (1967) J. Mol. Biol. *30*, 507.
WAGNER, A. F., R. L. BUGIANESI and T. Y. SHEN (1971) Biochem. Biophys. Res. Commun. *45*, 184.

WARSHAW, M. M. and I. TINOCO (1965) J. Mol. Biol. *13*, 54.

WATANABE, Y., L. PREVEC and A. F. GRAHAM (1967) Proc. Nat. Acad. Sci. *58*, 1040.

WELLS, R. D., J. E. LARSON, R. C. GRANT, B. E. SHORTLE and C. R. CANTOR (1970) J. Mol. Biol. *54*, 465.

WETMUR, J. G. and N. DAVIDSON (1968) J. Mol. Biol. *31*, 349.

WOOD, H. A. and G. STREISSLE (1970) Virology *40*, 329.

WUNDERLY (1961) Principles and Applications of Paper Electrophoresis (Elsevier, Amsterdam).

WYATT, G. R. (1955) *In*: E. Chargaff and J. N. Davidson, eds., The Nucleic Acids *1* (Academic Press, N.Y.) p. 243.

YOUNG, R. W. and H. W. FULHORST (1965) Anal. Biochem. *11*, 389.

ZACHAU, H. G., D. DUTTING and H. FELDMANN (1966a) Hoppe Seylers' Z. Physiol. Chem. *347*, 212.

ZACHAU, H. G., D. DUTTING and H. FELDMANN (1966b) D. Shugar, ed., Genetic Elements (Academic Press, N.Y.).

ZACHAU, H. G., D. DUTTING, H. FELDMANN, F. MELCHERS and W. KARAU (1969) Cold Spring Harbor Symp. Quant. Biol. *31*.

ZAITLIN, M. and V. HARIHARASUBRAMANIAN (1970) Anal. Biochem. *35*, 296.

ZAMIR, A., R. W. HOLLEY and M. MARQUISEE (1965) J. Biol. Chem. *240*, 1267.

ZAPISAK, W. F., A. G. SAPONARA and M. D. ENGER (1969) Biochem. *8*, 1170.

ZEIGER, R. S., R. SALOMON, C. W. DINGMAN and A. C. PEACOCK (1972) Nature New Biol. *238*, 65.

Subject index